Buddhism and Medicine

Buddhism and Medicine

❖

AN ANTHOLOGY OF MODERN AND CONTEMPORARY SOURCES

Edited by C. Pierce Salguero

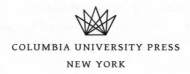

COLUMBIA UNIVERSITY PRESS

NEW YORK

Columbia University Press
Publishers Since 1893
New York   Chichester, West Sussex
cup.columbia.edu
Copyright © 2020 Columbia University Press
All rights reserved

Library of Congress Cataloging-in-Publication Data
Names: Salguero, C. Pierce, editor.
Title: Buddhism and medicine : an anthology of modern and contemporary sources /
edited by C. Pierce Salguero.
Description: New York : Columbia University Press, [2019] |
Includes bibliographical references and index.
Identifiers: LCCN 2019001088 (print) | LCCN 2019013093 (e-book) |
ISBN 9780231548304 (electronic) | ISBN 9780231189361 (cloth : alk. paper) |
ISBN 9780231548304 (e-book)
Subjects: LCSH: Medicine—Religious aspects—Buddhism—Sources.
Classification: LCC BQ4570.M4 (e-book) | LCC BQ4570.M4 B83 2019 (print) |
DDC 294.3/3661—dc23
LC record available at https://lccn.loc.gov/2019001088

Columbia University Press books are printed on permanent
and durable acid-free paper.
Printed in the United States of America

Cover image: Statue of Bhaiṣajyaguru from Unified Silla kingdom, ninth century.
Photo by the author, with permission from National Museum of Korea, Seoul,
and the National Research Foundation of Korea grant #NRF-20141342.

CONTENTS

CROSSING BOUNDARIES

BUDDHIST HEALING IN PRACTICE

ACKNOWLEDGMENTS

The editor wishes to express sincere gratitude to all of the contributors to this volume, who have taught him much about the complex and multifaceted connections between Buddhism and medicine in the modern and contemporary period. Their diligence and responsiveness made this volume a joy to produce. He especially wishes to thank Justin Stein, Bill McGrath, Mona Schrempf, Ben Joffe, and Katja Triplett for reading far beyond their own chapters and making contributions to the betterment of the volume as a whole.

ABBREVIATIONS

Anthology, vol. 1   Preceding volume of this series: Salguero, C. Pierce. 2017. *Buddhism and Medicine: An Anthology of Premodern Sources.* New York: Columbia University Press.

Ch.	Chinese
Jp.	Japanese
Kr.	Korean
MN	*Majjhima Nikāya*
Mong.	Mongolian
Skt.	Sanskrit
T.	*Taishō shinshū daizōkyō* (See www.CBETA.org)
Tib.	Tibetan
Vtn.	Vietnamese

Introduction

C. PIERCE SALGUERO

S ince its first emergence in northeastern India in about 400 BCE, Buddhism has provided billions of individuals with vital tools to understand health and deal with illness.[1] Throughout all periods and locations to which it has subsequently spread, Buddhism has played a role in shaping adherents' health-seeking behaviors in conscious and unconscious ways. A range of therapies intended to cure or prevent illness has developed within the context of all major branches of the religion. Textual traditions, material culture, and institutional structures have likewise evolved to deliver those therapies to monastics and the laity alike. Over the past two millennia, Buddhist ideas and practices related to health and healing have often played a major role in the popularization of the religion in new recipient cultures.

Contemporary scholars and practitioners often call these various Buddhist inventions and adaptations of healing "Buddhist medicine." Though it is a modern term coined only in the twentieth century,[2] this concept can be useful for certain types of analysis. It draws attention to the important role Buddhism has played historically as a vehicle or catalyst for cross-cultural exchange, and it reminds us that there have been some commonalities in how Buddhists have approached health and illness across time and space.[3] However, there is also a danger that the use of this term may lead some to believe that there is a single Buddhist system that persisted across these diverse geographic and cultural terrains. While there are indeed some widespread beliefs and practices throughout the Buddhist world, "Buddhist medicine" (if we choose to use that term) is in no way a monolithic, unitary, or unchanging tradition. Whatever shared orientations there are have continually been adapted and transformed across time and geography as they have intersected with the prevailing cultures, intellectual traditions, and social realities of different corners of the Buddhist world.[4]

It is true that Buddhists have tended to believe that there is a strong connection between the condition of the mind and the well-being of the physical body. They have tended to hold the belief that powerful enlightened beings (human or otherwise) can be ritually called upon to provide healing powers, energies, or interventions. They have tended to blame certain illnesses and physical conditions either directly or indirectly on the influence of karma. However, the ways that even such basic ideas as these have been articulated have diverged widely among different Buddhist cultures.

Rather than approach Buddhist medicine as a single coherent system that can be explained succinctly, it is better if we understand it as a complex and varied topic calling for our sustained investigation. It is a vast field of inquiry to explore. It is the sum total of the countless, ever-changing points of articulation between Buddhist and medical knowledge. It is the nexus at which the boundaries between "Buddhism" and "medicine" are bridged, blurred, or obliterated. And, at times, it is also the processes by which the two are cleaved apart and walls built between them.[5]

For many (perhaps most) readers of this book, the most familiar example of Buddhist engagements with health and well-being will be one particular intervention that has become increasingly popular in the West, and indeed globally, in recent decades. I speak, of course, of "mindfulness" meditation. The study of the health benefits of mindfulness has increasingly become a cause célèbre in international scientific circles, where debates continue over whether and how the practice benefits a range of health indicators, including stress hormones, telomeres, longevity, brain matter, and more. Meanwhile, the mainstream popular media trumpets the arrival of the so-called mindfulness revolution with breathless coverage. At the time of this writing, mindfulness has featured on the cover of multiple issues of *Time* magazine, is included in the titles of over ten thousand books for sale on Amazon.com, and results in 188 million hits on Google.[6] The ubiquity of the topic, particularly on the English-language internet, has ensured that, for many people today around the world, Buddhism is very closely associated with health and well-being (not to mention practically synonymous with meditation). At the same time that mindfulness has gone mainstream, there has also been much hand-wringing among scientists and psychologists who are proponents of mindfulness concerning the degree to which the practice should be considered Buddhist and, if not, where exactly the boundaries lie.[7]

As a point of articulation, mutual influence, and negotiation between Buddhism and medicine, mindfulness is a contemporary example par excellence of the concerns of this book. However, this is but one example out of many. In its typically myopic way, the popular media in focusing on mindfulness has tended to obscure the fact that there are countless connections between Buddhism and well-being going far beyond meditation, and that this has been true since the very beginnings of the tradition.

This book, and the three-volume series of which it is a part, investigates many aspects of this centuries-long interplay between Buddhism and medicine, from ancient times to today (from Sarnath to Silicon Valley, I like to say). By placing our contemporary interests in the health benefits of mindfulness within this wider context, it is my hope that this series will help us to better appreciate the rich spectrum of therapeutic repertoires and resources that Buddhism has created and makes available to its devotees beyond the buzzwords of the present moment. Guided through the material by eighty-five leading historians, anthropologists, religious studies scholars, researchers from other disciplines, and practitioners of both Buddhism and various branches of Asian medicine, I also hope that these books encourage us to approach developments such as mindfulness from a perspective that does not privilege an exclusively biomedical, Western, or even contemporary vantage point.

To those ends, the first volume of this series, *Buddhism and Medicine: An Anthology of Premodern Sources* (referenced throughout as "*Anthology*, vol. 1"), focuses on providing a wide-ranging overview of the diversity of Buddhist engagements with medicine in the premodern period. It covers developments in Buddhist thought and practice from the Pāli and Sanskrit sources of ancient India to the Tripiṭakas (Buddhist canons) and manuscript traditions of medieval China, Japan, Korea, Mongolia, Southeast Asia, and Tibet. The earliest texts included in that volume are thought to originate in Indian oral traditions during or shortly after the lifetime of the Buddha in about the fourth century BCE. The latest text was written in 1977 in Myanmar and is based on an early nineteenth-century lineage. In between, the volume showcases the diversity and innovation of centuries of historical intersections between Buddhism and medicine across Asia.

This second volume is intended to extend those themes of diversity and innovation through to the present day. However, the present volume introduces an additional emphasis on how Buddhist individuals and institutions have navigated the major disruptions, discontinuities, and disjunctures introduced by modernity. In particular, it explores how the relationship between Buddhism and medicine has evolved, transformed, persisted, or deteriorated in the face of encounters with Western colonialism, the challenges to traditional authority brought by science and modern political structures, and the opportunities and pitfalls of globalization.

The third volume in the series, which will be published shortly after this one, presents my overarching synthesis that weaves together the materials in the two anthologies into a global historical narrative.

CONTENTS OF THE VOLUME

The current volume includes English translations of historical and contemporary texts, as well as ethnographic interviews with living practitioners of various forms of Buddhist and Buddhist-inspired or -influenced medicine. It follows the same format as that of the first anthology. A short introduction leads off each chapter, giving the reader an overview of the historical and cultural context for the source texts included therein. These introductions point out some of the texts' unique features and provide reading lists for further exploration. Also like its predecessor, this volume includes a comprehensive list of references for all chapters at the end of the book, as well as a glossary to assist nonspecialists in understanding the key terms that appear frequently across chapters. The reader will also find a geographical appendix at the end of the volume to facilitate navigating the contents in that manner. However, like the first volume, this one is organized thematically with the assumption that it will be read cover to cover as an integrated whole.

The thematic sections, and a brief overview of the chapters contained within each, are as follows. The first section, "Early Modernity," consists of chapters that are in various ways emblematic of how Buddhists struggled in the transition to the modern era. Scholars have long debated the term "modernity" and what it might mean to call something "modern," "early modern," or "premodern." The current volume does not engage explicitly in these theoretical discussions but instead uses "early modern" in a general way, as a term of convenience to refer to materials from the sixteenth to the nineteenth centuries. The chapters in this section deal with how Buddhists weathered the major historical ruptures that took place in various parts of Asia during that time period. These include the challenges Buddhist healers faced when interacting with Christian missionaries, when falling under the gaze of colonizers and cultural imperialists, and when impacted by the increasingly global flows of medical knowledge.

Chapter 1 begins explosively, with a showdown between Buddhists and Christians in the sixteenth and seventeenth centuries in Japan. Using sources both in the Portuguese and Japanese languages, the author discusses how Buddhist healers were wrapped up in the confrontation between Jesuit missionizing and Japanese resistance. Also focused on Japan, chapter 2 analyzes part of a sermon by a seventeenth-century female Japanese Buddhist leader whose arguments about meditation and health seem to articulate a vision that presages modern developments in Japanese Buddhism. Chapter 3, which moves to China and focuses on the medical writings of a seventeenth-century doctor there, challenges our conventional wisdom that a shift toward modernity necessarily involved turning away from religion by demonstrating how Buddhism lies at the foundation of the most influential trends in early modern Chinese medical thought. (See *Anthology*, vol. 1, ch. 62, for a discussion of roughly contemporaneous transitions in Tibet). Chapter 4 moves forward to the eighteenth century and shifts to Mongolia, which was then part of the great Qing Empire. The authors translate a treatise on smallpox inoculation and unpack what this short text reveals about the Qing colonial context. Chapter 5 explores a complex text by a Meiji-era Japanese author trying to integrate newly introduced Western medical knowledge into a Buddhist framework. The sixth and seventh chapters present diatribes against Asian Buddhist medicine from the high colonial period of the nineteenth and early twentieth century. Chapter 6 translates a poem that mocks Sri Lankan popular customs associated with the *yakṣa* demons, while chapter 7 translates three treatises by Western authors that are highly critical of Siamese religion and medicine. Both chapters demonstrate how poorly European and American observers thought of Buddhist healing interventions.

The second section, "Ruptures and Reconciliations," highlights Buddhist attempts to mend the ruptures with tradition experienced in the modern period through various types of apologetics, accommodations, and reinterpretations. Significantly, this section includes several chapters focusing on Buddhists' engagements with, and attempts to integrate, scientific or biomedical concepts, institutions, and practices. All of these presented challenges to traditional Buddhist ideas and authorities that needed to be navigated and negotiated.

Chapter 8 translates three Tibetan Buddhist texts about the dangers of using tobacco. These range in date from the nineteenth to the twenty-first century, but they all call upon traditional Buddhist imagery, fears of karmic retribution, and concepts of pollution to condemn the modern habit of smoking. Chapter 9 explores two different approaches to reconciling Buddhism with science taken by Chinese modernizers in the print-rich culture of 1920s Shanghai. Chapter 10 jumps forward a few decades to the 1950s and looks at the writings of an influential Tibetan physician on the compatibility between modern surgery and Tibetan medicine. Chapter 11 introduces a portion of the oeuvre of a Japanese scientist who took up painting late in life. His artwork touched upon some of the most pressing issues in contemporary bioethics—including DNA, heredity, and abortion—but does so through Buddhist imagery and reverence of the *Heart Sūtra*. The last two chapters in this section take us back to the Tibetan context, though this time to Tibetan diasporic communities. Both provide a glimpse into the ongoing challenge of interpreting Tibetan Buddhist and medical practice in light of science and biomedicine. Chapter 12 focuses on mantras and chapter 13 on the features of the human body, both outlining attempts by Tibetan authors to bolster the legitimacy and relevance of traditional Buddhist knowledge in the eyes of a contemporary global audience. Chapter 14 presents the writings of a Taiwanese monk on vegetarianism and healthy eating. Grounded in traditional notions of karmic merit as well as modern discourses of Humanistic Buddhism, his writings argue that eating well is necessary for the well-being of the individual, the nation, and the world.

The third section of this volume is titled "Hybridities and Innovations." While the previous section focuses on discourses preserving and legitimizing traditional Buddhist practices, this section emphasizes novel approaches to health and medicine. These new practices developed in the modern period, emerging directly from dialogues and intersections between Buddhism and secularism, globalization, new media, and other facets of contemporary global culture.

Chapter 15, for example, begins this exploration with a discussion of the impact of globalization on the resurrection of Esoteric Buddhist healing in Taiwan. The author introduces a charismatic guru whose writings in the 1960s combined an interest in Esoteric practices with Daoism, Indian yoga, Japanese martial arts, and other therapies that had begun circulating internationally. Chapter 16 takes us to Thailand, where Jīvaka Komārabhacca (a venerable doctor from the Pāli scriptures discussed in Anthology, vol. 1, ch. 1, 20) was reinvented as a popular medical deity. This reinvention, occasioned by a monk at a Vietnamese temple in Bangkok, involved a spirit revelation that allowed for Jīvaka's facial features to be rendered in an ethnically accurate and lifelike way. Chapter 17 then takes us to the Himalayan kingdom of Bhutan, where the government began developing the notion of evaluating a country's "Gross National Happiness" in the 1970s. When the GNH index finally began to be implemented in Bhutan in 2010, both it and the government's health policy came to be articulated in terms resonant with Buddhist values. Chapter 18 looks at the creation of new categories of health care practitioners in Japan after the catastrophic tsunami and nuclear disaster of March 11, 2011. The chapter introduces the writings of an influential innovator who outlines how Buddhist-trained "Vihāra priests" and interfaith chaplains offered "spiritual care" in a largely secular context. In chapter 19, the last in this section, the innovation in question is the use of new media to publicly promote and discuss what were once the secretive ritual practices of the "medicine wizards." This chapter analyzes four recent Facebook posts for what they tell us about both the practice of Buddhist healing in contemporary Myanmar and changing patterns of textual authority and information circulation in the age of social media.

The next section, "Meditation and Mental Health," turns to the subject of the health benefits of meditation, including, but not limited to, the practice of mindfulness. This section introduces various modern reformulations of Buddhist meditation in light of twentieth-century psychology, psychiatry, and mental health movements. They also discuss the institutionalization of Buddhist or Buddhist-inspired meditation practices in various government, corporate, university, and clinical settings.

Chapter 20 discusses a secularized therapeutic meditation developed in Japan in 1941, decades prior to the development of mindfulness protocols in the 1970s in the United States. Naikan ("introspection"), a practice extracted from Pure Land Buddhism, has since been used in prisons, hospitals, clinics, training centers, and other secular spaces, particularly for the treatment of alcoholism. Chapter 21 discusses how a Shingon Buddhist priest employs various meditations in hospitals and other clinical settings in Japan. This chapter translates excerpts from books written by a leading innovator in the contemporary Japanese practice of "spiritual care." Chapter 22 takes leave of Japan—and of Asia altogether—bringing us into the chambers of the British Parliament in the Palace of Westminster. Providing an excerpt of a recent parliamentary report on the benefits of mindfulness, this chapter also gives an outline of the history of mindfulness as it has evolved from a manifestly Buddhist practice into a secular therapy mandated by in the UK National Health Service. Chapter 23 includes the first transcript of an ethnographic interview included in the book. This interview with a Korean Sŏn (Jp. Zen) monk reveals a feedback loop whereby Korean Buddhist practices are influencing the study and practice of meditation in the West at the same time that the mindfulness protocols and mediation science originating in Western countries are influencing the meditation programs and trainings being taught by Buddhist monastics in Asia. Finally, chapter 24 rounds out our tour of meditation and mental health with an influential critique of "McMindfulness"—that is, the overly commercialized, overly hyped appropriations of mindfulness in corporate, clinical, and governmental settings—that appeared in a widely read popular media outlet.

In the fifth and penultimate section of the book, "Crossing Boundaries," contributors interrogate the category of "Buddhist medicine" by introducing healers and practices that lie on the margins, where it becomes increasingly unclear whether the label "Buddhism" fits any longer. The main point in this section is that, as already discussed above, Buddhist medicine is not a clearly bounded entity but rather a field of inquiry, a thicket of articulations that calls to be explored and described in all of its diversity. This section explores various syncretic assemblages in which aspects of Buddhism are combined with different kinds of non-Buddhist healing. Some call the resulting amalgam "Buddhist," whereas others refuse to, and still others do not know or simply do not care.

Chapter 25 discusses the remnants of Buddhist mantra healing discovered in Bengal by an Indian folklorist in the 1970s. With the Buddhist roots of this area of India long forgotten, these healing traditions had been absorbed into local Hindu, Muslim, and animist practices. Nevertheless, their ultimate origins in Buddhist mantra practice can still be discerned. While chapter 25 is a translation of a published work, the remainder of the chapters in the volume present transcripts of interviews with healers of various types. In chapter 26, interviews with two Chinese folk healers reveal that the boundary between Buddhist and non-Buddhist ritual healing is irrelevant to their practice. One states that he is not sure whether they are "Buddhist-style Daoists, or maybe Daoist-style Buddhists" and is not in the slightest bothered by the contradiction. In chapter 27, sectarian lines are blurred again by a Chinese American healer in New York City who has created his own blend of Buddhism, Daoism, Chinese medicine, Reiki, qigong, feng shui, and other eclectic practices from reading books, watching YouTube videos, and what he describes as "automatic movement." Likewise, in chapter 28, a Korean shaman reports how she has incorporated the bodhisattva Avalokiteśvara into a pantheon of spirits and ancestors that she uses to heal clients. Initially torn between Buddhism and shamanism, the practitioner describes the détente her spirit guides eventually reached with one another and the role

Avalokiteśvara plays in keeping the peace among her spirit allies. A somewhat parallel scenario is presented in chapter 29, which provides an interview with a New Age spiritual channel from northern California. The interviewee describes how Avalokiteśvara first appeared to her, her ongoing personal relationship with the bodhisattva, and how the deity empowers her healing sessions. Like the shaman, the spirit channel refuses to specifically call herself or her practice Buddhist, although she freely draws inspiration, imagery, and elements of practice from Buddhism.

The final section of the volume, "Buddhist Healing in Practice," continues to focus on transcripts of ethnographic interviews. Whereas the earlier sections of the book tend to focus on didactic arguments, the last two sections offer more intimate views into the personal biographical details, subjective experiences, and emotional lives of individual practitioners and patients. In this last section, individuals describe their experiences of Buddhist medicine, offering a geographically diverse sampling from around the contemporary world.

Chapter 30 begins in Thailand with an unlicensed folk healer whose description of the practice of medicine without a license is couched in the language and imagery of northern Thai Buddhist political resistance. Chapter 31, which focuses on a healer in Myanmar, similarly concerns how the practice of alchemy becomes an act of resistance against authorities who would standardize traditional medicine nationally. Chapter 32 takes us to a Tibetan diasporic community in Northern India. In this interview, a doctor of Sowa Rigpa (traditional Tibetan medicine) discusses the causes, symptoms, and treatments of mental illness among both Tibetan and Western patients. Chapter 33 introduces a Bhutanese practitioner of "edible letters," a Vajrayāna Buddhist form of talismanic healing. It includes a translation of an interview with him concerning details of his training and practice, as well as a translation of a short mantra text he carries with him describing the origins and efficacy of his therapies. Chapter 34 is a study of the "Way of Healing" of a group of Japanese women. It discusses specific Buddhist practices used by the women to heal or protect from illness, with an eye toward an overall Buddhist "orientation to living" that allows the women to deal with the suffering and pain they have experienced throughout various stages of life. Finally, chapter 35 presents a series of short excerpts from interviews with a diverse range of practitioners and patients of Buddhist medicine from a major metropolitan area in the United States. Taken together, these conversations showcase the diversity of articulations between Buddhism and medicine in different ethnic, linguistic, and sectarian contexts in this diverse city.

SCOPE AND LIMITATIONS OF THE VOLUME

Together, the chapters in this book illustrate many of the ways that Buddhism and medicine have intersected in the past few centuries and how these intersections continue to be relevant today. The chapters deal primarily with Asia but also suggest something of the larger global context. Notwithstanding the fact that a wide selection of practices, perspectives, and voices are presented here, there are some limitations to the present volume that must be stated explicitly.

First, a general reminder about the limitations of sources is in order. Since historians' work is based solely on written texts—and, what's more, on only that subset of texts that have survived the ravages of time—we can only ever glean an extremely partial view of the history of the human experience. It is like trying to study a vast and deep ocean of practice by examining the flecks of froth that collect on top of the waves. Ethnographic interviews, such as those presented toward the end of this volume, offer more intimate glimpses into the actual practices of actual people than is possible for any historical era. But even these are still mediated documents. Authors and interviewees present a certain face to the outside world and a certain interpretation of practice. Thus, this book should be understood as presenting a number of different viewpoints about Buddhist medicine, as expressed by certain individuals in different times and places. It cannot speak for, define, explain, or capture the practice of Buddhist medicine as a whole.

Another limitation of the present volume is that, with a total number of contributions numbering less than three dozen, its geographical and temporal coverage cannot be comprehensive. As editor, my intention was not to commission a range of more general pieces with the goal of comprehensive coverage. Instead, I have invited scholars currently working on various aspects of Buddhism and medicine to contribute focused snapshots from their own research projects. Thus, the scope of both volumes in this anthology is inherently limited by the interests of scholars working in particular subfields.

Happily, the geographic scope here has been expanded in comparison with the previous volume. In addition to materials from Bhutan, China, India, Japan, Korea, Mongolia, Myanmar, Sri Lanka, Taiwan, Thailand, and Tibet (as well as diasporic communities), the present volume also includes accounts by missionaries, colonial authorities, practitioners, and commentators from Europe and the United States. Many of these contexts were underrepresented or even completely lacking in the premodern volume. However, the current volume still does not include perspectives from modern Cambodia, Laos, or Vietnam—which have significant traditions of Buddhist medicine, both historically and today—or from other parts of the world, such as Australia, Latin America, or Africa—where various aspects of Buddhism, mindfulness, and Buddhist-inspired healing have been enjoying enthusiastic support recently. It is not for lack of trying that geographic and temporal gaps persist within this volume. But, alas, so long as there are exceedingly few Anglophone scholars who research Buddhist healing practices in these regions, a project such as this one will necessarily remain incomplete.

Turning to a third related issue, another regrettable lacuna in this volume is the very small proportion of chapters that focus on women: no more than about one-fifth of the total. In some ways, this imbalance can be traced to the gender hierarchies inherent in the Buddhist tradition itself. Men have historically enjoyed—and, in most Buddhist societies today, continue to enjoy—a markedly superior position within monastic and lay power structures and a much more authoritative voice as authors. At the same time, the gender imbalance in this book surely also reflects the imbalanced interests of scholars. If only because they gravitate toward the more influential or celebrated figures within the historical and contemporary Buddhist world, scholars for the most part continue to be predominantly interested in the thoughts and activities of Buddhist men. The contributors to this volume can attest that I continually pressed for greater inclusion of female voices in these pages, and two of them (Arai and Triplett) even obliged me by submitting at the last minute additional chapters focusing on women, for which I am very grateful. Still, we in the nascent field of "Buddhist medicine studies" need to do more as a group to broaden our inclusivity.

Finally, in discussing the scope and limitations of the present work, it is also worth mentioning that, although the chapters included here approach their materials from many different methodological and disciplinary angles, by no means are all scholarly disciplines represented. Chapters have been contributed by specialists in Buddhist studies, religious studies, history, linguistics, gender studies, medical anthropology, and history of medicine. These authors have invariably focused on the particular aspects of their source texts or ethnographic works that are of most interest to them as scholars in particular fields, and have thus made choices regarding what to highlight or omit based on their own scholarly expertise and training. A number of the contributors are themselves practitioners of Buddhism, meditation, chaplaincy, Asian medical traditions, or allied practices. They therefore approach their chapters with both a scholar's rigor as well as a practitioner's sensibility toward the details of embodied practice. As editor, I have made suggestions here and there, but I have not attempted to force these contributors to conform to a common approach, perspective, or style. Rather, at the same time that I appreciate the broad selection of contributions collected here for what they say about many different aspects of the historical and contemporary practice of Buddhist medicine, I also appreciate the broad sampling the authors have provided us of the diversity of methods in the academic study *of* those practices.

ABOUT THE TRANSLATIONS

Not all of the chapters presented here are translations, but the great majority are. As with the previous volume, our primary concern while producing and compiling these translations in the current anthology has been to ensure their accessibility for the widest possible readership. Our goal has been to produce a collection that will be helpful and interesting for diverse audiences, with minimum barriers to understanding. We expect our readers to include specialist and nonspecialist scholars from across the disciplinary spectrum, students at both the graduate and undergraduate levels, as well as general readers without any particular scholarly background. We assume that some readers will be very knowledgeable about Asian medicine but know nothing about Buddhism, and vice versa, and that some readers will be new to both. To these ends, the translations included here are rigorous but readable. They accurately capture the meaning of the original texts while remaining devoid of the stilted style that has been called "Buddhist Hybrid English," which sacrifices fluency in order to preserve the original syntax and sentence structure as much as possible.[8] Instead, we have used natural English grammar and phrasing in all cases, as well as English equivalents for even the most technical Buddhist and medical terminology.

An important exception to this general policy has been made for a handful of key Buddhist and medical terms that are rendered here in the original (e.g., *dhāraṇī, qi, tridoṣa, yin-yang*). Influential concepts such as these are consistently given in the language from which they derive in order to explicitly demonstrate connections between the key doctrines discussed across multiple chapters. The general definitions of these common terms are given in the glossary, but where there are unique instances of local usage or shades of meaning in other languages, brief explanations have always been included in the endnotes.

Speaking of the endnotes, in the interest of accessibility for a wide audience, contributors were asked not to include extensive annotations or notes about Buddhist doctrinal concerns, details about their translation decisions, local terminological variations, or other points of specialized interest. Everyone who has contributed to the current project has either published, or is in the process of publishing, scholarly works that touch upon these aspects, and those already published have been cited in the Further Readings sections and endnotes in each chapter.

FURTHER READING

Each chapter in this volume includes a list of further readings on specific aspects of Buddhism, medicine, and their intersections in various historical contexts. These have been compiled by the chapter authors with the intention of introducing the reader to the most accessible literature related to each chapter's contents. Readers should be aware that these lists include only English-language publications, though scholarship that has been published in other languages is cited in the endnotes accompanying each chapter. Readers should also note that these lists of further readings exclude theses, conference papers, forthcoming works, and other unpublished materials—although all of these are cited in the endnotes as well.

The further readings listed in this introduction represent published works that are particularly focused on modern Buddhist medicine and that therefore can situate the reader within this field more generally. Leaving aside the scientific literature on mindfulness—which, as suggested above, has become a cottage industry of considerable size[9]—there is far less scholarly material published on Buddhism and medicine in the modern and contemporary period than there is for the premodern period. Works concerning Buddhism and medicine in the premodern period are listed in the introduction to the first volume of this anthology.[10] For further reading on the topic of Buddhism and medicine specifically concerning the modern and contemporary period, the reader should consult the major publications listed below. Note that this list focuses entirely on descriptive works by humanities and social science scholars (e.g., anthropology, history, philosophy, and religious studies) and does not include prescriptive works by scientists, clinicians, or practitioners.

EAST ASIA

Arai, Paula. 2011. *Bringing Zen Home: The Healing Heart of Japanese Women's Rituals*. Honolulu: University of Hawai'i Press.

Johnston, William D. 2016. "Buddhism Contra Cholera: How the Meiji State Recruited Religion Against Epidemic Disease." In *Science, Technology, and Medicine in the Modern Japanese Empire*, edited by David G. Wittner and Philip C. Brown. Abingdon, Oxon: Routledge, 62–78.

Josephson, Jason Ānanda. 2013. "An Empowered World: Buddhist Medicine and the Potency of Prayer in Japan." In *Deus in Machina: Religion, Technology, and the Things in Between*, edited by Jeremy Stolow, 117–41. New York: Fordham University Press.

Traphagan, John. 2004. *The Practice of Concern: Ritual, Well-Being, and Aging in Rural Japan*. Durham, N.C.: Caroline Academic Press.

Uhlmann, Patrick R. 2007. "A Buddhist Rite of Exorcism." In *Religions of Korea in Practice*, edited by Robert E. Buswell, 112–29. Princeton Readings in Religions. Princeton, N.J.: Princeton University Press.

Winfield, Pamela D. 2005. "Curing with Kaji: Healing and Esoteric Empowerment in Japan." *Japanese Journal of Religious Studies* 32 (1): 107–30.

HIMALAYAN REGION

Adams, Vincanne, Mona Schrempf, and Sienna R. Craig, eds. 2011. *Medicine Between Science and Religion: Explorations on Tibetan Grounds*. New York: Berghahn.

Dietrich, Angela. 1996. "Research Note: Buddhist Healers in Nepal, Some Observations." *Contributions to Nepalese Studies* 23 (2): 473–80.

Garrett, Frances. 2009. "The Alchemy of Accomplishing Medicine (*sman sgrub*): Situating the *Yuthok Heart Essence* (*G.yu thog snying thig*) in Literature and History." *Journal of Indian Philosophy* 37 (3): 207–30.

Gyatso, Janet. 2015. *Being Human in a Buddhist World: An Intellectual History of Medicine in Early Modern Tibet*. New York: Columbia University Press.

Hofer, Theresia, ed. 2014. *Bodies in Balance: The Art of Tibetan Medicine*. Seattle: University of Washington Press.

Pordié, Laurent. 2003. "The Expression of Religion in Tibetan Medicine: Ideal Conceptions, Contemporary Practices and Political Use." *Pondy Papers in Social Sciences 29*.

Samuel, Geoffrey. 2014. "Healing in Tibetan Buddhism." In *The Wiley Blackwell Companion to East and Inner Asian Buddhism*. Edited by Mario Poceski. Chichester, West Sussex: John Wiley, 278–96.

Yoeli-Tlalim, Ronit. 2010. "Tibetan 'Wind' and 'Wind' Illnesses: Towards a Multicultural Approach to Health and Illness." *Studies in History and Philosophy of Biological and Biomedical Sciences* 41: 318–24.

SOUTHEAST ASIA

Gosling, David. 1985. "Thailand's Bare-Headed Doctors." *Modern Asian Studies* 19 (4): 761–96.

Kapferer, Bruce. 1983. *A Celebration of Demons: Exorcism and the Aesthetics of Healing in Sri Lanka*. Bloomington: Indiana University Press.

Patton, Thomas Nathan. 2018. *The Buddha's Wizards: Magic, Healing and Protection in Burmese Buddhism*. New York: Columbia University Press.

Ratanakul, Pinit. 1999. "Buddhism, Health, Disease, and Thai Culture." In *A Crosscultural Dialogue on Health Care Ethics*, edited by Harold G. Coward and Pinit Ratanakul. Waterloo, Ont.: Wilfrid Laurier University Press, 17–33.

Salguero, C. Pierce. 2016. *Traditional Thai Medicine: Buddhism, Animism, Yoga, Ayurveda*. Rev. ed. Bangkok: White Lotus.

Salguero, C. Pierce. 2017. "Honoring the Teachers, Constructing the Lineage: A *Wai Khru* Ritual Among Healers in Chiang Mai, Thailand." In *Translating the Body: Medical Education in Southeast Asia*, edited by Hans Pols, C. Michele Thompson, and John Harley Warner. Singapore: NUS Press, 295–318.

Tambiah, Stanley Jeyaraja. 1977. "The Cosmological and Performative Significance of a Thai Cult of Healing through Meditation." *Culture, Medicine and Psychiatry* 1 (1): 97–132.

THE WEST

Numrich, P. D. 2005. "Complementary and Alternative Medicine in America's 'Two Buddhisms.'" In *Religion and Healing in America*, edited by Linda L. Barnes and Susan S. Sered, 343–58. Oxford: Oxford University Press.

Salguero, C. Pierce. 2019. "Varieties of Buddhist Healing in Multiethnic Philadelphia." *Religions* 10 (1), doi:10.3390/rel10010048. Accessed June 16, 2019. https://www.mdpi.com/2077-1444 /10/1/48.

Wilson, Jeff. 2014. *Mindful America: The Mutual Transformation of Buddhist Meditation and American Culture*. New York: Oxford University Press.

Wu, Hongyu. 2002. "Buddhism, Health, and Healing in a Chinese Community." The Pluralism Project, Harvard University. http://pluralism.org/wp-content/uploads/2015/08/Wu.pdf.

NOTES

1. For introductory overviews of the relationship between Buddhism and medicine, see (briefly) Kitagawa 1989, (more in-depth) Anālayo 2016, as well as the third volume in the current series. For works concerning the practice of Buddhist medicine in various specific cultures across the globe, see the Further Reading sections in the introductions to either volume of the current anthology and Salguero 2014a.

2. Salguero 2015a: 48.

3. This is a major theme in the third volume in this series, and see also Salguero 2015b.

4. For one example of how these processes of transmission and translation have worked in history, see Salguero 2014b on medieval China.

5. Whether certain medical ideas or practices qualify as "Buddhist" has been a source of consternation and negotiation in certain circles both historically and today. See, for example, the debates in early modern Tibet discussed in J. Gyatso 2015 and in *Anthology*, vol. 1, ch. 62. For contemporary debates in the field of psychology among practitioners who incorporate mindfulness into their practice, see Helderman 2016; Sharf 2015.

6. All searches were conducted on on April 29, 2019. The *Time* magazine covers featuring mindfulness or similar meditation practices include the August 4, 2003, and February 2, 2014, issues, as well as a special issue dedicated to mindfulness published in 2017. According to a Google search ("mindfulness site:time.com"), the word "mindfulness" currently appears over 3,100 times on the *Time* website alone. An overview of the meteoric rise of mindfulness is provided in J. Wilson 2014.

7. Helderman 2016; cf. Sharf 2015.

8. I borrow the term "Buddhist Hybrid English" from Griffiths 1981.

9. A recent search of PubMed, a database maintained by the U.S. National Library of Medicine, resulted in more than 5,200 articles with the word *mindfulness* in their titles or abstracts. This search, conducted on July 22, 2018, represents an increase of more than 1,100 titles since the author's last recorded search on February 28, 2017. For a recent meta-study providing an overview of the fast-moving research area of meditation studies, see Goyal et al. 2014. For a range of critiques and discussions of mindfulness from the perspectives of the humanities and social sciences, see also J. Williams and Kabat-Zinn 2011; Purser, Forbes, and Burke 2016.

10. For a more comprehensive list of highlights, see Salguero 2014a (updated 2018).

Early Modernity

1. Buddhist Monastic Physicians' Encounters with the Jesuits in Sixteenth- and Seventeenth-Century Japan, as Told from Both Sides

KATJA TRIPLETT

In 1540, during the period of the Counter-Reformation, Pope Paul III officially recognized the Jesuits (the Society of Jesus or Company of Jesus) as a religious order dedicated to combating Protestant reforms in Europe and establishing Christian missions worldwide. Under the leadership of Ignatius de Loyola (Íñigo López, c. 1491–1556), the Jesuit order grew to a group of about one thousand. The activities of Portuguese Jesuits in Japan commenced with the arrival of Francisco Xavier (1506–1552) in 1549. In Asia, Jesuits hoped to convert members of the elite, who presumably would then also have their subjects convert. Such a top-down conversion did in fact happen, resulting in a large number of conversions during the heyday of the Jesuit mission in Japan.[1]

Christian efforts to win converts included the establishment of colleges, churches, schools, orphanages, and hospitals in various parts of Japan, not only by the Society of Jesus but also, later, by other Christian orders, especially the Franciscans. For Japanese Buddhists, Christianity was therefore not just a rival religion but also represented new practical forms of knowledge such as astronomy, cartography using globes, and surgery. This influx of new ideas, tools, and practices particularly stimulated exchanges between Jesuits and Buddhist monastic doctors, who had been operating in Japan for nearly one thousand years at that point.

The texts presented in the first section below date from the period of intense Jesuit missionary activity in Japan. Such reports by the Jesuits stationed in Japan were revised and printed for a wider audience in Europe. However, owing to the severe persecution of Christians in later years, records about cooperation between local Buddhist doctors practicing medicine in the Sino-Japanese style and the Jesuits from Portugal are scarce. These texts must be read primarily as records propagating the successes of the Society of Jesus in faraway "heathen" lands. However, they provide valuable insights into the Buddhist–Christian encounters in Kyushu and other places in Japan.[2]

In several of these texts, it is apparent that the Jesuit hospital in Funai (in today's Ōita, on Kyushu, the southernmost island in the Japanese archipelago) became a site of encounter between Buddhist monastic physicians and the wealthy Portuguese surgeon and merchant Luís de Almeida (1525–1597), who had taken lay orders in the Society of Jesus in 1556. After founding an orphanage in Funai, he established a large hospital and a pharmacy that dispensed medicines, some of which were imported from the Portuguese trade base in Macao.[3] The surgery that Almeida performed left a lasting, if low-level, impression on the Japanese, becoming known as "southern barbarian-style surgery" (nanban-ryū geka).[4] The first two translations below show that among the medical staff at Almeida's hospital was a Buddhist monastic physician, Kyōzen, who was renamed Paulo. Whether he was primarily interested in the imported creed and converted to Christianity, or whether he concentrated on medicine in order to study surgical methods in his capacity as doctor, remains unclear.

The first text translated below is an excerpt from a letter by Father Balthazar Gago (1520–1583) that describes the new hospital in Funai and the accomplishments of the convert Paulo. The Jesuit father reports on the usefulness of the Chinese medicines and books found among the doctor's possessions after he had died. The second text is from the History of Japan (História de Japam), a compilation by the Jesuit Luís Fróis (1532–1597) that was itself based on letters sent by the author. Here, Fróis recounts the relationship the Jesuits had with two "bonzes" (Japanese Buddhist monastics) who came from a prestigious monastic institution. Paulo makes another appearance in this account as an important supporter of the Jesuit mission in Japan.

The third passage translated below recalls the conversion to Christianity of the famous Buddhist monastic physician Manase Dōsan (1507–1594), who treated a Jesuit missionary in Kyoto. This abridged translation includes a compelling conversation between Dōsan and Belchior de Figueiredo (c. 1530–1597), the rector of the college in Funai, on ideas of the body and the soul, which took place in 1584. This account, also written by Father Luís Fróis, is also drawn from his extensive history of the mission in Japan.

In 1612, it was decreed that members of the Society of Jesus were prohibited from learning and practicing medicine or surgery, ending the Jesuits' official involvement in medical matters.[5] The Jesuit mission itself ended with the Japanese central military government's 1639 prohibition of all Christian activities in the Japanese empire, which was strictly enforced. A few years later, in 1644, the last foreign Christian missionary was executed, thus bringing to a close Japan's "Christian century."[6]

While European perspectives on encounters with Japanese religions, science, and customs are accessible and have been well studied, the study of the opinions of Japanese Buddhists about European culture in this period is limited owing to the volatile political circumstances in Japan. The fourth section below contains an abridged translation from the Japanese from *The Rise and Fall of the Temple of the Southern Barbarians* (*Nanbanji kōhaiki*), which relates the story of the Jesuit Church in Kyoto and depicts doctors as sorcerers.[7] Populist anti-Christian texts such as this circulated widely in Japan in the decades after the persecutions, peaking in the 1660s. While these texts provide some insight into the medical activities of the Christian missionaries, they use polemical and dehumanizing language aimed at discrediting both the foreigners and the Japanese individuals with whom they interacted.[8]

FURTHER READING

Bowers, John Z. 1970. *Western Medical Pioneers in Feudal Japan*. Baltimore, Md.: Johns Hopkins University Press, 2–19.

Cooper, Michael, ed. 1965. *They Came to Japan: An Anthology of European Reports on Japan, 1543–1640*. Berkeley: University of California Press, 239–42.

Reff, Daniel T., Richard K. Danford, and Robin Gill, eds. 2014. *The First European Description of Japan, 1585: A Critical English-Language Edition of* Striking Contrasts in the Customs of Europe and Japan *by Luis Fróis, S. J.* London: Routledge, 175–83.

Vos, Fritz. 1991. "From God to Apostate: Medicine in Japan Before the Caspar School." In *Red-Hair Medicine: Dutch-Japanese Medical Relations*, edited by H. Beukers, Antoine M. Luyendijk-Elshout, M. E. Van Opstall, and Fritz Vos, 19–26. Amsterdam: Rodopi.

ACCOUNTS BY PORTUGUESE JESUITS IN JAPAN

1. Excerpts from a Letter from Father Balthazar Gago to the Brothers of the Company of Jesus in India, Written in Japan on November 1, 1559[9]

Because of the hospital's fame, people flock to it from all these places. Since last summer, two hundred people have been healed from all kinds of diseases by surgery and physic. The father admitted all those who were suffering, however lost and desperate they were, and they were healed more by the Lord's grace than by medicine. Among them [was someone who had been suffering from] cancer for as long as sixty years, another who had been suffering for more than twenty years, and others with various kinds of tumors.

Our beloved Luís de Almeida, who has received a great talent from our Lord in surgery, has trained several members of staff and made them specialists. Among them is Brother Duarte da Silva who applies two kinds of therapy: with preaching for the soul and with powders, ointments, and cauteries for the body.

We had a Japanese man who conducted surgery and provided physic. He came from Miyako to Yamaguchi to meet the father [Cosme de Torres] who converted him and christened him Paulo. The man had originally trained as a bonze and in pagodas. As he appreciated communal life, he lived with the father when he came to Bungo. When in the company of the father, he was much given to penances, and he always mortified himself.[10] Father Mestre Belchior[11] saw his ability. [Paulo] practiced physic and used books and some medicines of his own. After he died[12] of an illness, a man named Miguel followed him, but he also died soon after. Both died in the Christian faith.

The father took the medicines and used them. The medicines came from China (and Chinese men studied the two books) and [thus the medicines] could easily be prepared and worked to great effect. He used one of the medicines to treat all kinds of diseases [that subject one to] fevers of three or four days. This medicine cured Guilherme Pereira[13] and the entire ship's crew when they all arrived in Bungo ill. Everyone was very pleased [about the cure]. Some took [the medicine] with them to China. After witnessing its effect, the father ordered that it should be distributed among them.

2. Excerpt from the *History of Japan*: "On the Conversion of Paulo and Barnabé, Two Famous Bonzes, and How Father Cosme de Torres Sent Brother Lorenço with Barnabé to the University of Hie-no-yama"[14]

Two years before [Father de Torres[15]] took the decision [to proselytize in Miyako], two bonzes came to him in the city of Yamaguchi from the kingdom of Yamato.[16] They came from a very famous monastery called Tōnomine. One of them was called Kyōzen and the other Sen'yō. They were men of great intelligence and great prowess, and one of them was very learned in the sects of Japan and an excellent physician. They listened carefully to the preaching of the sermons about the catechism. Then they spent several days presenting their doubts and pondering the answers given to them, and they did this with such intelligence, moderation, and decency that all who heard them were astonished. Finally, after they had both reached complete understanding, they became Christians.[17] The more learned of the two, who was more advanced in all matters, was given the name Paulo. He was a rare and excellent man of virtue. The other was given the name Barnabé.

3. Excerpt from the *History of Japan*: "The Conversion of the Best Scholar and Leading Doctor of Japan, Residing in Miyako" (Abridged)[18]

Among the physicians of the sixty-six domains of Japan, the three best reside in Miyako, and the most excellent of those three is called Dōsan.[19] This man is not only famous for his medical skills, but he has other rare skills, and, because of those, he is honored and venerated by the kings and princes, and he is given the utmost preference everywhere.

There are two [skills] that make him stand out: (1) He is the best scholar in all of the Japanese kingdoms, well versed in Chinese characters and knowledgeable in all the arts; and (2) he is the most eloquent person there is, and his parables and aphorisms are a great pleasure to the gentlemen when they converse with him. He has eight hundred disciples in Miyako whom he teaches the art of medicine, letters, and rhetoric. He is famous for healing, and for many years he has set up his house in Miyako for lecturing publicly on medicine. He was past seventy years of age, a man with a good complexion, of a prudent nature, living an orderly and moral life, and being kind when conversing with others.

Last year, Father Belchior de Figueiredo,[20] the rector of the college in Funai, had a grave and troublesome illness, so he went to Miyako because he was better accommodated there, especially in terms of physicians. Settled in Miyako, he was overwhelmed with so much pain that he wanted to visit the aforementioned doctor. But there was a difficulty: Because [the doctor] had such a great reputation, he made excuses about his age and never left the house to see any patient. Although other physicians were recommended to him, the father kept asking to see Dōsan, and, because the father could not stand, they carried him in a palanquin to [Dōsan's] house.

The father talked about [his health], and after Dōsan had given him some remedies, they started a conversation discussing medicines that could prolong life, both being elderly men. Reaching the topic of religion and what we do, Dōsan said something about himself: "For the health of my body, I have lived in chastity for sixteen years, despite having an old wife [i.e., being married for a long time]."

The father used this as an occasion to share some thoughts. The doctor was hard of hearing, so, leaning toward his ear, he said that bodily health, which lasts only for such a short time, as experience shows, forces men to toil and sweat to conserve it. Much more attention and diligence should be invested to conserve the health of the soul, which will lead to eternal life.

Dōsan replied, saying, "Is there life in men that abides?"

The father responded, "Yes, there is. Above the entire universe is a principle of immortal and glorious life; it is the Creator and absolute Lord of both Heaven and Earth. By his grace, souls live forever and are saved. This principle, which is superior and has infinite wisdom and kindness, gives each creature in the universe, and humans in particular, their being, life, and abilities."

The father knew that he [Dōsan] belonged to the Zen sect,[21] which does not recognize the immortality of the soul. Knowing that the Zen sect believes neither in the renunciation of glory nor in suffering torment in the future life, but rather that when the life of a man expires all his things end up [expiring] as well, that man becomes chaos in which there is neither life nor death, and that the Zen sect calls this *fombun*,[22] the father said, "Such a Creator of the universe is by no means to be compared with the Zen primary principle of everything. The Zen sect believes that all humans are created and become one and the same substance.

Such chaos has neither wisdom, life, nor kindness. We cannot tell the created what they do not have."

Dōsan replied, "While I have studied the sects of Japan, I have never yielded to any of them, not even the Zen sect, because I am not at all satisfied [by any of them]. I also have my way to get by, though."

The father said, "It is not enough for me to cure considering only medicine for [physical] health. Just so, being obliged and entrusted to you as a doctor and professor of [medicine], your consideration is not enough without commending us. We are preachers and professors of the divine and supernatural science and of the salvation of men, ordered to Japan many thousand leagues [away] to propose this for this purpose."

Dōsan smiled, showing that he was satisfied with the comparison but still disappointed the father by saying, "Why should old Dōsan get into new considerations now?"

"Now more than ever," said the father, "you are aware that you are already near your last moments."

[Dōsan] thought of another excuse, saying, "I have no physical strength anymore to go to your church, which is far away, and hear your sermons."

[In the end,] Dōsan kept his promise [to visit the church] and brought two presents as was customary in Japan, one for Father Organtino,[23] who was [our] superior in these parts, and the other for Father Belchior de Figueiredo. He visited him in his cell, took his pulse, using words of much love, and offered to cure him free of charge out of love and the sense of obligation that he felt toward him.

Following preparation, [Dōsan] asked for baptism. Father Organtino baptized him and named him Belchior. Dōsan received the holy baptism with gratitude, and after he was joined with the Lord, and the Fathers and brothers had cheered, he bade them farewell.

The news of Dōsan's conversion reached the ears of the Vô,[24] the supreme king of all of Japan. The heathen enemies of the law of God maligned [the event] in such a way that he [the Vô] sent a message about it, saying, "It is unworthy for Dōsan to become a disciple of the law of the Christians, an enemy of the law of the *camis* [i.e., *kami*],[25] whom he calls demons, a law which will certainly provoke their wrath."

Dōsan responded prudently, saying, "Having only been a Christian for a very short time, I had not heard that the law of God calls the *camis* demons. The priests should know that the *camis* were men and princes of the past and [belong to] the royal generation of the Vô and the nobility of Japan, but I have heard a doctrine of virtues and of righteousness."

The message Dōsan sent was soon made known to the Church, and he sent a message to the Japanese brothers who preached. The message stated that if, by chance, they had referred to the *camis* in this manner [i.e., as demons], they should now always refer to them [differently] out of respect for the Vô and the nobility of Japan so as not to anger the hearts of the Vô and the gentile lords with this [and turn them] against the Christians. Instead, they should describe the *camis* as dead men, whose strengths and merits did not grant them salvation or help them in the problems of this life, and they should [say] this with moderate words, not offending the gentiles.[26]

A Japanese Anti-Christian Polemic[27]

4. Abridged excerpt from *The Rise and Fall of the Temple of the Southern Barbarians*

So, the stranger, having arrived at Azuchi, took a three-day rest at Myōhōji Temple. Nobunaga[28] asked him, via [the interpreter] Inoko Hyōnosuke, for the reason he had come to Japan. The interpreter transmitted the conversation between the two sides.

Organtino[29] replied, "I have made this journey for the single reason of spreading Buddhism.[30] I have absolutely no other desire than realizing this wish."

This was the information he gave. After the meeting, Nobunaga lodged him at Myōhōji Temple and designated Nakaizumi Tōzaemon to oversee the stranger's care. Now, among those who came from Organtino's homeland were brothers and fathers including Brothers Gregory and Luís.[31] The two brothers were admirable medical doctors and surgeons. [They] sent a request to Nobunaga saying, "The religion of the Emperor of Heaven saves the sick, the poor, and the suffering in all countries. It gives peace to the people in every situation and through its teachings fulfills their wish to live in peace in the present, as well as their wish to enjoy felicity in the future. In order to attend to this care, we would like to have a garden in which to cultivate all kinds of medicinal plants." Nobunaga approved of this idea and told them to choose a place in the provinces bordering Yamashiro.

The people of the temple [the Jesuit church in Kyoto], far from being concerned by the multitude [of inquisitive people coming to see the church], sent men to all corners of the capital and beyond. They went to the crossings of mountain paths or country paths with their little wayside shrines and to places under bridges. The task was to find the most degraded, beggars and those who suffered from the most serious illnesses. They took them back with them, gave them a hot bath and clothing, kept them warm, and cared for them in all sorts of ways so that yesterday's beggar was today a gentleman clad in Chinese silk.

The joy experienced by these poor people resulted in the healing of many of their illnesses. In particular, leprosy and other serious afflictions disappeared within a few months and were healed entirely by the strangers' medical treatment. In all kingdoms, near and far, news of all kinds about them [the strangers] was spreading. They were treated as veritable buddhas and bodhisattvas who had appeared here on Earth to rescue and save the world. Those who were afflicted with terrible pain, without resources, who found themselves without strength, or those who could not be healed despite the care of all the doctors, people of the noble class as well as of the lowest came from everywhere to gather in front of the temple.

The two brothers, Gregory and Luís, brought them all in and gave them good remedies, and then, having gathered the half-cured ill, they told them thus, "Now, our care can heal the illnesses of this life, but not the terrible illnesses in the time to come. The defilement of the body can be washed off, the one of the heart cannot, even with the waves of an ocean. If people who, without having done anything bad in their present life, fall ill or experience misery, this is the effect of bad deeds in their former life.[32] As a consequence, it is impossible to escape eternal pain before ending this former existence. Let everyone, whether or not they are protected from eternal pain by the purity of their heart, glance into this mirror!"

Having said this, they reverently hung up a mirror called the Mirror of the Three Worlds[33] and had them [their audience] look into it. Their audience felt faith blossom in their hearts. They said to themselves, "What an admirable and rare thing, surely, to see what will happen in our next life."

And they looked into that mirror. Now, images appeared in it, and some looked like a cow, some like a horse, a bird, a beast, and others just looked like hideous figures. The people were frightened, shed tears, and pleaded that the two brothers call down the mercy of the King of Heaven on them and save them from the punishments to come. The brothers replied, "You are all in deep trouble. We can tell you the mantra (shingon) for worshiping the King of Heaven. Purify your hearts, and, with all the power of your soul, repeat the sacred words while holding a rosary. With each repetition, move one bead."

With this, they gave them [their audience] rosaries called contas, which are composed of forty-two beads. This is the content of the mantra: "Let me be born in the heavenly paradise in my future life, and give me a happy life, Maria!" These methods served the two fathers and the two brothers to abuse those with simple spirits and attract them to their evil teachings.

The sick kept coming in great numbers to the temple [the church]. There were those who came to recover and others whose illnesses were difficult to cure so that they came to succumb to them. There were about thirty who were very seriously ill and, after all previous treatment had proved ineffective, recovered their health there. That is how the number of converts never ceased to increase. There were three in particular who, by their intelligence and their talents, became close disciples of the fathers and ended up taking part in the propaganda for the ignorant. The first one, originally from the province of Kaga, had been a bonze of the Zen sect, and he was called Eshun. The second one was once a merchant in the province of Izumi, and he was called Anzaemon the cloth merchant. The third one was also a native of the province of Izumi, a farmer called Zengorō from the village of Sumimura, born with a harelip. The two fathers saw with joy the religious progress of the three men, who were very gifted and remarkably well educated. They gave Eshun the name Fabian, Anzaemon the name Cosme, and Zengorō was called Simon.

The fathers and brothers rejoiced [over their success in propagating their creed], and the fathers taught them [the three men] some magical arts in secret in the interior of the temple [the church]. The three converts devoted themselves to these arts with untiring perseverance. They took towels, and in place of the towels one saw a horse. They threw dust into the air, and it turned into a bird. They caused a dried-up tree to flower and turned a handful of pebbles into precious pearls. They sat suspended in midair, hid underground, and made black clouds appear all of a sudden, or let it rain or snow. They had all these kinds of magic tricks in their power.

[After Nobunaga's death, Fabian's attempt to win the support of the new ruler, Hideyoshi, came to Hideyoshi's attention.][34] This great general, who was quick of mind and very perceptive, immediately understood what had happened and said, "Nobunaga had been the official protector of this sect. After his death by an unexpected and fatal blow, it is now me who has this power. It is true that I do not care about any of what the Buddha preached. But at least it is because of Buddhism's morality that the people believe and follow its practices, whereas the extraordinary way of these strangers consists of converting people by seducing them with their generosity. In particular, I remember now that some of the local rulers (daimyōs) started to participate in this creed. We must immediately abolish the Temple of the Barbarians!"

Fabian, Cosme and Simon, without waiting until all the streets were filled with soldiers, which would make escape impossible, ran away without even taking anything with them: Fabian to Kyushu; the second to the province of Tōtōmi, where he had acquaintances; and the third hid himself in the province of Echizen.

Four years later, Cosme returned from Tōtōmi to Izumi and started living secretly in Sakai at a place called Nakanohama. He had taken the name of Ichibashi Shōnosuke and practiced surgery. Simon also returned to Sakai at about the same time, establishing himself in the eastern valley, and called himself Shimada Seian. He earned a living practicing medicine. In 1588, when Hideyoshi resided in Fushimi castle, two men from Sakai visited him there and, talking about this and that, recounted the following: "Recently, a certain Ichibashi Shōnosuke, a surgeon, and Shimada Seian, a physician, have established themselves in Sakai. It appears that they practice an extraordinary kind of magic. They let a piece of paper cut into the shape of a flower float in a great basin filled with water, and the paper slip changed into a fish, which we saw swimming around in the water. Or, even better, they put one end of a string into their mouth and blew it up so that it became as thick as a rope and, throwing it across the hall, turned into a large serpent."

Hideyoshi did not so easily accept those supernatural arts and asked, "I have never yet seen any ghostly apparitions. Could they not show some to me as well?" They replied that they would bring them to him to show him ghosts that evening at dusk and left.

The two were summoned at the agreed hour. They first asked for help extinguishing all the lights; then they opened the panels, and in the garden one could see a classical landscape, illuminated by the moon of the seventeenth day of the ninth month; nothing was missing, neither the mysterious light nor the sudden gusts, the torrential rain, the flickering lights in the leaves on the trees and plants, the cold air. A strange apparition came out from among the trees: a young woman dressed in white, her hair all astray, looking like someone who had experienced great suffering. She remained in the garden without moving. The ladies and gentlemen gathered in the hall exclaimed, "Enough; this is not funny anymore!"

The apparition, however, came closer, and when it was near the veranda, Hideyoshi, who could see it better, recognized Chrysanthemum, his former mistress from the time when he was still called Kinoshita Tōkichi. After Hideyoshi rose to power, Chrysanthemum had come to him, requesting that she be placed in the service of the Imperial Palace. She had previously served there but had been driven away by people throwing insults. The palace refused to take her back, and Chrysanthemum turned on Hideyoshi in rage. Hideyoshi had then killed her with his own hands. The two men could not possibly know of this event. "How did fate make them show this woman, and how cruel of them!" everyone thought.

Finally, Hideyoshi, his face a picture of anger, made the two sorcerers leave. He then said, "These people possess extraordinary, unheard-of skills. This is probably nothing more than something left over from the faction of the Christian temple. Arrest them and question them!" They confessed that they were the men called Cosme and Simon, and consequently they were tortured by crucifixion at Kuritaguchi on the nineteenth day of the ninth month of 1588.

NOTES

This chapter was drafted with the support of a grant from the Humanities Center of Advanced Studies "Multiple Secularities—Beyond the West, Beyond Modernities" at Leipzig University, funded by the German Research Foundation. For further information, please consult www.multiple-secularities.de.

1. Depending on the source, there were between 300,000 and 750,000 Christian converts out of an estimated population of twelve million in early seventeenth-century Japan.

2. This Christian–Buddhist encounter is both the earliest and the best documented in letters, diaries, and other texts, even when compared with encounters in Sri Lanka (Hirota 2014: 412).

3. In fact, Almeida invested heavily in trading ventures, and, after he had joined the Society of Jesus, profits from his trading activities, which included trade in silk, were used to finance the Catholic mission (Schilling 1931: 18, 27–28). In 1585, the Holy See ordered the Society of Jesus to cede all mercantile enterprises, as these were not deemed befitting of a religious order.

4. See Michel 2001: 7.

5. See Boxer 1951: 202–204, on medicine.

6. For an overview of the "Christian century" in English, see the classic studies by Boxer 1951 and Elison 1973.

7. For a translation of a similar narrative, see Leuchtenberger 2013.

8. Buddhists such as Suzuki Shōsan (1579–1655) published anti-Christian writings after the eradication of Christian practices and the Christian mission in Japan. See Elison 1973; King 1986; Paramore 2009: 61–64.

9. Translation of the letter as printed in *Cartas*, f. 63r–64v, the modern Portuguese edition (Garcia 1997) of the 1598 publication. Eglauer provides an abbreviated and somewhat faulty German translation of Gago's letter (1794, vol. 1: 157–59). Balthazar Gago, a Jesuit from Portugal, landed on Kyushu in 1552. Not long after his arrival, he had an audience with the ruler of Bungo, Ōtomo Yoshishige, through an interpreter, Brother Juan Fernández (c. 1526–1567), who was sent by de Torres from Yamaguchi to Bungo for the express purpose of making a favorable impression on the powerful "King of Bungo." However, Ōtomo Yoshishige, who was broadly supportive, did not agree to provide funds for building a hospital in Funai. In the end, Almeida financed the hospital himself.

10. The practice of mortification aims at subduing the body. It often involves self-flagellation.

11. Father Mestre Belchior Nunez Barreto (c. 1520–1571) arrived in Japan in 1556 but left after only a few months, journeying to China and Cochin.

12. A letter written by Almeida on November 1, 1557, states that Paulo has just died (Garcia 1997: f. 52v–53r).

13. Guilherme Pereira (c. 1537–1603) was one of five orphans travelling on the same ship with Mestre Belchior Nunez Barreto in 1556. Guilherme was there to help with the mission in Japan. He later joined the Society of Jesus.

14. The Portuguese Jesuit Luís Fróis came to Japan in 1563, where he remained. Hie-no-yama is Mount Hiei, a mountain near Kyoto where the center of Buddhist learning was located. The following is a translation from the Portuguese of his letter, as printed in the modern edition of Fróis's *Historia de Japam* (Fróis and Wicki 1976, vol. 1: 81–82). I have referenced the German translation of the first part of Fróis's work (1549–1578) by Fróis, Schurhammer, and Voretzsch (1926: 39–40). The entire *History* comprises three parts and covers the work of the mission from 1549 through 1593.

15. Cosme de Torres (1510–1570), Balthazar Gago (c. 1520–1583), and Gaspar Vilela (1525–1572) were, at the time, the only fully ordained Jesuit fathers in Japan. Several lay brothers supported them, however. Cosme de Torres led the mission in Japan from 1551 to 1570.

16. Yamato is the area around Nara, not far from Kyoto.

17. Although the *História de Japam* describes this episode as occurring in 1554, the two Japanese men were most probably baptized in the summer of 1555; see the discussion in Laures 1951: 22–23n7. Brother Duarte da Silva (1536–1564) wrote a letter from Bungo on September 20, 1555, reporting on the two monks from Miyako; see also Eglauer 1794, 1: 59–60; Haas 1904: 47n10.

18. Translation of the text as printed in Fróis and Wicki 1976, vol. 2: 195–201. Chapter 26 is a slightly revised letter written by Fróis in Nagasaki on August 27, 1585, which is printed in Garcia 1997: f. 152r–159v.

19. Manase Dōsan was the personal doctor of Oda Nobunaga at the time. Oda Nobunaga (1534–1582) was a formidable general who planned to gain power over all of Japan. Nobunaga succeeded to a large extent but was then forced to commit suicide by an opponent. Manase Dōsan's encounter with the Jesuits is not mentioned in Japanese documents.

20. Belchior de Figueiredo (c. 1530–1597) was born in Goa, India, and entered the Company of Jesus in 1554. He first worked in Goa but came to Japan in 1564, where he worked in various places, including Funai, for several decades. He ultimately returned to Goa for health reasons and died there.

21. Fróis called it "seita dos jenxus."

22. Jp. honbun. The Jesuits followed the commentary on Aristotle's "On the Soul" ("De Anima") by the medieval Christian author Thomas Aquinas (1225–1274). In "On the Soul," Aristotle shows that the soul must be immortal. According to Thomas Aquinas, Aristotle held the soul to be the primary principle (see book II§§271–75 and the commentary in Foster and Humphries 1954: 193). In his report on the conversation between Father Belchior and Dōsan, which he did not witness himself, Fróis wants to refer to a Japanese Buddhist equivalent for the primary principle. In Buddhism, the term honbun does indicate an original state but actually means that every human being is originally (hon) endowed with the Buddha nature; the beings literally "share" (bun) in the Buddha nature.

23. Gnecchi-Soldo Organtino (1530–1609), an Italian Jesuit, came to Japan in 1570.

24. The Vô is Ōgimachi, the heavenly ruler (tennō) or emperor of Japan. He reigned from 1557 to 1586. Vô in Portuguese means "grandfather."

25. The kami, local Japanese deities, are the object of worship and devotion at shrines and inside homes. The numerous kami (usually the number of eight million is given) have different functions and attributes and are revered in a system called the "Way of the Gods," or Shintō. Combinatory forms of worship involving Shintō, Buddhism, Daoism and Yin-Yang divination, as well as the mountain cult of Shugendō, evolved in early and medieval Japan and prevailed until the end of the nineteenth century, when the traditions were separated from one another by the government.

26. While many Japanese researchers, including Ebisawa (1944: 264), maintain that Dōsan did convert to Christianity, Hattori contests this. Not long after the encounter, it was alleged that a conversion had taken place; Toyotomi Hideyoshi (1537–1598) rose to power and issued an edict to abolish Christianity. However, Dōsan remained in high favor and continued to treat Hideyoshi as his personal doctor. Had Dōsan been as devout a Christian as Fróis states, he likely would have fallen from grace. Hattori assumes that the doctor, had such an encounter occurred, was merely interested in the Europeans' medicine and sought out the Jesuits' company for this reason. In 1608, Dōsan was posthumously elevated to a high rank of honor. This would not have occurred during a period when Christians were being persecuted had Dōsan been a Christian (Hattori 1971: 424–29).

27. Translation of selected passages from the Anonymous 1970, vol. 10: 281–308; referencing the French translation by Millioud 1895a, 1895b. See a short discussion of the content of this "heathen source" in Schurhammer 1928: 111–14; for a translation into modern Japanese, see Ebisawa 1964. Because the Portuguese and Spanish arrived in Japan from their colonies located somewhere to the south, they were called "southern" barbarians.

28. Nobunaga resided at his castle in Azuchi, not far from Miyako (Kyoto), among other places.

29. The text renders his name as "Urugan."

30. Here, "Buddhism" may simply denote "religion." It could also be mentioned because Catholicism was initially thought to be a form of Buddhism in Japan. The Japanese word for Christianity (*Kirishitan*) would have been more logical here, but the source text rarely uses loan words from the Portuguese to describe Catholic missionary matters.

31. It is probable that the names in the tale are meant to be generic Christian names and thus cannot necessarily be interpreted as representing particular historical persons.

32. The sermon of the two brothers clearly contains Buddhist teachings about karma and the cycle of births.

33. This is again reference to Buddhist terminology, the "three worlds" meaning past, present, and future. In popular Japanese tales and pictures, the king of the underworld uses a large mirror to show the deceased what they have done in life; if a person has killed an animal, his or her next birth will be as that particular animal.

34. In an extensive passage omitted here, Fabian tries to approach one of Hideyoshi's protégés via that favorite's mother. He manages to meet the old woman and engages her in a lengthy debate on religious matters. Fabian's attempt to convince the woman of the superiority of Christianity fails because of the astute intelligence and craftiness of his female interlocutor, who sets him up in a public debate with an uneducated man dressed as a monk. Of course, Fabian fails pitifully. Fabian in the tale likely represents the well-known historical figure Fukan Fabian (1565–1621), a Japanese Jesuit who was cherished by the Christians as an orator and author. In the first decade of the seventeenth century, however, he left the Society of Jesus and engaged in anti-Christian activities. On Fabian's writings, see Paramore 2009: 11–33.

2. On Sickness, Society, and the New Self in Early Edo Japan

Soshin's *Dharma Words* (Seventeenth Century)

KATJA TRIPLETT

M any scholars agree that, in comparison with earlier periods, Japanese
Buddhism was relatively static in the early modern era (1600–1868). After a
series of military battles and governmental policies curbed the power of some of
the most formidable temples, Buddhist institutions were organized more rigidly
into schools and branches to improve administration and control. In a move to
eradicate Christianity, Buddhist temples assisted the new military government of
the Tokugawa shoguns in registering the entire Japanese population as Buddhist.

A closer look at early Tokugawa-period Buddhist thinkers such as Soshin
(1588–1675), however, reveals an intellectual dynamism that conflicts with the
image of early modern Japanese Buddhism as static. Evidence of this dynamism
can be found in Soshin's anti-authoritarian and anticlerical statements. As Soshin
herself worked at the military court of the Tokugawa shogun, her statements can
also be read, paradoxically, as a demand to maintain the social status quo of
"high" and "low" society and to concentrate on nonmundane matters. These
two seemingly contradictory trends would later come to characterize modern
Japanese Buddhism. They can be seen in the formation of powerful lay Buddhist
organizations in the nineteenth and twentieth centuries and in the active participation of Buddhist priests in ultranationalist politics. The second half of the
twentieth century also saw the emergence of Critical Buddhism,[1] a movement
within Zen Buddhism that deplored such political participation and discussed
doctrinal matters raised by Soshin and others many centuries before.[2]

The translation below, an excerpt from Soshin's *Dharma Words* (*Soshin-ni kōhōgo*), comes from a dynamic era of transformation into a new social order following a long period of civil strife and war in Japan. Soshin, born Nā, reached a high-ranking position at the court of the military ruler in Edo (today's Tokyo) and mentored members of the household on matters of Zen Buddhism. While she can be regarded as one of the most powerful lay Buddhists of the time, remarkably few extant records exist to shed light on her life and work. She is referenced in the early nineteenth-century official chronicle of the Tokugawa clan,[3] as well as in other texts.[4] In addition, records of Soshin's teachings— including the text partly translated below[5]—have survived.[6] Manuscript copies of *Dharma Words* are held in several Japanese libraries, as well as the archive of Saisōji, the temple established for Soshin by her patron, the shogun Tokugawa Iemitsu (1604–1651).[7]

The excerpt of *Dharma Words* introduced here is organized in a question-and-answer format. Soshin answers the questions with a series of "items" that convey her main arguments, while also drawing on a range of Buddhist and Daoist texts. Instead, everyone can experience liberation by focusing on their own minds and by engaging with this world. The passage translated below, from the beginning of Soshin's sermon, lays out the problem of sickness and its causes.[8] Soshin argues that one's mind is identical to an "original mind" that is free from sickness. She writes that the obstacle to realizing the identity of one's own mind with the original mind is the illusion of a separation of body and mind. Interestingly, Soshin links the notion of an illusory separation of body and mind to spatial hierarchies of "high" and "low" and to human society. When one regards body and mind as separate, members of the high society copy the low, and the low hope to rise. Thus, the individual is caught up in constant preoccupations with social standing and forgets to concentrate on what really matters, thereby suffering from sickness. With her belief that even ordinary laypeople could or should strive to reach awakening, Soshin demonstrates an anticlerical stance suggesting that awakening is not the preserve of the ordained.

Soshin's *Dharma Words* are also of particular interest when studying the early modern period because it is a rare example of writing by a woman from a period during which women were increasingly dissuaded from openly engaging in learning and politics. Education was deemed a private pursuit for women, and they were actively discouraged from publishing their work and giving lectures.

Soshin's in-depth knowledge of Buddhist scriptures and her close acquaintance with the teachings of the Zen Buddhist tradition (which customarily included a familiarity with Daoist ideas) are the result of time spent with her paternal uncle, the abbot of a subtemple of the great Myōshinji temple in Kyoto. Her Buddhist name, Soshin, meaning "Ancestral Heart," was used with the affixed character *ni* indicating her status as a monastic woman, although she was likely never formally ordained. Soshin is thought to have studied with the influential Rinzai Zen Buddhist master and physician Takuan (1573–1645).[9] After the shogun's death in 1651, Soshin, already widowed by that time, retired to Saisōji temple.

After Soshin's death in 1675, her teachings do not appear to have reached a wider circle because her enemy, the influential Hayashi Razan (1583–1657), who rose to power at the shogun's court, thoroughly opposed her views. In a text from 1651, Razan calls Soshin an arrogant "witch-nun" and accuses her of having "felicitous meetings"[10] with the ringleader of a thwarted rebellion. Soshin, who had a warrior class (samurai) background and had been introduced to the military court by the head of the shogunate's women's quarters, the powerful Lady Kasuga (1579–1643), was unscathed by these allegations.[11]

FURTHER READING

Bernstein, Gail Lee. 1991. *Recreating Japanese Women, 1600–1945*. Berkeley: University of California Press.

Cogan, Gina. 2014. *The Princess Nun: Bunchi, Buddhist Reform, and Gender in Early Edo Japan*. Harvard East Asian Monographs 366. Cambridge, Mass.: Harvard University Press.

Seigle, Cecilia Segawa, and Linda H. Chance. 2014. *Ōoku: The Secret World of the Shogun's Women*. Amherst, N.Y.: Cambria.

Williams, Duncan Ryūken. 2005. *The Other Side of Zen: A Social History of Sōtō Zen: Buddhism in Tokugawa Japan*. Princeton, N.J.: Princeton University Press.

Yonemoto, Marcia. 2016. *The Problem of Women in Early Modern Japan*. Asia: Local Studies, Global Themes 31. Oakland: University of California Press.

SOSHIN-NI'S DHARMA WORDS[12]

QUESTION: Do the various diseases come from outside, or is their ultimate cause in the mind?[13]

ANSWER: The various diseases enter from nowhere but break out when the mind has become stagnant inside by [excessive] eating and drinking, and also when Wind from outside has a strong effect on the interior, and also when the Wind itself is very strong. That is why we have the saying of Laozi: "Disease appears after acquiring fame or shame."[14] However, until the moment we contract "cold *ki*" [i.e., a disease caused by cold], it is not painful while the cold is slight. The same thing is also true for the Wind, as long as you think that the Wind is slight.

ITEM: The ultimate cause of disease in the mind is the essential point. Our original mind[15] is free from sickness anyway. We must consider oneness with the body[16] as an underlying principle of Heaven and Earth. In the classical [Buddhist] writings it says, "The body is the root of the eighty-four thousand diseases of affliction. If the mind itself is clear within, rather like space, then the mind, which was separate from the body, emerges to become one with it."[17] Or, it is also said, "The perfect body of truth[18] is fundamentally free from disease."

ITEM: Sickness arises from delusion and from illusory thought.

ITEM: Delusion is when we regret not being able to return to the past and when we constantly grapple with the future, which we cannot know. It is present in the mind without interruption. Worry about things—this is all because of delusion. In other words, we cannot even guess what our concerns will be on any given day. If we can bring each concern, one by one, to a close, then we have the original mind that is free from sickness. As a matter of course, there will be no single obstruction anymore. Hence it is said, "The perfected do not plan before and do not think about it after. They remain unchanged in the now. With every thought, they return to the Way."[19] The mind is full of regretting what we cannot return to and full of grappling with the future that we cannot know. It gets tied up deep in worries that are without limit. This is called the malady of the mind. Those who have resolved to see the truth as it is should accept this teaching and immediately search for the delusion that torments the mind. When they find the delusion, the mind will be free from sickness. Furthermore, they will fulfill the principle of Heaven and Earth and will not encounter any calamities. Fulfilling this is the actual realization of one's peace of mind that they used only to imagine. As Zhuangzi once said, "The perfected use their mind like a mirror. [It grasps nothing. It refuses nothing. It receives but does not keep]."[20]

ITEM: The foolish also worry about their bodies[21] without understanding the impermanence of all bodies. Hence it is said, "The ancients suffered in their bodies; when the body disappears, they obtain the Way."[22] Those who resolve to [see] the truth as it is experience the healing of their real body. When this happens, they spontaneously reach the state of freedom from sickness.

ITEM: As I noted above, *illusory thought* means thoughts that arise about not being able to return [to the past] and not being able to see into the future. From this, all kinds of concerns arise ceaselessly. When we look at these concerns carefully, we simply see that being in the now, we cannot bring anything to a close. Our immediate concerns all split into many kinds of assumptions. Finally, there is nothing that brightens the mind anymore. Everything becomes convoluted. When we resolve to return our mind to the original mind, it is like a storm that disperses the clouds and brings clear weather. The resolve is thus like a fresh breeze that sweeps away the clouds. The principle of oneness with all gods and buddhas comes true.

ITEM: Even if various kinds of illusory thoughts arise initially, each single thought has its own origin, and that is the deluded mind that [wants to see] the distant future.

ITEM: Since each single thought has an origin, the mind that pursues the wish not to respond to the body becomes the origin of a single thought. When we do not comply with what we think and when we do not get rid of thoughts in the mind, the number of various kinds of different ideas will increase in the "mind of attachment."[23] These keep us from resting during our whole life. Hence Zhuangzi said in his "Nourishing the Lord of Life," in which he reveals to us the origin of disease, "There is a limit to our life, but to knowledge there is no limit. To pursue what is unlimited with what is limited is a perilous thing; and when, knowing this, we still seek the increase of our knowledge, the peril cannot be averted."

ITEM: Ignoring this, in the present we foolishly forge plans as a matter of course. A single thought arises with doubts and speculations. Those [of you] who follow this teaching have already discovered your deluded minds. You do not hide it. But, when there is nothing that the mind can attach itself to, the mind becomes light and free from sickness. When it wants to grasp at things and you do not let your resolve waver, this will be commendable conduct!

ITEM: As soon as we separate body and mind, there will be all kinds of complications, and the mind will become heavy. This means that we forget the place of our body. Those people up high imitate those below; those below hope to rise up high. Hence, body and mind become separated. If you follow the natural principle diligently, body and mind become nonexistent, and this nonseparation in effect turns into nonthought and nonmind,[24] which will become nonsickness.

ITEM: If you do not clear up the doubts about all matters, the heart becomes heavy. The speculations about all these things will turn into mere conjectures. When we do not feel like ever clearing up our doubts, we will become confused. In contrast, those who have resolved to see the truth as it is see their reflection in the mirror of immutable wisdom. The mind that has learned the errors resulting from one's own delusion becomes the mind that does not know the myriad doubts. This is the (state of) freedom from sickness and peace of mind. Hence Bodhidharma said, "Those [who free themselves from all appearances without effort] cure all diseases without treatment."[25] Furthermore, such a mind is like the fulfillment of the principle of Heaven and Earth.

NOTES

This chapter was drafted with the support of a grant from the Humanities Center of Advanced Studies "Multiple Secularities—Beyond the West, Beyond Modernities" at Leipzig University, funded by the German Research Foundation. For further information, please consult www.multiple-secularities.de.

1.   On Sōtō Zen Buddhism, see Bodiford 1996.

2.   Sharf 1995; Victoria 2006.

3.   See Kuroita and Kokushi taikei henshūkai 1982: 217–18.

4.   See, for example, Hayashi Razan's *First Report on the Kusa Bandits* (1651) in Hayashi 1979. For an introduction to and analysis of the text, including references to Soshin, see Paramore 2009: 90–91.

5.   Sueki 2006: 352.

6.   *Dharma Words* is a collection of sermons accessible via two prominent printed collections of early modern Buddhist writings, both published in the early twentieth century; see Soshin-ni 1916, 1925.

7.   For an introduction to Soshin's work and thought, see Sueki 2006, which also lists the available manuscripts. Biographical details are also given by Shoshin-ni 1916; Shiba 1994.

8.   For more on the context of Soshin's ideas regarding the Buddhist ideas of sickness and healing, see Shinmura 2013: 43.

9. Takuan is known to have cultivated the medical tradition of Manase Dōsan (discussed in chapter 1 of this volume); see also Shinmura 2013: 265–73. On Takuan's medical ideas, see Ahn 2012.

10. See Paramore 2009: 91.

11. A modern Japanese writer has made Soshin's life story into a novel; see Nomura 2000.

12. The translation is based on the modern edition of the sermon in Soshin-ni 1916: 266–68.

13. Jp. *isshin,* "one mind," meaning the ordinary is one with the absolute. The term can also signify absolute reality. In her sermon, Soshin refers to the "one mind" only in the first two sections. She then uses other compounds or simply the character for "heart" or "mind" (Jp. *shin, kokoro*), the place where thoughts and feelings arise.

14. Soshin quotes the saying of sages active in ancient China, usually by mentioning only one phrase. Her audience must have known the citations by heart so that they could complete these quotes in their minds and follow the sermon at the same time. In some places, I have added further elements of a quotation in brackets to better convey its meaning.

15. See glossary. Soshin uses *honshin* primarily to signify the perfect body of a Buddha, which is free from disease (Sueki 2006: 355).

16. Jp. *ittai,* "single body," meaning a single substance or "oneness." Although the phenomena are externally different, in nature they are the same. The term describes the fundamental unity of the universe. Soshin refers to a well-known saying ascribed to the Chinese sage Laozi: "Heaven, Earth, and [I] have the same root; all things are one body with me."

17. In this excerpt from the sermon, Soshin frequently quotes from the *Six-Section Collection from the Small Room* (*Shaoshi liumen ji*, T. 2009), a short, anonymous text from China on the six teachings of Bodhidharma, the putative founder of Chan (Jp. *Zen*) Buddhism who lived in the fifth or sixth century.

18. Jp. *hosshin, hōshin,* "Dharma body," signifying the perfect body of the Buddha, who is free from disease.

19. This passage is found in the *Six-Section Collection from the Small Room*.

20. The passage is a quote from Zhuangzi's *The Normal Course for Rulers and Kings*.

21. The character used here (Jp. *shin* or *mi*) means not only "body" but also "oneself." Here, it signifies the concern about one's body and one's place in society.

22. This passage is found in the *Six-Section Collection from the Small Room*.

23. Jp. *chakusuru kokoro* is a colloquial synonym for the more formal Buddhist term for the attached mind (Jp. *jakushin*).

24. Jp. *munen mushin* denotes the state of absence of deluded thought, a major aim in Zen Buddhism.

25. This passage is also found in the *Six-Section Collection from the Small Room*.

3. Buddhism and Scholarly Medicine in Seventeenth-Century China

Three Prefaces to the Work of Yu Chang (1585–1664)

VOLKER SCHEID

The transition between the Ming (1368–1644) and Qing (1644–1911) dynasties is sometimes referred to as China's early modern period. In the eyes of some historians, during this period Chinese society underwent economic, social, and cultural changes that appear to be similar to those that historians characterize as early modernity in Europe and elsewhere.[1] Medicine was one domain in which these transformations played out. As human subjectivity and the emotions, for instance, emerged as important resources for understanding and acting within the world, they also became objects of new medical ideas and practices.[2] A critical philological engagement with canonical texts and historical artifacts engendered a different relationship with the past, as intellectual orientations, more widely than before, shifted from the metaphysical search for the principles behind things to a more empirically focused interest in things themselves.[3] Socially, physicians mixed more easily than ever with the country's elite. Prominent physicians worked hard to establish medicine as an occupation built on the same moral foundations and scholarly attitudes espoused by their literati peers (i.e., those from the class of scholars and bureaucrats).[4]

By and large, historians of science in late imperial China subsume medicine into a broader field of natural studies that had been dominated ideologically and socially by a literati class working within a broad and multifaceted Neo-Confucian tradition. Although seventeenth-century literati also engaged widely with Daoist and Buddhist ideas and practices, modern scholars have perceived such interests as supplementary to more conventional literati concerns. Historians of the period examining literati medicine thus tend to view Daoist and Buddhist therapeutic practices as essentially religious in nature and leave their study to historians of religion, who often ignore them.[5]

This chapter challenges this division of academic labor and the interpretation of history on which it rests by examining the work of the influential seventeenth-century physician, teacher, and medical author Yu Chang. The historical literature invariably depicts Yu as a prototypical scholar-physician (*ruyi*) who, having passed the provincial exams, was accepted by literati as one of them.[6] His ideas were consistently innovative—iconoclastic even—and it is not difficult to depict him as a leading exponent of a hypothesized early modern turn in Chinese medicine. He was one of the first authors to employ the new critical philology (*kaozheng*) in examining medical classics. He sought to base the study of medicine on clear principles and stipulated precepts for judging actual practice. He valued observation over the search for the true meaning of canonical texts; and, much as he sought to commune with the ancient sages, he insisted that his own judgment was of equal value. His work laid the foundation for the two currents of practice that dominated Chinese medicine between the eighteenth and twentieth centuries: cold damage (*shanghan*) and warmth disorder (*wenbing*) therapeutics.[7] At the same time, he was the most important influence on the group of physicians that would eventually bridge the tension between these two currents. He also influenced the development of medicine in Japan, as well as in twentieth-century China.[8]

Yet, his most important sponsors perceived Yu Chang as a Buddhist physician first and foremost. Popular accounts portrayed him as an enlightened if somewhat eccentric doctor, while Yu Chang himself consistently linked his medical practice to Buddhist beliefs and the Chan meditative practices in which he had trained. His influence on the development of East Asian medicine over subsequent centuries calls into question current assumptions about the decline of Buddhist influence on the development of medicine in the late imperial and early modern periods. Given also that his "early modern" attitude—his critical interrogation of the past, his belief in the gradual accumulation of knowledge over time, his emphasis on the individual self as the ultimate source of authority, and his efforts to model medical education on transparent principles of practice—explicitly developed out of, and not against, his Buddhist religious beliefs, Yu Chang forcefully challenges assumptions about the relationship among religion, critique, and science, not only in China but everywhere.[9]

Yu Chang studied in the Cao-Dong tradition of Chan Buddhism. He became a Buddhist monk in 1645 in the wake of Manchu penetration into Southern China. The texts I have translated in this chapter are the prefaces to some of Yu Chang's most important medical works. The first selection is the author's own preface to a critical edition of Zhang Zhongjing's *Treatise on Cold Damage*, one of the key texts of Chinese pharmacotherapy dating from the late second century BCE. Entitled *Communing with the Ancients*, this piece was published in 1648. The second and third translations below are prefaces to *Methods and Precepts for Physicians* by Yu Chang and his friend Qian Qianyi (the seventeenth century's most famous poet but also an infamous official serving under both the Ming and the Qing governments), published in 1658. Both texts clearly reflect Yu Chang's deep commitment to Buddhism.

The reader will notice that, collectively, these pieces reframe the *Treatise on Cold Damage* and its venerated author within a Buddhist framework. They establish Buddhist ethics of compassion for all beings as a rationale for the practice of medicine and uphold the figures of the Buddha and bodhisattvas as ultimate sources of superior medical knowledge. They also firmly locate Yu Chang's practice of medicine within a context of Buddhist morality and practice, even comparing him to the most celebrated physicians mentioned in the Buddhist *sūtras*. Finally, it is notable that Yu Chang explicitly employs Buddhist practices and ontologies to advance Chinese medical practice.

FURTHER READING

Elman, Benjamin A. 2005. *On Their Own Terms: Science in China, 1550–1900.* Cambridge, Mass.: Harvard University Press.

Hinrichs, T. J., and Linda L. Barnes. 2013. *Chinese Medicine and Healing: An Illustrated History.* Cambridge, Mass.: Harvard University Press.

Leung, Angela Ki-che. 1997. "Medical Learning from the Song to the Ming." In *The Song-Yuan-Ming Transition in Chinese History*, edited by Paul Jakov Smith and Richard von Glahn, 374–98. Cambridge, Mass.: Harvard University Press.

Schäfer, Dagmar. 2011. *The Crafting of the 10,000 Things: Knowledge and Technology in Seventeenth-Century China.* Chicago: University of Chicago Press.

1. YU CHANG'S PREFACE TO *COMMUNING WITH THE ANCIENTS*[10]

In the beginning, when the boundless chaos opened, the sage rulers first emerged. The common usage [of things] had not yet been established. So, when medicinal herbs were prepared for the first time, how was the connection between the Way of medicine and life established? The Yellow Emperor honored his minister Qibo as his heavenly teacher. Every time he listened to [Qibo's] refined and distinct [discourse] on medicine, he made sure to have it recorded in writing, bowed down to respectfully receive [the instructions], and stored these texts in a golden chest and jade casket. This led to the emergence of divine craftsmen who, from Chunyu Yi and Bian Que onward, from generation to generation continued to pass on their knowledge. Whether through the development of formularies or the formulation of pulse doctrine, their writings illuminated the entire universe.

However, since that incomparable time, it has become near impossible to find people able to extend their spirit to comprehend what came before the establishment of the Spirit Orchid [Hall], those who investigate the secrets of the primordial chaos on their own, or those who can explain the symbols [lit., "the trigrams before brushstrokes"] left by a culture without writing, in which the reader inferred meanings solely from images and from those meanings attained the numinous. [People] would enter the boundless darkness robed like Faxian [the Buddhist monk who traveled on foot from China to India in search of Buddhist texts]. In later periods, [knowledge of] the Way declined and was replaced by mere techniques, and this decline of vitality in medical affairs has by now been long lasting.

Hence, with only my words and actions to rely on and no one to resonate with, I was ignorant and naïve. As all the principles [of medicine were] obscure [to me], it was as dark as for someone walking at night with his heart in secret anguish. Therefore, I shut myself away to satisfy my [intellectual] hunger with the books of the ancients in an effort to go back [in time] and commune with them. However, if one studies too broadly, [one's knowledge] remains too superficial to gain a complete picture of things. A single life is insufficient to learn it all. Still, by focusing on the essentials, one can seek out the dark pearl[11] and the subtle truth behind deceptive appearances. I wonder if both the ancients and I have been limited by the Dao, for we are the same in that we solemnly decipher and pick out life's mysteries in quiet contemplation without definite clues. What the ancients say is intrinsic to me. Beholding the Dao of Heaven and my own life, one may not pass responsibility from one to the other when it comes to the crucial points. The ancients have long gone, and now I carry the burden of the scriptures they bequeathed. They need to be dissected, and their many disorderly tangles need to be organized. This is a duty that is difficult to shirk.

In former times, Ānanda asked the World-Honored One, "In the past, who did the Buddha take as his teacher?" The World-Honored One replied, "I took myself as teacher." This is why, when he was born, he pointed up to Heaven and down to the earth, declaring that "I alone am the Honorable One." From that, one can see the measure of "I": Between Heaven and Earth, past and present, what can be obtained is without limits. Yet, this is not something I dare to make a point of. My sole intention is to use spirit and breath to truly commune with the ancients in secret union, as when seeking enlightenment of one's ignorance or receiving commands in a face-to-face audience.

Expounding a topic is like using a burning-glass to make fire or a cool glass sphere to condense water. It happens by spontaneous resonance that obviates thought. I swiftly achieved my original intention of communing with the ancients. Now, the drawback of scholarly excellence is that, in explaining the canons,[12] it frequently oversteps its authority; while a drawback of dull conservatism is that, in adhering rigidly to established meanings, it frequently merely plagiarizes. Whether overstepping one's mark or plagiarizing in the pursuit of fame that lasts for only a moment, the consequences endure for a long time. Appraising these disastrous approaches, how could one not dread both?

I could not bring myself to merely dabble in [Zhang] Zhongjing's *Treatise on Cold Damage*, which, covering all under Heaven and Earth, is the model of all treatment methods and the ancestor of all formulas. [However, the original text] has become mixed up with later interpretations, rendering it unusable, like when rice is mixed up with dust or soup with dirt. [My book's] special feature is that it employs natural principles and extends them to analogous things, elucidating [Zhang Zhongjing's] divine understanding even as it also opens new facets, all of which the reader can grasp quickly without regret.

With respect to the manifestations of spring warmth, I have taken a different view [to that of others], building on the example of the *Inner Canon*. I investigated the main ideas thoroughly but, in my research, did not dare to stray from [Zhang] Zhongjing's *Treatise* or add even a word [to what he said]. Thanks to this, future authors will no longer need to search in darkness or approach [the topic] obliquely. At any time, they can put the ideas [I outline] into practice and achieve effectiveness immediately. That, at least, is my hope.

I have thoroughly investigated a myriad of sources and have considered the *Spiritual Pivot, Basic Questions*, the *Classic of Difficult Issues*, and the *A-B Classic*. The ideas expressed in these texts are vast, and it is difficult to distill an essence from them. What I have therefore done is to study what is left of [Zhang] Zhongjing's *[Essentials of the] Golden Casket*,[13] carefully analyzing the categories in their different branches and establishing ten chapters of strategies and precepts for treating miscellaneous patterns [of illness]. Pondering deeply for nine years, I drafted this manuscript to penetrate the mysteries and profundities [of the text] and enable readers to gain fresh perspectives. Combined with the *Treatise on Cold Damage* it is designed [as a useful tool,] like a boat for crossing a river or a big cauldron for cooking fish. Even if what I present here should be mocked by the experts, I would not therefore disengage from the duties of my life for a single day.

Now individuals worry about not having enough natural disposition and intelligence, but they do not worry about not having principles and [obtaining] the Way. Generations worry about losing principles and the Way but do not worry about not knowing the self. In ancient times, gentlemen who executed their affairs without fault and mastered the Way without abusing it were called *Gates to the Country in the Mountains*. I hope to encounter [such gentlemen], because similar people resonate naturally with each other, and past and present are the same. Through this compilation, I hope to ignite many [other] torches and wait for the perfectly penetrating superior wisdom possessed by the bodhisattvas to radiate its splendor so that it may illuminate the profoundest subtleties in complete agreement with the Yellow Emperor, Qi Bo Qibo, and Zhang Zhongjing. Untalented as I am, useless as chaff, I feel nevertheless honored to offer [this work].

Written just now in the first month of summer 1648
by Yu Chang (courtesy name Jiayan) from Xichang.

2. YU CHANG'S PREFACE TO
METHODS AND PRECEPTS FOR PHYSICIANS[14]

The path of medicine is vast, and its obligations are heavy. Over the centuries, physicians who are better than middling have never been easy to find, while the truly excellent physicians that ever lived under Heaven can be counted on one hand. [This being the case,] who then are the groups of people that are called physicians in our own times?

There are those who rely on intelligence and wit. The mind of these masters is haughty, but their choice [of formulas] is not precise. So, while it is true that they often hit the target, they miss it just as often. Then there are the gatekeepers who paint a mark at the door to prevent anyone else from entering, presenting themselves as able to stop the turn toward death; even where the cause is not yet lost, they are already to blame for delaying action. There are also those who work using heterodox ways. Careless and possessing poor knowledge, they go after danger without a solid foundation. If by chance one is entrapped by their arts, the outcome will be as sad as when a child wields a knife.

Patients suffer when too many physicians assemble in their households claiming to have the talent of sages. Shallow ones, false ones, and slick ones all peddle [their wares and in doing so] experiment with the bodies and lives of their patients. Physicians are troubled by the complexity of their patients' cases, and whatever action they take ends up [with the patient] in dire straits. Finding it difficult to rely on formulas, the pulse, or what else they have learned from their teachers, they use their patients' bodies and lives for their experiments. It is said that people's lives can be harmed by water and fire, assault and war, wild animals and the laws of the land. Yet, none of these is as pervasive as illness. [Among the reasons for] people's deaths, whether due to evil spirits, heretics, hungry ghosts, or beasts, none is as pitiful as those deaths [that land people] in Hell. Physicians who entrap their patients by practicing to a standard that is without clarity of mind and ignorant of skills eventually create a worldwide entrapment that covers the sun and creates a living hell. Its causes and effects are obvious.

The [Buddhist] scriptures state that ignorance is the seed of all hell. With layer upon layer of darkness and no way of salvation, how would one not pity [those trapped within it]? I also had my eyes closed, only seeing darkness. However, seeing darkness does not mean there is no light at all. Like a fishing lamp on a wild shore or the shine of glowworms in a deserted village, even a crack of weak light may enlighten a thousand years of ignorance among physicians. The methods and precepts I have formulated [in this book] constitute a straightforward path to follow and are an aspect of my carrying out the Buddha's work.

Bathing one's shallow understanding in the deep understanding of the Yellow Emperor, Qi Bo, and Zhang Zhongjing clears the senses. One builds one's chariot behind closed doors, but when one goes out, one keeps to the [common] road; [hence,] one can take a stance without fault. Even if one is ignorant and ill informed, as long as one knows that nothing gets by the law of cause and effect, if one is worshipful, careful, and deliberate, one extends oneself by the day and the month, [eventually] lighting up one's courage, smashing through unclarity, and gradually filling up one's knowledge. Given the original clarity of mind [i.e., the purity of one's true nature], if one consults earlier [texts and authors] and relies on their judgment, why should ignorance not be illuminated?

The former sage Zhang Zhongjing lived and served toward the end of the Han dynasty and wrote the *Treatise on Cold Damage and Miscellaneous Disorders*. This was also the time when Buddhist doctrine was first transmitted to China and when the division of Buddhist meditation schools into five houses was not yet at its height. Gathering the light of his inner nature, [Zhang Zhongjing] joined hands and worked together with the sages of past, present, and future, all the buddhas and all the ancestors. He is therefore the physicians' Medicine King Bodhisattva and Supreme Medicine Bodhisattva of Healing [i.e., the healing bodhisattvas Bhaiṣajyarāja and Bhaiṣajyasamudgata].

But his blessed circumstances had only one-hundred-millionth of the blessings of our Buddha, the Tathāgata himself. After another hundred years, the transmission [of his works] became dormant and ended. Later generations with inferior fortune had to turn back toward the [original] sources. Eagerly competing, they guessed how much or how little knowledge each [source] possessed, even as they themselves had assimilated only a minute amount of the limitless true essential illumination.

Our Buddha, the Tathāgata, tired himself through many eons[15] as the King of Medicine, establishing methods for [treating] illness and dispensing medicine in accordance with their dynamics to thereby deliver salvation to all sentient beings. By the last of his lifetimes, after continually improving his eighty-four thousand complete and perfect teachings, each of these teachings [or dharma gates] was filled with the bright illumination [of enlightenment]. All sentient beings who receive this illumination through but a tiny crack can seize the opportunity to enter deeper through that gate to perfect their own buddha path.

Past, present, and future, in the void as well as the immeasurable phenomenal world, the light of the countless millions of buddhas and bodhisattvas shines, radiantly reflecting each other. Each of these buddhas and bodhisattvas has his own personal vow and calling. They disseminate scriptural invocations and versified utterances unceasingly throughout many eons. There is no one in their light to whom is not revealed the subtlest wonders [of the universe] and who is not furnished with what is necessary to extinguish worries and an ocean of grief. Later, when the Venerable Ānanda was enlightened to the path of "no more learning" (*wuxue*), which did not differ from the informed view on nonduality of the Buddha himself, he was able to compile the canonical scriptures of the Tripiṭaka and the twelve canons, so that they might forever function as essential teachings for humans and *devas* and create a bridge to provide salvation to all creatures. All the final authentic truths of all the buddhas' and bodhisattvas' understandings have thus been transmitted from the Tathāgata's own mouth and were collected in the hands of Ānanda.

If my own inner nature has glanced the unlimited and unimpeded light of Amitābha Buddha, the writing that flows from this will be sufficient to illuminate those who wish to learn. For why should not a man of clarity, his guts filled from many carefree banquets, permeated with the universe's splendor, attain the measure of enlightening the present with the past? Having truly assimilated the illumination of both the *Inner Canon* and [Zhang] Zhongjing, making public their subtle meanings, without being either excessive or leaving anything out, I can act as a daily guide through the thorny thicket of the many knotted problems. Comparing the shortcomings and strengths of my own text with [the writings of] the ancient sages is like comparing fifty steps with a hundred steps; we are that far apart.

The manuscript for printing has gone through ten drafts, and the printing blocks were changed four times for fear of mixing the insights of an ordinary mortal with those of sages and spirits, which is like using cotton waste to repair beautiful brocade. But, in the end, this could not be avoided. Especially with respect to improving on the different categories of the six *qi* [disorders]—wind, cold, summer heat, dampness, dryness, and fire[16]—and the miscellaneous illnesses, the efforts of an entire lifetime would not be enough to complete the task. Even exhausting the effort of a thousand life times, one would still be unable to complete the task.

When I have exhausted all thought and have cut myself off from thinking consciousness (*yishi*), I enter directly into a meditative state, my whole body drenched in sweat. How dangerous this is! How dangerous this is! For how could I carelessly claim that different paths lead to the same destination? This is an important *koan*: Wait for when something can be improved and [only] then improve it.

3. QIAN QIANYI'S PREFACE TO
METHODS AND PRECEPTS FOR PHYSICIANS[17]

[Yu Chang] from Xinjian, a man of learning who elaborated on the secrets that the Yellow Emperor, Qi Bo, and Zhang Zhongjing did not transmit, is the author of the book *Communing with the Ancients*. When I composed a preface for it, I identified as its core theme that his seeking out of the original ways and arts of medicine is comparable to a Confucian scholar's comprehensive understanding of Heaven, Earth, and Man. To the people of our times, his words are the Milky Way; they echo each other in astonishment. Two years later, when, at the age of seventy, this man of learning set out to publish *Postscript to Communing with the Ancients* and *Methods and Precepts for Physicians* as instructions for students, he again turned to me for my comments.

I have read the texts on *śamatha* and *vipaśyanā* in the Tiantai tradition, which discuss the Four Great Elements and the Five Viscera, the increase and decrease of which lead to disease [see *Anthology*, vol. 1, ch. 37]. As the origins from which each arise differ, the diseases that eventually manifest are [even more] manifold. Therefore, to treat disease, one must be aware of its causes. As for the essentials [of medical practice], there are the four skillful means from the *Yogācāra* [see *Anthology*, vol. 1, ch. 6§2] and the seventy-two secret methods from the *Saṁyukta Āgama* [referring to a text partly translated in *Anthology*, vol. 1, ch. 36]. The extraordinary depth and subtlety of these texts have never been matched by the secular canons of the two schools of medical classics and classical formulas.

One should understand that our Tathāgata who came into this world is also the great King of Medicine, the bodhisattva of the five realms, and [the provider of] skillful means for saving sentient beings. He employs excellent formulas and medicinal therapies for the treatment of all illnesses. The Buddha, had he not amassed vows through eons of time, made offerings of the purest and best herbs to all buddhas, and taught enlightenment to all living beings, would not have been able to manifest himself as the King of Medicine to convey the Dharma, nor would he have been more exceptional than the Confucians who understood Heaven, Earth, and Man.

[Yu Chang], our man of learning, dressed and comported himself like a Confucian on the outside, but, in his heart, he hid Chan Buddhism. With the help of the Cao-Dong school's teaching of the five positions of ruler and minister, he gained enlightened insight into the principles of medicine, which he employed when deciding on the methods for composing medical formulas. In his "Treatise on Yin Disorders," he broadened their original foundation in the Four Great Elements to the three realms [of *saṁsāra*] by drawing on the subtle teachings of the three realms from the Tiantai and Dilun schools [of Buddhism]. This is what is meant [when we say] that the King of Healing Herbs and Trees heals all the diseases of the body.

The narrowminded people of our age, who focus on the precise measurement of medicinals and the composition of prescriptions in black ink have as much insight as oxen and sheep. When someone deviates from the norm, is it not appropriate that they repeat it to each other in astonishment? In my own view, there is no clearer account of the Tathāgata's teaching on medicine than the story about the old physician and the visiting physician in the Mahāyāna *Mahāparinirvāṇa Sūtra*, or *Nirvāṇa Sūtra*.[18] In this story, when the old physician treated a disease, he did not differentiate among wind, heat, cold, or warm pathogens but instructed all [his patients] to take only milk [as medicine]. The guest physician, instead, appropriately advised that [when the king became ill] milk should be strictly forbidden to him. The guest physician's recommendation was followed, and the king's disease was cured. The country had been spared a violent death; from this, we can infer the effectiveness of the prohibition against milk. The king subsequently suffered from a fever from which he could not recover without taking milk. In this case, the milk that the guest physician employed to get rid of the disease was nothing but the previously interdicted old physician's milk as medicine. If you were to reject the old physician's milk and seek the guest physician's milk, even if you were to ask for it in the *deva* Śiva's heaven, how could you obtain it?

Judging from this, given that the causes of disease are manifold, diseases themselves also are quite different from each other. It is not always possible to employ old formulas for new diseases. Observing change and judging between life and death lies within nothing more than the three fingers [when feeling the pulse] in the course of a single breath. As when two armies face each other, winning or losing is determined within a short space of time. One may insist on studying ancient military techniques and lining up battle formations based on the illustrations [in these texts]. But this is not what a good general would do. The Cao-Dong teachings states, "Move and you are trapped; diverge and you fall into doubt and vacillation. Turning away and touching are both wrong, for it is like a massive fire."[19] Do not the books written by this man of learning indicate that he was on the point of attaining precisely this?

The Buddha says that selecting medicines like the old physician is like worms eating up wood. Just because the [marks left behind by the] worms appear to trace out [written] characters, those who know would never propose these [as words] that were speaking [to us]. Today, texts like *Communing with the Ancients* are like the guest physician's medicinal milk. The spirits of those who study them will be illuminated, for these are not words formed by worms and laughed at by the wise. People will not turn their backs on the trouble taken by this man of learning who has provided us with skillful means.

NOTES

I am grateful to Nalini Kirk, Nathan Sivin, and Dolly Yang for their invaluable help in translating the prefaces in this chapter.

1. For a critical review of the relevant literature, see Clausen 2000; Ng 2003.
2. Messner 2000, 2006a, 2006b, 2016.
3. Elman 2001, 2005, 2011, 2015.
4. Chao 2009.
5. For examples and useful introductory overviews of science and medicine in late imperial and early modern China, see Chao 2009; Elman 2005; Hinrichs and Barnes 2013: 129–208; Leung 1997; and Sivin 2015, whose monograph is exceptional for the space it accords to nonelite and religious practices.
6. For a comprehensive biography of Yu Chang, see Lü 1984. For typical examples of the representation of Yu Chang as a scholar-physician in the sinophone literature, see Mao Juntong and Ding Guangdi 1992; Liu Zuyi and Sun Guangrong 2002: 835–48. There are no works dedicated to Yu Chang in the anglophone literature. However, he and his works invariably appear in studies of early modern China as influential exemplars of scholarly medicine. See, for example, Elman 2005: 25, 232–35, 284; Furth 2007: 143–45; Hanson 2011: 110–17, 124, 155.

7. Hanson 2011.

8. I discuss Yu Chang's influence on the development of medicine in China in Scheid 2013, 2017, forthcoming.

9. One may want to compare, for instance, the importance of Buddhism in Yu Chang's thinking with Janet Gyatso's (2015) analysis of the relationship between Buddhism and medicine in seventeenth-century Tibet. There, the author suggests that modernity as a universal historical category is characterized by the separation of religion and a critical epistemology to which physicians are inclined by way of their engagement with bodily reality.

10. Yu Chang 1999a: 3.

11. This is a metaphor for the Dao.

12. The literal translation here refers to the explication of the *sūtras*, but it can be assumed that Yu Chang extends this meaning to the explication of the medical canons.

13. Yu Chang is referring here to the *Canon of the Golden Casket and Jade Case* (*Jingui yuhan jing*), which circulated in the Song dynasty as an alternative version of Zhang Zhongjing's *Treatise on Cold Damage and Miscellaneous Disorders* (*Shanghan zabing lun*).

14. Yu Chang 1999b.

15. *Kalpa* (Skt.), an eon or world period. An eon is defined in Indian cosmology as a day of Brahmā, or one thousand *yugas*, equating to 4,320 million human life years. A *kalpa* therefore also describes an unimaginably long period of time.

16. The six pathogenic *qi* of Chinese medicine distinguish heat from fire. The former is continuous, sweltering, and unabating, just like the heat of summer, and hence commonly referred to as "summer heat." The latter comes and goes more quickly, like the flushing of a hot flash.

17. Qian Qianyi 2001.

18. See translation of this text in Blum 2013.

19. The text and a translation of the "Song of Precious Mirror Samadhi" (*Baojing sanmeige*) by Dongshan Liangjia (807–869), from which this quote is taken, is available at http://www.sacred-texts.com/bud/zen/hz/hz.htm.

4. An Eighteenth-Century Mongolian Treatise on Smallpox Inoculation

Lobsang Tsültim's "The Practice of Preparing Medicine for the Planting of Heaven's White Flower" (1785)

BATSAIKHAN NOROV, VESNA A. WALLACE,
AND BATCHIMEG USUKHBAYAR

A short text called "The Practice of Preparing Medicine for the Planting of Heaven's White Flower" is contained within the medical treatise *The Method of Preparing Oil-Based "Basam"[1] Medicine*.[2] The treatise was composed in the Tibetan language by the well-known Mongolian Buddhist scholar Chahar Géshé Lobsang Tsültim (1740–1810).[3] It is also mentioned in his biography, written by his disciple Lobsang Samrübnima.[4] Smallpox inoculation was already in practice in Mongolian Buddhist temples before the text was written in 1785, but this was the first independent work on smallpox inoculation that appeared in Mongolia during the colonial rule of the Qing dynasty (1636–1912).

It is probable that the method of inoculation outlined in the text was brought to Mongolia from Tibet in the seventeenth or eighteenth century. The fundamental text of Tibetan medicine, *The Four Medical Tantras*, mentions smallpox but does not speak of any preventive measures against it. However, *A Supplement to the Third Tantra*, composed by Desi Sangyé Gyatso in 1691, mentions a "secret" medicine for smallpox, which consists of scabs caused by smallpox infection. Lobsang Tsültim himself was an influential figure in Mongolian Buddhism and had studied Tibetan medicine and authored many scholarly treatises in the Tibetan and Mongolian languages. According to his biography, he was the only survivor of a smallpox-infected family.[5] When local authorities sought his medical advice during an epidemic, he developed the inoculation procedure for smallpox described in the text.

Lobsang Tsültim's treatment is closely connected to Buddhist meditational and devotional practices, as well as to the Mongolian nomadic lifestyle. At first glance, it appears to be a ritual text that could date from a much earlier era.[6] However, a closer investigation of the treatise reveals a confluence of Mongolian, Tibetan, and Chinese medical knowledge facilitated by the Qing colonial context. During the seventeenth and eighteenth centuries, the emperors Kangxi (r. 1662–1722), Yongzheng (r. 1723–1735), and Qianlong (r. 1736–1796) became important patrons of Mongolian monasteries and medical facilities.[7] The reasons behind the Qing state's investment of such extensive resources in Mongolian institutions were predominantly political, as openly stated by the Qing emperors themselves. In Emperor Kangxi's own words, the main goals were to appease the "tenacious and belligerent" Mongols by inspiring their faith in Buddhism and teaching them obedience.[8]

Although Mongols were introduced to Tibetan and Chinese medicine during the period of the Mongol Empire, it was during the Qing rule that Mongolian medical knowledge and institutions truly flourished; for example, the first medical college in Mongolia was established in 1685 during the reign of Emperor Kangxi.[9] Eventually, a large number of Buddhist medical colleges were established, which subsequently trained thousands of physicians. The most important Tibetan medical works of the time were translated into Mongolian, and a large body of original Mongolian works and commentaries on Tibetan medical treatises were produced. However, the Qing colonial period presented a double-edged sword. Along with the medical benefits of the Qing's patronage of the Buddhist medical tradition came new diseases, such as gonorrhea, smallpox, and syphilis, which were spread in Mongolia by the Qing soldiers and Chinese traders who were allowed by the Qing administration to settle in Mongolia's capital.[10]

Lobsang Tsültim's treatise below contains information on the treatment of syphilis and infectious diseases causing chills,[11] as well as smallpox inoculation. It also mentions general preventive and hygienic practices for common infectious diseases. Mongols believed that the outbreak of smallpox, which they called "Heaven's White Flower" (Mong. *tngri-yin čaġan čečeg*), was the result of demonesses who induced a heat disorder of the bile, which entered the blood, affecting the bone marrow and causing skin rashes. According to the text, smallpox medicine involved a number of medicinal substances for treating pathological heat in the blood and for preventing the excess of heat in the body. The mention of Chinese names for medicinal ingredients and diseases in this text suggests that the author had access either directly or indirectly to some Chinese medical sources, as well as Tibetan ones. Additionally, the text incorporates traditional Buddhist therapeutic approaches, such as mantras for various manifestations of the goddess Tārā, as well as of one's own tutelary deity (Tib. *yidam*), for healing and for protection against hostile spirits and spells.[12]

The text is divided into three sections. The first discusses the necessary preparations for the procedure, which both the person who is to be inoculated and the inoculator must follow. The second gives an account of the preparation and administration of the medicinal powder used for smallpox inoculation, which contains smallpox scabs, particular herbs, and "precious pills."[13] The last section focuses on the importance of chanting mantras for the efficaciousness of the treatment and on the necessity for the patient to adhere to the prescribed behavioral and dietary restrictions that follow the inoculation. Notably, owing to the fact that the smallpox epidemic was brought from China to Mongolia, the visits of Han Chinese and other foreigners were obligatorily limited.

FURTHER READING

Chang, Chia-Feng. 2002. "Disease and Its Impact on Politics, Diplomacy, and the Military: The Case of Smallpox and the Manchus (1613–1795)." *Journal of the History of Medicine and Allied Sciences* 57 (2): 177–97.

Hopkins, Donald. 2002. *The Greatest Killer.* Chicago: University of Chicago Press.

Perdue, Peter. 2005. *China Marches West: The Qing Conquest of Central Eurasia.* Cambridge, Mass.: Harvard University Press.

Wallace, Vesna A. 2012. "The Method-and-Wisdom Model of the Medical Body in Traditional Mongolian Medicine." *Arc—The Journal of the Faculty of Religious Studies, McGill University* 40: 1–22.

"THE PRACTICE OF PREPARING MEDICINE FOR THE PLANTING OF HEAVEN'S WHITE FLOWER"[14]

OṂ, may there be well-being!

With compassion and the blessings of the Guru and the Three Jewels, for the planting of Heaven's White Flower, clean the residence [where the inoculation will be carried out], and pay homage to the Three Jewels. Throw away any filthy items, dress both the inoculator and the patient with clean clothes, stay away from impurities such as smoke, and provide a clean environment. The inoculator must meditate with an intensive spiritual practice and express his reverence in chanting. Imagine a continuous white light, like offering water, shining from the realm of the Supreme Guru to the ten directions, illuminating the patient for the sake of healing and medicine for the sake of blessing. Recite the "Twenty-One Verses" of praise to Tārā three times, [make] an offering to the Dharma Protector, present a sacrificial cake offering[15] to the local spirit,[16] and wish and pray [for a successful inoculation]. [The person who is to be inoculated] must be washed or cleansed with holy water and censed with *guggul* smoke.[17]

While chanting many times for the assistance of the compassion and blessing of the Guru and Three Jewels, trust that the medicine will have potency in the same way that the *devas*' holy water, the *nāgas*' jewels, and the sages'[18] elixir for rejuvenating do for every being. Visualize a golden mountain that brings prosperity, and speak of the best of days. Create [in your mind] a scene in which, owing to the blessed words of the Guru, of the tutelary deity, and of the Guardians [of the Four Directions], countless white lotus flowers bloom everywhere, and everlasting peace abounds. Pay homage to the Supreme Guru.

Protect with the fearless *vajra* the benefit that happiness bestows.

Method of Preparation

For the preparation of the "Sacred Collection of Seven Pills," scabs of the smallpox patient are taken as a fundamental medical ingredient. A gallbladder stone[19] and "Six Good Medicines" are mixed in. For that, seven [parts] of a gallbladder stone are taken; two of *Bambusa arundinaceae*; four of saffron; two each of nutmeg, clove, green cardamom, and black cardamom;[20] nine of smallpox scabs; and precious pills are added. Ground them all into a powder. With regard to hygiene, the patient needs to take a bath and must pay homage to the Guru, the Three Jewels, the tutelary deity, and the Guardians. Let the medicine be inhaled through the right nostril in the case of boys and through the left [nostril] in the case of girls. After that, pay homage to the Guru and to the Three Jewels.

Obedience and Restrictions After Inoculation

Do not speak unethically, and do not create bad odors, such as [from] alcohol and smoke, around the inoculation place. Events such as causing bleeding, producing impure odors, the loud noise of livestock, visitations from strangers, trading goods such as clothes and bedding, and shaking and dusting off clothes outside [the home] must be avoided, especially when it is windy. Also, having a visitor from among the Han Chinese, speaking negative words, uttering the names of grains such as rice, and [eating the meat of a] camel[21] are prohibited. These abovementioned inappropriate foods must not be consumed [by the patient]. Noisy activities, such as worshiping and playing musical instruments, are also forbidden. The patient must be kept only in the inoculating place, and chanting near the patient [must be done] softly. Constant cleaning and dusting are required. Mantras, especially [those] of Dolma, Loma Gyon ma, and Palden Lhamo, must be chanted many times.[22]

Blessings!

NOTES

1.   *Basam* is the name of a Mongolian medicine that contains many plants and other compounds mixed with clarified butter.

2.   Lobsang Tsültim 1785. Copies of this text are kept in several collections in the city of Ulaanbaatar, including at the National Library of Mongolia. In this chapter, we have used a copy from our own private collection.

3. Chahar is his birthplace, and Géshé is his monastic title.

4. Lobsang Samrübnima, a disciple of Lobsang Tsültim, composed Lobsang Tsültim's biography in the Tibetan language after Lobsang Tsültim's death in 1817. The biography was translated into Mongolian by Jürmeddanzan the following year. According to the biography, a book titled *The Practice of Preparing Medicine for the Planting of Heaven's White Flower* was written in 1785. We have been unable to find this book as an independent text but have found its content included as a part of a more extensive medical treatise called *The Method of Preparing Oil-Based Basam Medicine*, which is included in this chapter in English translation.

5. His uncle and four siblings died from the smallpox epidemic in 1754, when he was fifteen years old.

6. See examples in *Anthology*, vol. 1. A Mongolian ritual text is translated in chapter 35 of that volume.

7. Elverskog 2006.

8. Jinkhene Dagaj Yavakh Khuuly 2004.

9. Baigalma 2006; Bold 2006.

10. R. Andrews 1921; Pozdneyev 1971, 1980.

11. *'Dar ba'i nad* is the name of an infectious disease with periodic symptoms of shivering, cold, and heat, resembling malaria.

12. Healing rituals involving Tārā are introduced in *Anthology*, vol. 1, ch. 40.

13. "Precious pills" (Tib. *rin chen ril bu*) usually contain precious substances, such as gold, silver, and the like, and are prepared through a complex pharmaceutical procedure and empowered by a lama's mantras and meditation. For more information, see *Anthology*, vol. 1, ch. 60.

14. Lobsang Tsültim 1785: 6–8.

15. Tib. *tor ma*, Skt. *bali*.

16. Tib. *gzhi bdag*.

17. *Commiphora mukul*, also known as "Indian beddelium."

18. Skt. *ṛṣis*.

19. Tib. *giwang*, bile that is solidified and stone-like. This is extracted from elephant gallbladder, but, owing to its rarity in Mongolia, a substitute is used.

20. *Amomum sabulatum*.

21. In traditional Mongolian medicine, camel meat is thought to aggravate the Wind Element.

22. These are the goddesses Tārā, Śabarī, and Śrī Devī.

5. Psychosomatic Buddhist Medicine at the Dawn of Modern Japan

Hara Tanzan's "On the Difference Between the Brain and the Spinal Cord" (1869)

JUSTIN B. STEIN

Hara Tanzan (1819–1892) was a polymath who rose to prominence in the Buddhist circles of nineteenth-century Japan. Tanzan is primarily known as a Sōtō Zen priest in the decades spanning the Meiji Restoration of 1868 and is remembered in several well-known stories that cast him as a man of great humility and preternatural insight. He is renowned for being the first lecturer on Buddhist texts at the University of Tokyo, for framing Buddhism as a form of Indian philosophy and a science of consciousness, and for being an early proponent of empiricism and experimentalism in Japanese Buddhism during a period in which Western philosophy and psychology were increasingly gaining ground in Japanese intellectual circles.[1]

In contrast to Tanzan's renown in intellectual histories of modern Japanese Buddhism, scholars have paid little attention to Tanzan's innovative combination of Buddhist theories of consciousness with elements of Eastern and Western anatomy to propose physiological explanations of physical illness and mental unease.[2] His "On the Difference Between the Brain and the Spinal Cord" summarizes his conception of two substances at the heart of his psychosomatic understanding of physical and mental health: enlightenment, located in the brain as an energetic form he calls "brain *ki*," and unenlightenment, a physical fluid associated with the spinal cord.[3] The nerves connecting the brain and spinal cord cause unenlightenment to mix with enlightenment, resulting in a fluid Tanzan calls "mixed consciousness."[4] Mixed consciousness, Tanzan writes, must be regularly excreted from the body as mucus and phlegm, as it causes physical disease when its circulation becomes blocked. He argues that meditation practitioners can consciously extract the nerves that allow unenlightenment to flow from the spinal cord into the brain. Doing so keeps mixed consciousness from forming, allowing the practitioner to both purify enlightenment and achieve perfect health. He supports these theories with experimental data drawn from his own experiences, concluding that his training in both Buddhism and medical science has allowed him to demonstrate the shortcomings of each. Until the time of his studies, he argues, Buddhism's ignorance of the physiological constraints on enlightenment had handicapped its profound philosophy of mind and its program of liberation, whereas medical science's blindness to the underlying relationship among physiology, consciousness, and the roots of disease (both physical and mental) had similarly limited its ability to promote human flourishing.

Tanzan's embodied vision of the awakening process incorporates elements of Sino-Japanese medicine, Daoist inner alchemy, Japanese translations of European anatomical texts, and various aspects of Buddhist doctrine, particularly Tanzan's interpretation of Yogācāra philosophy and The Awakening of Faith (Daijōkishinron). He taught these ideas and associated meditation practices through an organization called the Buddhist Immortal Society (Bussensha), which was active from 1878 until his death in 1892. Some of his methods survived into the early twentieth century, when subsequent generations of students adapted them for popular audiences in increasingly secularized forms that eventually had little if any recognizably Buddhist content.[5] Tanzan's interpretations of Buddhism (if not his unorthodox meditation practices) were also influential through his role as an instructor at the University of Tokyo, although some of his students reacted against his teachings on the cognitive roots of disease and the potential to purify the body's enlightenment through meditative practice.[6]

Tanzan's idiosyncratic theories had their acolytes and their detractors in their time, but they offer historians of Buddhism and of medicine a unique, creative synthesis of Buddhist doctrine with local Sino-Japanese and localized "Western" anatomies that in some ways anticipate later biomedical and neuroscientific explanations of meditation as therapeutic. His Daoist-inflected self-cultivation techniques recast "original enlightenment" (hongaku), a central category of Japanese Buddhist thought since the medieval period, in terms of a fluid circulatory model of health that incorporated biomedical research into the anatomy of the nervous system. By proposing an explanation of the origins of physical disease and mental suffering, as well as solutions to these human ills, Tanzan's "On the Difference Between the Brain and Spinal Cord" situates Buddhism as a means to knowledge that is as valid as, and complementary to, biomedical science. Through his idiosyncratic readings of both Buddhist psychology and early East Asian medical anatomy, Tanzan produced what he considered innovative, effective psychiatric interventions to eradicate disease, calm distress, and produce authentic understandings of ultimate reality.

FURTHER READING

Johnston, William D. 2016. "Buddhism Contra Cholera: How the Meiji State Recruited Religion Against Epidemic Disease." In *Science, Technology, and Medicine in the Modern Japanese Empire*, edited by David G. Wittner and Philip C. Brown, 62–78. Abingdon, Oxon: Routledge.

Low, Morris, ed. 2005. *Building a Modern Japan: Science, Technology, and Medicine in the Meiji Era and Beyond*. New York: Palgrave Macmillan.

McVeigh, Brian. 2017. *The History of Japanese Psychology: Global Perspectives, 1875–1950*. London: Bloomsbury Academic.

Yoshinaga, Shin'ichi. 2015. "The Birth of Japanese Mind Cure Methods." In *Religion and Psychotherapy in Modern Japan*, edited by Christopher Harding, Fumiaki Iwata, and Shin'ichi Yoshinaga, 76–102. New York: Routledge.

"ON THE DIFFERENCE BETWEEN THE BRAIN AND THE SPINAL CORD"[7]

I discovered something important about the human anatomy and heart (and when I say *heart* here, I do not refer to the anatomical heart but rather to consciousness and psyche) in terms of Buddhist doctrine. Yet, I am not satisfied keeping my discovery to myself but venture to inform those of great learning and virtue and ask [for their thoughts].

We Buddhists teach that there are three kinds of consciousness. The first is the true mind of excellent enlightenment and pure cognition. The second is the mind-essence that gathers, creates, and grasps. (By this I mean the Sanskrit *ādāna*-consciousness, this mind that gathers together various qualities to create the form of the body, to which it grasps tightly before it disintegrates.[8] This is close to what Western doctors call the vital force.) The third is the mundane cognition[9] of unenlightened beings (i.e., the consciousness of ordinary mind, the deluded mind, the hindrances, etc.).

Based on this truth, I conducted decades of observation and study to explain this reality [of the three kinds of consciousness]. To that end, I read the standard medical texts (and found that, while ancient Chinese medical texts have lots of mistakes, so do the anatomical texts used by contemporary Western physicians). While these texts are correct in saying that the brain is the seat of consciousness and mind, they make a grave error in considering the spinal cord to be part of the same system with the same function (saying it is like the end of a branch, spilling out of the brain).

Rather, the brain is the seat of the consciousness of excellent enlightenment, with nine pairs of fibers. [. . .][10] While [the brain] has the subtle faculties of listening, seeing, understanding, response, activity, and memory, the spinal cord is equipped with the mind-essence of gathering, creating, and grasping tightly, without consciousness. (This theory has not been developed by anyone else in the past or present, so there will certainly be those who doubt it. Refer to my *Theory of Consciousness*.[11]) [The spinal cord] has thirty-one pairs of fibers that produce fluid [. . .] that nourish and help the entire body. These two types of fibers (the brain *ki* fibers and those of the spinal fluids) weave a net through the whole body, so it is difficult to distinguish between the two.

The nine pairs of fibers coming out of the brain allow the spinal fluid to influx into the brain *ki* (in other words, excellent enlightenment and wisdom), causing the two to mix. This is why Buddhists call this "mixed consciousness" (what I earlier called the consciousness of mundane cognition). This consciousness spreads throughout the body, so that unenlightened people's bodies do not contain the pure enlightenment of pure cognition. This is why Buddhists have observed and studied that, when the consciousness of mundane cognition comes an end, the essence of the pure consciousness of true mind manifests itself. No one but Buddhists can perform this method of study (this is explained in the *sūtras*), though I will not go into that here.

This is conclusive evidence that mixed consciousness is the sole source of disease. Fevers, malaria, headaches, tuberculosis, abdominal pains, beriberi: They are all caused by the influx of spinal fluids into the brain where they mix with brain *ki*, which then spreads to various parts [of the body]. (This spreading of the nine pairs [of fibers extending from the brain] goes beyond the [description offered in] Western medical texts, which just explain that they spread like ivy.) Excretion of that fluid [of mixed consciousness] out of the body creates a healthy

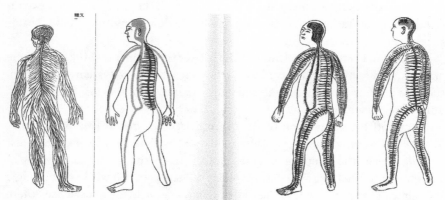

FIGURE 5.1 HARA TANZAN'S ILLUSTRATION OF HIS CIRCULATORY THEORY OF ENLIGHTENMENT (SHADED) AND UNENLIGHTENMENT (BLACK). IN THE DIAGRAM ON THE FAR RIGHT, THE BRAIN IS LABELED "SOURCE OF ENLIGHTENMENT" (*KAKUGEN*).

Source: Akiyama 1907: 108–109.

body, free of disease. (There is no significant way of excreting the mixed fluid out of the body except as nasal mucus and as sticky phlegm. [As someone who has] escaped disease for a long time, I can therefore say that distress and disease have a single cause.)

If the fluid is obstructed and [then] all starts to moves at once, it causes fever. (Medical texts say fever is normally caused by external factors or is dependent on time and place, but these are just indirect causes and not the true cause of disease). When that circulation is a little weak, it becomes malaria. When it becomes obstructed in the brain, it causes headache; when it is obstructed in the abdomen, it becomes abdominal pains; when it is obstructed in the lungs, it becomes tuberculosis; when it is obstructed in the legs, it is called beriberi. (Roughly, [the mixed fluid becomes] the sticky phlegm of the respiratory system and rich nasal mucous. [It can also cause] skin diseases, such as scabies and abscesses. Overall, phlegm and pus are both produced by fluctuations in the production and movement of mixed consciousness. Western physicians differentiate between phlegm and pus, but I cannot agree. Phlegm is only [the mixed consciousness] that is spoiled, whereas pus is that which is putrefying.) All these diseases have a single cause, although they can appear differently.

In general, Western anatomical theory is based on two thousand years of experimental research, so if I want to criticize it solely based on Buddhist principles of inner observation, people will not believe me. Thus, I [also] want to argue from my own experiments, intimate evidence, and numerous experiences.

When I first gained the power of *samādhi*[12] [. . .], it was because I was able to cut off the abdominal consciousness.[13] [. . .] I experienced a sudden expansion and filling up of the consciousness in my chest and brain. Once I cut off [the circulation from] the chest, that area became empty and pure, and there was a sudden expansion in my head. When I cut off [the circulation] from my brain, my head and chest both became empty and pure, after which there was a sudden expansion both in the back part of my brain and in the flow of my spinal fluid. This is the first piece of evidence.

Also, when I cut off the pathway at the base of the brain, my thinking became empty and pure. If the spinal cord were a branch of the same system as the brain, the nine pairs of nerves would all suddenly expand, but it was just the opposite. This is the second piece of evidence.

To cut off the connection to the top of the brain means [the practitioner achieves] wise insight into exquisite reality,[14] as well as the power of steadfast *samādhi*. This is the complete extraction of the fibers that grow from the top of the spine into the brain. (As *The Awakening of Faith* says, the wisdom of a single thought can instantly remove the root of ignorance.[15]) [In my experience,] there was not even a tremble in the spine or hip, but only at the point where spinal fluid would normally enter the brain did it turn back and flow elsewhere [i.e., back into the body]. Thus it is obvious that this consciousness of grasping tightly is at the top of the spine, and it is the brain that is at the end of the branch. (The neck is like a root and the spinal cord is like the tree trunk. The head is like a stem, but the brain is the most excellent because it is the source of enlightenment.)

And yet, the fibers that go from the top of the spine into the whole brain are more than just one or two. Thus, to extract them all is quite difficult. (When there is a surplus of spinal fluid, a little may influx [into the brain], causing mixed consciousness and the disturbing hindrance of moving thoughts. Thus, it is very difficult to completely extract [the fibers].) Unless one meets a virtuous teacher, various anxieties will arise, but if the spinal cord were the end of a branch of the brain and one were to cut off this passage, the thirty-one pairs [of nerve fibers coming out of the spinal cord] would certainly be desiccated. And yet, when this passage is cut off, at first the parts of the body to which the spinal fluid flows do experience distress, but soon after they get plump[16] [and flourish] like wild grass grows on manure. This is the third piece of evidence.

In general, Buddha's doctrine of consciousness is pure and subtle, but its lack of a detailed explanation of this part [described in this essay] is still a defect. [On the other hand,] the experiments of Western science misunderstand the fundamentals of consciousness. (To provide details [about consciousness, science has] missed cultivation-realization and mistaken its branches for its roots. This is why it is unaware of the reality of enlightenment and unenlightenment.) But, as it's said, everything [i.e., both Buddhism and science] has its advantages and disadvantages.

NOTES

This chapter was drafted with the support of a grant from the Japan Society for the Promotion of Science.

1. Furuta 1980; Kanamori 1990; Kimura 2001; Yoshinaga 2006, 2015; Klautau 2008, 2012; K. Inoue 2014; Takemura 2017.
2. The notable exception is Shin'ichi Yoshinaga, whose work inspired this chapter.
3. The terms *enlightenment* (Jp. *kaku*) and *unenlightenment* (Jp. *fukaku*) are key categories in *The Awakening of Faith*, a foundation of East Asian Buddhism, and the locus classicus of the concept of "original enlightenment" (Jp. *hongaku*); that is, the potential for enlightenment in unenlightened beings. See Stone 1995: 18. Tanzan taught courses on *The Awakening of Faith* at the University of Tokyo and later published a commentary on it. See Hara 1988 [1885]; K. Inoue 2014.
4. Jp. *wagōshiki*. Tanzan also refers to this as "mixed heart-mind" (Jp. *wagōshin*).
5. See Yoshinaga 2006: 9–11, 2015: 95–96.
6. For example, the prominent Buddhist reformer Inoue Enryō (1858–1919) studied under Tanzan at the University of Tokyo and agreed with his teacher's monistic philosophy that Buddhism is a rationalistic philosophy of the mind. See K. Inoue 2014; Yoshinaga 2015; Takemura 2017. However, Enryō critiqued Tanzan's analysis of the origin of physical illness as overly psychosomatic, citing the cholera epidemic of 1858 that ravaged "the worldly and the saints alike." See E. Inoue 1901.

7. Akiyama 1907: 98–102. I would like to sincerely thank Shin'ichi Yoshinaga for his generous assistance with the translation of this text, as well as Dylan Luers Toda and Erik Schicketanz for their assistance with some terms and references, and Michel Mohr for his prior assistance with Tanzan's work.

8. *Ādāna*-consciousness (Jp. *adana-shiki*; Skt. *ādāna-vijñāna*) is a Yogācāra term that can be translated as "appropriating consciousness" or "clinging consciousness." Most Yogācāra schools associate it with the eighth consciousness called "storehouse consciousness" (Skt. *ālaya-vijñāna*), but some associate it with the seventh consciousness of "mind-consciousness" (Skt. *mānas-vijñāna*), which seems to be how Tanzan uses it here. See Lusthaus 2004: 919; Muller 2018, s.v. *adana-shiki* (comments by Lusthaus and Yamabe).

9. Jp. *nensō shiryō*. These are the opposites of the Zen Buddhist expressions of enlightenment, "no thought, no mind" (*munen musō*) and "nonthinking" (*hishiryō*). The latter phrase is particularly prominent in the writing of Dōgen (1200–1253), the founder of the Sōtō Zen sect to which Tanzan belonged.

10. Some of Tanzan's copious parenthetical statements have been omitted from the translation in order to improve its readability. Such cases have been marked with "[. . .]."

11. Akiyama 1907: 85–92.

12. Jp. *jōriki*; Skt. *samādhi-bala*.

13. Tanzan's attention to circulation among the triad of the head, chest, and abdomen suggests some awareness of Daoist inner alchemical meditation practice on the *dantian*. For more about the anatomy of Daoist inner alchemy, see Esposito 2008; Pregadio 2008. Elsewhere, Tanzan maps Yogācāra theories of consciousness onto these three centers, associating the six sensory consciousnesses (Skt. *mano-vijñāna*) with the abdomen, the seventh "mind-consciousness" (Skt. *mānas-vijñāna*) with the chest, and the eighth "storehouse consciousness" (Skt. *ālaya-vijñāna*) with the head. See Yoshinaga 2006: 7.

14. Jp. *hōmyō nyojitsu*.

15. T. no. 1666, 32: 581b14. This reference is to a section in *The Awakening of Faith* regarding those bodhisattvas who aspire to enlightenment through insight.

16. This is said in a positive way, as a sign of health.

6. No Sympathy for the Devils

A Colonial Polemic Against *Yakṣa* Healing Rituals (1851)

ALEXANDER McKINLEY

T he *yakṣa* has a long and winding history in Buddhism. Historians argue that *yakṣas* were deities in a pre-Buddhist nature cult who were subsequently tamed and absorbed as servants of the Buddha.[1] Although the Buddha and powerful Buddhists could control *yakṣas*, using them as guardians or for labor, *yakṣas* also developed reputations for nefarious chicanery, and many caused illness. This resulted in the evolution of elaborate healing rituals in Sri Lanka meant to drive away the influence of *yakṣas* and restore mental and physical well-being to patients exhibiting symptoms of sicknesses ranging from gastritis to hysteria.[2] Many extant Sinhala palm-leaf manuscripts from the nineteenth century concern these *yakṣa* arts, especially the power of Buddhism to alleviate their ill effects.[3]

This connection among *yakṣas*, the Buddha, and health went unappreciated by most Christian observers, who saw only dangerous devil worship in *yakṣa* song and dance. Christian encounters with Sri Lankan *yakṣa* cults began with the sixteenth-century Portuguese, who decried what they saw as demonic heathenry. Yet, even as missionaries sought to displace these traditions, they also legitimized *yakṣas* by sympathizing with victims and by believing in and exorcising devils. Thus, early missionaries were essentially competing in the same market as *yakṣa* healers: one of curses and cures. This set Catholics apart from their Dutch Protestant successors, who were less interested in the supernatural.[4] The Dutch Protestant missionary movement classified *yakṣas* as pure superstition but feared them for other reasons. While the Dutch sought to regulate all non-Protestant activities in their territory, they seemed particularly concerned with stopping *yakṣa* rituals and singling out "devil dancers" as a rebellious threat.[5]

The British colonial project inherited these prejudices and added its own biases. After deposing the last Sri Lankan king in 1815, the British became the first European power to take control of the entire island. This gave them an unprecedented ability to intervene in Sri Lankan religious affairs, and the treaty they signed with native chiefs to formalize their power stipulated that the British were the new royal stewards of Buddhism. The British interpreted *yakṣa* cults as a dark underbelly of Buddhist practices, a remnant of animism that obscured the value of real Buddhist philosophy. While calm monastic scenes were an acceptable vision of the Orient, *yakṣa* rituals were everything that was considered wrong with lived Buddhism. The colonial surgeon Henry Dickman represented this in the language he used to describe a Buddhist monastery versus a *yakṣa* exorcism. The former involved "a room or hall . . . tastefully decorated with leaves, fruits, and flowers, in the usual oriental style," whereas the latter had "horrible-looking beings, with immense eyes and noses . . . frightful in the extreme."[6] Some early colonial authors did show scholastic interest in *yakṣa* rituals,[7] and the first Sinhala text to be published in English translation in London was in fact a *yakṣa* ritual book.[8] But missionary opinion dominated, which, by the mid-nineteenth century, was bolstered in its anti-*yakṣa* stance by the potent ally of modern medicine.

British colonial agendas made *yakṣa* rituals a public health concern.[9] Merging medical and missionary motives, the Ceylon Religious Tract Society published the four-page pamphlet translated below as part of their overall goal of publishing proselytizing Christian literature in the Sinhala language. *The Advantages of Devil Ceremonies* (*Yak piḷivetvala prayojanaya*) was originally printed in 1851,[10] and it proved to be one of the Society's more widely disseminated tracts. By 1896, the book was in its fourth edition, and another twenty thousand copies were printed that year.[11] The work may have been repeatedly printed because of its popularity among Sinhala readers, which may have been because it was one of the goofiest works the Ceylon Religious Tract Society ever produced.

Of course, despite the title of the tract, it recognizes no advantages of devil ceremonies. That joke was the whole point, rephrased in different ways over twenty-seven quatrains, using the same poetic mode of composition by which Sinhala *yakṣa* knowledge had traditionally been transmitted. The translation of this poem below attempts to preserve some of the original form of the Sinhala quatrain, which uses a unique poetic grammar with relatively terse articulations of ideas. This occasionally results in some unusual English phrasings; to help with comprehension, therefore, some punctuation and bracketed words have been added.

In the poem, *yakṣa* activities, denoted by the word *yakkama*, are seen to be advantageous only for people who wish to waste all their money feeding thieving exorcists (*yakāduran*), employing phony self-aggrandizing doctors, and watching their relatives perish in pain. The author makes no reservations about insulting patrons of *yakkama*; such a person was an "idiot" or an "ignorant savage." This critique lumps *yakkama* with all sacrificial offerings (*bali*), planetary rituals (*graha piḷivet*), and the larger system of Āyurveda practice (*vedakam*). The doctors who prescribed *yakkama* are contrasted with "intelligent doctors" who prescribed modern medicine (*behet*). While Āyurvedic doctors and exorcists might take credit, only modern medicine was considered a legitimate way to treat illness.

The poet who authored the tract sought to shame *yakkama* patrons for not being urbane, warning that all-night ceremonies would prevent workday productivity and that people from other countries would learn of their ignorance. It is implied that foreign *yakṣa* experts, likely from South India, were sometimes brought to Sri Lanka. In contrast, the poet points to the many Sinhala, English, and Moorish people who had already rejected *yakkama* in favor of modern medicine. By the end of the poem, however, the missionary voice has overshadowed the modernizing and the medical. *Yakkama* endangers the eternal soul. Hell is certain for devil worshippers, but the possibility of God's forgiveness always remains through the mercy of Jesus, who assures a comfortable afterlife for those too ill for medical salvation. Combining bodily and heavenly health, *The Advantages of Devil Ceremonies* thus sought to bring Buddhists into a modern medical and religious world by trading *yakṣa* treatment for the panacea of Christian imperialism.

FURTHER READING

Kapferer, Bruce. 1983. *A Celebration of Demons: Exorcism and the Aesthetics of Healing in Sri Lanka.* Bloomington: Indiana University Press.

Scott, David. 1994. *Formations of Ritual: Colonial and Anthropological Discourses on the Sinhala Yaktovil.* Minneapolis: University of Minnesota Press.

Wirz, Paul. 1954. *Exorcism and the Art of Healing in Ceylon.* Leiden: Brill.

THE ADVANTAGES OF DEVIL CEREMONIES[12]

1.
Friend, if you would like to see what an idiot is,
when a relative becomes ill,
old women have *yakkama* done for the cure,
not considering how many doctors have failed to heal.

2.
If there is a strong desire for you to give
your possessions to exorcists, then this is for you.
When those people's skill is spoken of,
you should lend an ear and listen to that.

3.

If [you are] of a mind to receive an unskilled doctor,
who speaks lies as though living in ignorance,
always doing rituals, then a person who speaks no wisdom
will always be satisfactory for you to seek.

4.

Do you desire to always display to the world
the ability of thieves to cheat you?
When the *yakṣa* dance and sacrificial ceremony is done,
everyone will quickly realize that.

5.

For plantain bunches, rice, oil, coconuts, and similar stuff,
without giving a justification of there being any result,
if [you are] of a mind to spend money in vain,
have the *yakṣa* dance done, friend.

6.

Like this, sleep is ruined at the time of nighttime dewfall,
so that the next day one becomes unable to work.
If you'd like to become ill all the time,
you should do the *yakṣa* rituals without delay.

7.

Doctors who have not tried to become skilled
when seeking other avenues to make a living,
if you'd like to give good support to them,
do the *yakṣa* dance and other rituals without delay.

8.

Like a drunken, frenzied person taking and drinking a lake or a pond,
someone roughly dances. Thinking that illness and pain will be cured by this,
if you'd like to appear to be that much of an idiot always,
do the *yakṣa* dance and other rituals without delay.

9.

"Having erected a platform made of clay, reciting poetry
when one roughly dances, once spoken, the illness will be cured."
    Thinking this,
would you like to appear as an emaciated ascetic now?
Then happily commence the sacrificial ceremony to realize for yourself.

10.

Friend, here you appear as an ignorant savage.
If you prefer that, do *yakṣa* rituals always.
Likewise, if you'd like to receive disrespect from the wise, and praise from
the ignorant, have *yakkama* done always.

11.

For people from distant countries to discover your ignorance,
spend money to bring exorcists from those countries.
To always do Āyurveda when life is running short, *yakkama* done
to enter death, no meaning spoken—that's a good Āyurveda teacher.

12.

Friends and relatives who live with illness, cold wind striking night and day,
while remaining silent and alone, fall asleep and die.
Thus, on the day you wish to increase their illness and pain,
do the *yakṣa* dance and other rituals without skimping.

13.

A loss, having been idiotic, your relatives and friends are going to die.
If you would like to be at fault always for this which you have done,
spend a bit of money, and conduct *yakkama* for them.
Without any doubt, that fault will thereby be able to be received.

14.

To have people with rough traits dawdling around your home,
happily consuming rice and betel, to sit and watch the dances
night and day, to destroy the fruits of you and your neighbors,
and to allow it—if of such a mind, have *yakkama* done, dear friend.

15.

The Lord God's protection, too, so as to lose,
like a queen who spent time in myriad suffering,
removed from a king of commanding virtue and married to an outcaste.
If you want to appear the same as this, have *yakkama* done, dear friend.

16.

These beautiful friends and relatives of yours, in hell for all time.
If there is any such intention to cast them down, you, too, will fall.
If they always desire for you to do these *yakkama* and *bali* rituals,
those things will occur certainly.

17.
Yakṣa and planetary rituals happen like this.
Realize the special fault in this way.
Without insight, people with stubborn mental darkness,
without delay, do *yakṣa* rituals without end.

18.
Giving medicine to the person who became ill,
after various *yakṣa* rituals are done fully.
After that illness is healed by the medicine,
that exorcist receives the thanks for that.

19.
Doctors like this have a mind to do *yakkama*.
[When] the illness of an ignorant person is healed, they always say,
"With these verses I made another person's state well."
To you all, they always need to speak as such.

20.
Not having those rituals performed further, Sinhala
people, along with English people and Moorish
people, not having those things done at any time,
heal illness with medicine every time.

21.
When one baby and another baby cry from hunger,
a clay cake is put in their hands, so as to soothe those babies.
Instead of a medicine, as though giving a poison to an ill person,
these *yakṣa* rituals are done for ill people out of love.

22.
Friend, like this, without gaining a result from *yakṣa* rituals,
mind, body, wisdom, and wealth will diminish definitely.
Furthermore, people with Lord God have mental courage, but
the ever-burdening *yakṣas'* blessing sadly makes thick suffering arise.

23.
Though *yakkama* and other such rituals are done to protect us,
the Lord God is angered, and those who do it receive hell.
After *yakkama* is done, on the day of death and arrival in the afterworld,
for those people arriving from here, there will be suffering without end
    dreadfully.

24.

Because of that, friend, when your relatives or a friend become sick,
without taking them to do *yakkama* as [some] doctors still say,
take them to intelligent doctors with wisdom and receive reward.
According to what those doctors say, medicate those sick ones.

25.

Like that, if without health, bring [the patient] to different skilled doctors,
and, according to what they say, medicate without delay.
After, if still without health, to see comfort in the next world,
that person [should] turn their heart to Eternal Heaven.

26.

Because of words against Lord God the Creator, in body and mind
countless people had sinned; for those people exists
forgiveness in the name of noble Lord Jesus, Lord God the Father, removing
from suffering the people who ask him with devout hearts.

27.

Readily offering to always give forgiveness and health,
if one faces the faultless Lord God, that health is given.
If not, that ill person will be taken from this world, and in the blessed
city of Heaven will arrive in eternal comfort most high.

NOTES

1. DeCaroli 2004; Sutherland 1991.
2. Some of the vast scholarly literature on Sri Lankan *yakṣas* includes Gooneratne 1865; Wirz 1954; Obeyesekere 1969, 1970; Kapferer 1983, 1997; D. Scott 1994.
3. See, for example, Rīri Yak Kavi, Colombo National Museum Library manuscript 22/C1, leaf 2b.
4. Zupanov 2006: 197.
5. Arasaratnam 1996: xviii, 22–23; Tennent 1998: 54.
6. Dickman 1863: 143–44.
7. Upham 1829.
8. Anonymous 1829.
9. Anonymous 1891.
10. Whitney 1856: xxvii.
11. Of these tens of thousands of pamphlets that circulated for half a century, only one 1896 copy remains in the Colombo National Museum Library (call number 104/U24).
12. Though first published in 1851, this translation was made from the 1896 edition (Anonymous 1896).

7. "Enveloped in the Deep Darkness of Ignorance and Superstition"

Western Observers of Buddhism and Medicine in the Kingdom of Siam in the Colonial Era

C. PIERCE SALGUERO

The first European ships to arrive in Southeast Asia in the early sixteenth century were Portuguese, followed by Dutch, Spanish, British, and French. With the influx of merchants and missionaries to the area, competition for power and resources between the European countries intensified. These foreign powers graduated from controlling trade ports to occupying larger and larger tracts of land. By the late nineteenth century, few patches of land were left that had not been annexed by a Western nation.

The sole territory on mainland Southeast Asia that avoided European colonization was the kingdom of Siam.[1] Though forced to open its doors to European trade in the 1850s and '60s, Siam successfully engaged in what has been called "survival diplomacy" in order to stave off colonization. As was the case in other independent Asian states at the same time—most notably in Meiji Japan—the Siamese ruler, King Mongkut (i.e., Rama IV, r. 1851–1868), initiated programs of modernization and Westernization designed to strengthen the state's military, education, science, technology, and infrastructure. The modernization of public health and medicine were part and parcel of these efforts.[2]

Although Siam succeeded in avoiding being absorbed by a colonial power, reforms proved insufficient to preserve the kingdom intact. Attacked by France in the Franco–Siamese War in 1893, the country was forced to concede a significant portion of its territory in modern-day Laos. With Siam now encircled by colonizers, the French to the east and north and the British to the west and south, a treaty was negotiated to recognize the kingdom as an independent buffer state in 1896.[3] This agreement notwithstanding, both imperial powers continued to chip away at Siamese territories over the ensuing years, resulting in the loss of additional territory through 1910.

The three texts included below, dated between 1865 and 1907, are excerpts from English-language tracts written during this period of high colonialism by Western observers living in Siam. Neither British nor French, these authors enjoyed support from the Siamese royal family and were affiliated with elite institutions in the kingdom. Nonetheless, these authors were freely and vocally disdainful of the Siamese people, especially of their medical, religious, and cultural traditions.

The author of the first piece below was the American Dan Beach Bradley (1804–1873), a Protestant missionary doctor who lived in Siam for nearly four decades starting in 1835.[4] Closely associated with the royal family, Bradley enjoyed their patronage as a successful medical doctor and publisher. His name is known to this day in Thailand for having performed the kingdom's first recorded surgical operation, introducing vaccination, and advocating Western obstetric practices. Bradley also introduced the printing press to Siam, created the first typeface for the Thai language, and founded the first Siamese newspaper. His article on Siamese medicine excerpted below was first published in his self-published annual almanac, the *Bangkok Calendar*. It proved to be an influential piece, cited whenever the topic of medicine in Siam came up over the ensuing century, and was even reprinted in 1967 in the Thai journal *Sangkhomsat parithat* (*Social Science Review*).

The author of the second selection below was another American missionary doctor, Ernest Adolphus Sturge (1856–1934). Though most well known for his missionary activity in Japan, he was first assigned to Siam in August 1880. He published several reports on the state of Buddhism in the kingdom (which he perceived to be in decline), education at the mission schools, and local customs in Petchaburi where he lived. The piece included below, on the matter of Siamese medicine, was considered highly newsworthy. Originally published in a biweekly medical journal from Philadelphia, it was later recopied or excerpted in various other outlets, including in the prestigious medical journal, the *Lancet*.[5]

The final selection below is by C. Beyer, a German engineer who was involved with building hospitals in Siam. His essay was submitted to the Siam Society, a scholarly organization founded in Bangkok in 1904 under royal patronage, of which Beyer was a member and for which Beyer later served on council. Beyer's paper, which the author acknowledges was inspired by Bradley's abovementioned publication, was presented formally at a society meeting on February 7, 1907. It was published in the society's journal later that year, along with many accolades and positive responses from the other members.

Taken together, the selections below give the reader a sense of the "state of the field" of the Anglophone study of Siamese medicine between the late nineteenth and early twentieth centuries. All three articles indicate how Western observers encountered religious and medical ideas, such as reincarnation, the Four Elements, and the bodily Winds. These pieces are also quite obviously laden with the blatant ethnocentrism characteristic of the colonial period.[6] Representing the conventional wisdom of the leading doctors, missionaries, and scholars, they belittle and scoff at native religious and healing traditions, seeing both as indications of the overall ignorance and backwardness of the people of Siam. While the doctors concentrate most on lamenting the deplorable and "practically useless" state of Siamese therapeutics, they also theorize about the source of this deficiency. Beyer, for example, points to the "Indo-Siamese" fascination with "transcendental philosophy" and the Buddhist doctrine of nonviolence as reasons for the inability of the people of Siam to engage in empiric observation. Both he and Bradley mention the innate qualities of the Siamese people as a limiting factor, Beyer citing the closeness of their "race" to nature and Bradley comparing them with animals.

While scholars of the post-colonial era would eschew such blatantly racist and Orientalist positions as are expressed in the passages below, the notion that Buddhism is inherently inimical to empirical investigation continued to influence Western perceptions of the relationship between Buddhism and medicine through much of the twentieth century.[7] It is only recently that these overwhelmingly negative characterizations have given way to the generally positive value placed on Buddhism common in mainstream North America today. As discussed in numerous other chapters in this anthology, this new view sees the Buddha as an empirical scientist of sorts and approaches Buddhism as a valuable potential source of healing practices—the complete opposite of the perspectives expressed here.

FURTHER READING

Lord, Donald C. 1969. *Mo Bradley and Thailand*. Grand Rapids, Mich.: Eerdmans.

Puaksom, Davisakd. 2007. "Of Germs, Public Hygiene, and the Healthy Body: The Making of the Medicalizing State in Thailand." *Journal of Asian Studies* 66 (2): 311–44.

Salguero, C. Pierce. 2016. *Traditional Thai Medicine: Buddhism, Animism, Yoga, Ayurveda*. Rev. ed. Bangkok: White Lotus.

Wyatt, David K. *Thailand: A Short History*. 2nd ed. New Haven, Conn.: Yale University Press.

1. EXCERPTS FROM DAN BEACH BRADLEY'S "SIAMESE PRACTICE OF MEDICINE" (1865)[8]

It may be truthfully stated, in general terms, that the Siamese practice of medicine is enveloped in the deep darkness of ignorance and superstition. Keen and studious observation, which is so indispensable to safe and successful practice, is exceedingly rare in the profession. What is written in their medical books of the virtues and powers of particular medicines is received by native physicians as true of course; and their own powers of observation are so obtuse that however wide from the truth those descriptions may be, they would not be likely, on a trial of their virtues however long continued, to detect their falsity. If any article of their *materia medica* does not produce the effect it was written that it would, it is attributed, not to the want of that power in the medicine, but to some counteracting influence beyond human ken to foresee and human power to avert. There is a similar air of sanctity thrown over Siamese medical books as there is over their religious books, and almost as soon would they discredit the latter as the former. Every medical writer professes to acquire his knowledge from the original and infallible source—viz the Primitive Teacher [i.e., the Buddha]. And every practitioner professes to have some extraordinary gift of healing directly from the same fountain. If he would gain the confidence of his patient, he must put on the air of some prophetic wisdom and be able to say, from the most cursory observation of the case, whether it be Wind, Fire, Water, or Earth that is at fault, where the seat of the disease is, and what medicines will certainly cure it.

The Cunning of Native Physicians

It is amusing to witness how many ways a Siamese physician can take to run clear of discredit. No matter how confidently he has expressed his opinion of the nature of a disease and named the remedial agent that will cure it, no matter how wide the result may seem to prove him to have been incorrect, he can show his patient, and all concerned, that the failure was not at all from the want of an accurate diagnosis, or other adequate medical knowledge, but solely from some extraordinary obstacles that no man could have foreseen, as for example some sudden change of the internal Wind, or some blast of Fire, or mist of darkness from Earth or from Water, or some angel or devil, that has counteracted his well-laid plans. Deception and craft would appear to be their native air and medium of vision. Everything seems to look wrong to them unless it be wrapped up in superstition, which of course is chiefly made up of error. This remark is as true in relation to their science of medicine (if such it can be called) as to their religion.

Native Medical Recipes

They have great confidence in medical recipes, which are supposed to have been copied from their standard works on medicine. So much are they in repute, that the builders of Boodhist temples will be at the trouble and expense of engraving great numbers of them on marble tablets, and having them permanently fixed in the walls of buildings attached to the temples, in conspicuous and convenient places, so that whoever will may freely copy them and treat their diseases accordingly.[9] In doing this, they conceive that they are conferring great blessings on the poor and will reap a rich reward for it in some future state of transmigration. The benevolent phase of the idea is certainly good, however little benefit the poor may realize who follow the prescription. It would seem to be an incipient step toward the full expansion of a similar but a less selfish idea, which is now seen developed in Christian lands in the form of hospitals and infirmaries.

Siamese Obstetrics

Superstition has invested the whole subject of native midwifery with the most silly and ridiculous notions, and some very pernicious and cruel. In accordance with the teachings of Boodhism, the Siamese believe that there never have been any new creations of animal or intelligent beings and hence that all living creatures that ever have been, or ever will be born, are simply and only transmigrations from previous states of existence—that all mere animal beings have once been in a higher state in some previous life, in the form of men or women on Earth, or as angels in Heaven or devils in Hell, and that mankind have all transmigrated to their present state either from some of the many heavenly worlds or from some of the many infernal abodes.

The native books on midwifery make an earnest business of teaching parents how they may know whence their newborn infants have come and soberly state certain signs by which they may know whether their expected child is to be a son or daughter. [...] There are a thousand other superstition observances connected with this subject that tend greatly to enslave and dwarf the mind of the mother. Happy should Christian mothers be that they have not been brought up under such chains of ignorance and consequent misery. [...] Nevertheless, facts seem to prove that parturition is both shorter and easier to Siamese mothers than is usual to Europeans and Americans. Certainly this cannot be attributed to good treatment, but rather to the fact that they are more animal in their natures, and consequently share with the animal creation more liberally than the latter, in the animal immunities of parturition.

Happy would it be for these poor deluded mothers if they would allow their animal simplicity to govern them more than they do immediately after the birth of their children. Just at this point commences their most unnatural, cruel, and destructive custom of having the mother lie by a hot fire from the time the child is born constantly for a period varying from five to thirty days. [...][10]

Now it seems quite appropriate that such a monstrous custom as this among the Siamese should be drawn out and exposed to the Christian world in the pages of the *Bangkok Calendar* for the purpose not of ridiculing these unhappy native mothers, but with the view to excite Christians to tender sympathy for them. [...]

The writer, from long observation of the working of this treatment of Siamese mothers and their infant children, is fully persuaded that it is a tremendous evil upon the Siamese race, a prolific cause of dyspepsia, dropsy, barrenness, and consumption of the bowels and the lungs in the mother, and of convulsions, diarrhea, dysentery, cholera-infantum, and hydrocephalus in their offspring. In short, it is not too much to say that it opens floodgates of disease, impotency, and constitutional weakness, which, more than any other cause, prevents their increase as a people and crushes them down to inferior grades of physical and mental stamina.

Siamese Ignorance of Anatomy

The most learned among the native physicians have the least possible knowledge of human anatomy. They have some vague notions of a few of the bones but no idea of their number. As to distinct muscles of the human body, they know absolutely nothing, regarding them all as an indistinguishable mass of flesh. With a few of the more superficial tendons, they are of course somewhat acquainted and can call them by appropriate names. But of the nerves, they are the most profoundly ignorant, and hence there is no word, or set of words, in the Siamese language by which to designate any one of them. They cannot avoid seeing some of the most superficial veins, and knowing that they contain blood, but whether it flows within outwardly or the reverse they seem not to have had a thought about it, only so far as to take it for granted that it runs in all directions.

Concerning the arterial circulation, they have the most ludicrous notions, supposing the pulse, wherever felt, to be a conductor of Wind.[11] The writer once upon a time, being in company with a chief physician of the kingdom, and he withal a prince, in endeavoring to convey some correct ideas of the circulation of blood, put a finger on his pulse at the wrist and asked him the question, "What is it that bounds there under the finger?" He promptly replied, "*Pen lom*; it is Wind." And whenever the writer has endeavored to explain to the native physicians what disastrous effects the least volume of Wind would produce if injected into the arteries, they have invariably stared at him with the blankest incredulity.

2. EXCERPTS FROM E. A. STURGE'S "SIAMESE THEORY AND PRACTICE OF MEDICINE" (1884)[12]

All nature, according to the Siamese, is composed of Four Elements, namely Earth, Water, Fire, and Wind. The human body is supposed to be made up of these same Elements, which are divided into two classes: visible and invisible. To the former belongs everything that can be seen, as the bones, flesh, blood, etc.; to the latter, the Wind and the Fire. The body is composed of twenty kinds of Earth, twelve kinds of Water, six kinds of Wind, and four kinds of Fire.[13]

The varieties of Wind are as follows: The first kind passes from the head to the feet and the second variety from the feet to the head; the third variety circulates in the arteries, forming the pulse; the fourth variety resides in the abdomen outside of the intestines; the fifth resides in the intestines; and the sixth enters the lungs in the act of inspiration.

The four kinds of Fire are first, that which gives the body its natural temperature; second, that which causes a higher temperature, as after exercise or in fevers; the third variety causes digestion; and the fourth causes old age.

The Siamese divide the body into thirty-two parts, as the skin, heart, lungs, etc. The body is thought to be subject to ninety-six diseases, due to disarrangement of the Earth, Wind, Fire, and Water. An undue proportion of Fire causes fevers, and dropsies are caused by too great a proportion of Water. Earth is supposed to produce disease by invisible and impalpable mists and vapors, and Wind can cause all manner of complaints. Nine out of every ten natives, when asked what is the matter with them, will answer, "Wind." (Not long ago, on our way to Bangkok, we found a man dead upon the riverbank. The boatmen were speculating as to the cause of the man's death, but the oldest man in the company soon settled the matter by gravely remarking that, in all probability, it was due to Wind.) It is thought that the external Elements are constantly acting upon the Elements composing the body, causing health or disease. Thus, in the hot season, the Siamese believe, we are more liable to fevers, and in the rainy season to dropsies due to too great an absorption of Water. Spirits are also supposed to have great power over our bodies, deranging the Elements and thus producing all manner of maladies. One of our young men remarked not long ago, while travelling in a rather lonely portion of country, "I am not afraid of tigers, but I do fear spirits." The Siamese have numerous spirit-doctors, and many are the propitiatory offerings made to the immaterial beings that fill the air.

In the time of Buddha lived one still worshipped as the Father of Medicine [i.e., Jīvaka Komārabhaccha; see *Anthology*, vol. 1, ch. 1, 20; vol. 2, ch. 16, and below in §3]. To him, it is said, the plants all spoke, telling their names and medical properties. These were written in books and have become sacred. If they fail to produce the results ascribed to them, the fault is never theirs but is due entirely to want of merit in either doctor or patient. The natives use almost everything as medicine; the bones and skins of various animals occupy a large part of their pharmacopoeia, while the galls of snakes, tigers, lizards, etc. are among the most valuable of their medicines. Most of the Siamese remedies are very complicated, being composed of scores of different ingredients. The following is an absurd recipe for snake bite: A portion of the jaw of a wild hog, a portion of the jaw of a tame hog, a portion of the jaw of a goat, a portion of goose bone, a portion of peacock bone, a portion of the tail of a fish, a portion of the head of a venomous snake; these, being duly compounded, form a popular remedy when the venom has caused lockjaw. Burnt human bones, powdered and mixed with an equal portion of powdered alum, form a favorite medicine for sprinkling on ulcers. The eyeteeth of tigers, bears, lions, and various other animals (the more the better), ground up together, form the most popular remedy for fevers. The ashes of earthworms and human hair, mixed with coconut oil, are frequently used for cuts. Every native physician has an image of Phra Ruesi [i.e., Venerable Sage (Skt. ṛṣi)], the father of arts, in his house. All drugs are first placed in this idol's hand and receive his blessing; afterward they are taken to the patient's house and boiled in earthen pots, a wickerwork star always being placed above and below the drugs to prevent the spirits from tampering with them. In all fevers, the doctor fills his mouth with some concoction and squirts it over the naked body of the patient in a fine spray, exactly as the Chinese laundrymen sprinkle clothes.

Dissection is never practiced among the Siamese; consequently, they are grossly ignorant in regard to the science of anatomy. The writer has not infrequently seen them hew a body in pieces with a cleaver at least two feet long, but very little is ever learned from these rough postmortem examinations. They are usually made with the expectation of finding one or more tumors in the abdominal cavity, which they suppose to be the work of witchcraft. They usually are successful in finding what they look for. Sometimes the spleen, at other times a kidney or some other normal organ, is mistaken for an abnormal growth inserted in the body by superhuman agency. The functions of the different organs are not at all understood. In the heart is supposed to be a cavity about the size of an almond. This cavity is thought to be filled with a fluid that changes its color and consistency with our passions. When we are calm and peaceful, this fluid is perfectly clear, like water; when we are angry, it is turbid; when very angry, it turns dark; and when we are in love, it is red. In stupid persons, the apex of the heart is rounded, while in those possessing the usual amount of wisdom, it is pointed. It is not known that the heart has anything to do with the circulation.

3. EXCERPT FROM C. BEYER'S "ABOUT SIAMESE MEDICINE" (1907)[14]

Siamese medicine has its origin in Indian medicine. Siamese tradition says it was first taught by Komārabhacca, who lived at the time of Buddha. As the name implies, he was the son of a courtesan and was put away by his mother and was adopted by King Bimbisāra [see Anthology, vol. 1, ch. 20]. He fled from Bimbisāra and studied medicine for seven years with a teacher in Taxila. After seven years, he was sent out by his teacher to collect plants that had medical properties. He came back with the answer that all plants could be used in medicine, upon which his teacher declared that he had completed the studies. Komārabhacca is the author of the old Indian writings on medicine, which are considered as sacred, and which even to this day are kept translated into Siamese in temples. Thus, both Indian and Siamese medicine show the characteristics of Indian culture; I mean the culture of the mind, not that which we have got by technical development, which in my opinion cannot satisfy mankind, who have higher and nobler aspirations.

The culture of India was from the very beginning an abstract culture, directed toward philosophical speculation, against which the study of the concrete, the observation of nature, and practical utility were kept in the background, and it was the characteristic of Indian culture that the study of the concrete was neglected. Indian philosophy, mathematics, [and] Indian religious symbolism are so abstract that it is difficult for the Western mind to follow them entirely to their highest aspirations, but this splendid talent for speculative philosophy, this talent for getting familiar with the most abstract things, caused the more positive side of the human mind to be absolutely neglected. Indian science is a philosophic, theoretical science; instead of sober observations, the collecting of facts, of experiments, we find, as we shall see presently in Indo-Siamese medicine, speculative ideas that, starting from a preconceived idea, tried to adapt it to medicine and its therapeutics. [. . .]

But is it not strange that Indian culture—and everything in Siam is Indian culture—which, in philosophy, religion, and folklore, as well as in architecture, has attained a high standard, should have been with regard to the science of medicine practically useless? In the first instance, transcendental philosophy and medicine are difficult to reconcile. Medicine is occupied in collecting facts by objective observation and by experiment. It must not put aside those facts for vain speculations if it will continue its victorious course through centuries. This fact has not been recognized by Indian medicine; it has thus done nothing for the progress of medicine. A physician may be a philosopher, but medicine has nothing to do with philosophy.

It must not be forgotten that the easy way of life enjoyed by people in the tropics is not favorable to serious scientific investigations. The Indian race being brought into constant contact with nature has little opportunity for empiric observations.

Finally, religion is also responsible. It is one of the first tenets of Buddhism not to take life, not even that of an animal. How should he then approve of experimenting on animals? But as he contended that his doctrine contained all science, he simply based all science on religious philosophy. This is the reason why Indian, and consequently Siamese, medicine did not enter into details about anatomy. The nature of illness was based on phantastic and wrong ideas and consequently misunderstood. Medicine is, it may be said, in some regards in a similar state to medical science in Greece in the time of Hippocrates—who lived some two thousand four hundred years ago, about 450 BC—especially with regard to this idea of the Four Elements. But we must do justice to Hippocrates, whose ethics, whose knowledge of anatomy and surgery, was far superior to anything that I have found in the Siamese books of medicine.

NOTES

1.   Brief histories of Thailand are offered in Terwiel 1984; Wyatt 2003.

2.   The modernization of the public health system is described in Puaksom 2007.

3. On Anglo–French competition in Siam, see Kratoska 2001, vol. 2: 80–91.

4. Feltus 1936; Lord 1969.

5. See *Lancet* 124 (3196): 985, published November 29, 1884.

6. For a discussion of Burmese medicine with a similar tone, see Macdonald 1879.

7. Some Western scholars, for example, still see Buddhism's "otherworldly" philosophical stance as having stood in the way of the development of empirical medicine in certain historical contexts. See the discussion in Salguero 2018: 238; cf. Unschuld 2010: 132–53.

8. Excerpts from Bradley's 1865 article in the *Bangkok Calendar*, reprinted in Bradley 1967. This piece has been edited for inclusion in this volume, including minor changes to punctuation and capitalization, for readability. None of these edits have affected the meanings of the passages.

9. On this practice at the royal temple, *Wat Pho*, in Bangkok, see Salguero 2016: 8–16.

10. For a more detailed, and more neutral, description of these and related practices, see Wales 1933.

11. See the glossary and *Anthology*, vol. 1, ch. 41–43, for a discussion of Buddhist concepts of various Winds in the body.

12. Sturge 1884. This piece has been edited for inclusion in this volume, including minor changes to punctuation and capitalization, for readability. None of these edits have affected the meanings of the passages.

13. This formula is common in Buddhist sources, such as in the Pāli scriptures *Majjhima Nikāya* 28, 62, and 140. Its usage in Thai medicine is described in Salguero 2016: 41–44.

14. Beyer 1907. This piece has been edited for inclusion in this volume, including minor changes to punctuation and capitalization, for readability. None of these edits have affected the meanings of the passages.

Ruptures and Reconciliations

8. Three Tibetan Buddhist Texts on the Dangers of Tobacco (Late Nineteenth to Twenty-First Century)

JOSHUA CAPITANIO

This section presents three texts from the Tibetan Buddhist tradition that discuss the dangers of tobacco consumption. Each piece presents one or more narratives describing the emergence of tobacco into the world as the result of some sort of demonic activity and then goes on to explain the harms of tobacco use for Buddhist practitioners. Each also details methods to quit using tobacco.

Tobacco was introduced to East and South Asia around the late sixteenth and early seventeenth centuries,[1] and evidence of tobacco consumption in Tibet can be found by the early seventeenth century.[2] Tobacco was brought to Tibet from neighboring countries, and the different myths of the origins of tobacco discussed below include accounts of its spread to Tibet from India, China, and Mongolia. Tibetans smoked tobacco in pipes, by itself or mixed with other substances, and also consumed it in the form of snuff.[3] Smoking tobacco has traditionally been forbidden for Buddhist monks in Tibet, but the use of snuff was sometimes allowed.[4] The first text below is mainly concerned with prohibiting the use of snuff rather than the smoking of tobacco. Tobacco was also sometimes mixed with opium, and several of the sources cited in the texts below discuss tobacco and opium together and even appear to conflate the two at times.[5]

The three texts presented here represent different genres and were produced during different periods between the late nineteenth and early twenty-first centuries. Although each presents a slightly different perspective on tobacco use and different methods for addressing this problem, they all agree on the extreme danger it poses for practitioners. The first piece is a type of revealed text known in Tibetan Buddhism as a "treasure" (*terma*),[6] revealed by Tutop Lingpa (1858–1914).[7] The second text was composed by Jikdrel Yeshe Dorje (1904–1987), commonly known as Düdjom Rinpoche,[8] and contains a collection of quotations on the dangers of tobacco use taken from a number of treasures and prophetic texts revealed by some of the most well-known treasure-revealers in the history of the Nyingma school.[9] The third text is a transcript of a lecture given to a Chinese audience by Khenpo Sodargye (b. 1962), an ethnic Tibetan who belongs to the Larung Gar monastery in western China and is one of the most well-known Buddhist figures in the People's Republic of China.[10]

These three texts share a number of common points. Each presents one or more narratives describing the origins of tobacco, and these narratives contain many similar themes. All present tobacco as a plant that was created by *māras*, a class of demonic being portrayed in Buddhist literature as single-mindedly focused on the destruction of the Buddhist teachings.[11] In most stories, it is a female *māra* who is responsible for the creation and dissemination of tobacco, and the production of tobacco—from a *māra*-woman's womb, her menstrual blood, or her egg—is connected to these *māra*-women's reproductive systems. Therefore, the texts establish a clear connection between tobacco and Buddhist notions of impurity: of desire, sexual intercourse, and the female body. Finally, in many of the stories, tobacco is represented as a foreign substance that came to Tibet from one of its borderlands.[12] Thus, all three texts present tobacco as a foreign and impure substance whose very existence is a threat to the Buddhist teachings.

These pieces are also alike in the way their authors avoid or downplay certain topics. For example, the dangers of tobacco are seldom discussed from the general standpoint of Buddhist ethics. The texts do not present tobacco consumption as a violation of any particular Buddhist precepts; rather, they claim that the karmic damage done by tobacco consumption results from its demonic origins. Those who consume the substance are helping to fulfill the vow(s) of the *māra*-demons who produced it and are thereby contributing to the ultimate destruction of the Buddhist teachings.

Because of its polluting influence, tobacco use is seen as particularly harmful for practitioners of the Vajrayāna, the form of Tantric Buddhism common in Tibet. Vajrayāna practitioners are subject to particular rules of conduct known as *samaya*, which are accepted during esoteric rites of tantric empowerment. These rules are commitments whereby the practitioner agrees to abide by certain restrictions in exchange for the blessings and aid of the deity or deities invoked in the empowerment, who may impose weighty punishments if *samaya* are violated. These commitments are subject to contagion, so that association with one who has broken his or her commitments constitutes a breakage of one's own *samaya*.[13] Thus, each of the three texts emphasizes that any contact with tobacco smoke or with people who consume tobacco will result in a downfall of *samaya*, with the consequence that one's tantric practice will be significantly hindered.

In these three texts, concern with the damage that tobacco consumption poses to the Buddhist teachings in general and one's practice of Tantric Buddhism in particular seems to greatly outweigh any discussion of the physical damage caused by smoking. Certain afflictions caused by tobacco are mentioned, such as headaches, wind disorders, lung diseases, and so forth. However, tobacco consumption is framed primarily as a spiritual issue, and the techniques recommended for addressing it—making vows in the presence of spiritual beings, requesting the aid of spiritual beings in quitting the addiction, and practicing methods of repentance to purify the negative karma accumulated from smoking—are all religious techniques.

In these texts, we thus see that the use of tobacco, largely seen as a public health problem in the modern West, is framed within Tibetan Buddhism as an issue of spiritual contamination that has implications for the very survival of the Buddhist teachings. Tobacco is a demonic substance created by the *māras* for the explicit purpose of destroying Buddhism. As such, it certainly has the power to affect one's bodily health, but as these texts emphasize, the threat it poses to one's spiritual well-being is far more significant. The threat introduced by tobacco therefore must be met with a rededication to sincere Buddhist practice.

FURTHER READING

Benedict, Carol. 2011. *Golden-Silk Smoke: A History of Tobacco in China, 1150–2000.* Berkeley: University of California Press.

Berounský, Daniel. 2013. "Demonic Tobacco in Tibet." *Mongolo-Tibetica Pragensia* 6 (2): 7–34.

Düdjom Rinpoche Jikdrel Yeshe Dorje. 1991. *The Nyingma School of Tibetan Buddhism: Its Fundamentals and History*, translated by Gyurme Dorje and Matthew Kapstein. Boston: Wisdom.

Laufer, Berthold. 1924. *Tobacco and Its Use in Asia.* Anthropology Leaflet no. 18. Chicago: Field Museum of Natural History.

1. "Pith Instructions on Forcefully Eliminating the Powerful *Māra* of Tobacco for Persons in These Degenerate Times"[14]

I bow to the Guru, the Great Glorious Heruka.

As an obstacle on the path of liberation for migrating beings in these degenerate times,
The powerful *māra* of tobacco is the embodiment of all negative omens,
An inauspicious force that obstructs the paths and stages.[15]
Formerly in the sacred land, the exalted realm of India,

The unsurpassed, unequaled teacher, Lord of Subduers,[16]
Turned the Dharma-wheel of the fourfold collection of scriptures.[17]
At that time, the king of *māras*, the Lord of Desire,[18]
Maliciously tried three successive times to send down obstacles.
Then, where the peerless Lord of Subduers and his heirs and retinue were
    abiding,
That very embodiment of wisdom and compassion ignited the flames of
    primordial wisdom,
Thereby causing the *māras'* harmful efforts to fail.
All the powerful *māras* were utterly defeated in their hearts,
And, overwhelmed, shed tears of blood on the ground.
As the seventh tear fell, they made this vow:
"As a result of this, in the realm of Vaiśālī,
May a plant arise with flat, green leaves, just a forearm's height.
It will be unfit for consumption, but when placed in the nose,
It will bring along with it the afflictive emotions of the five poisons.
The eighty-four thousand [afflictions] will flourish,
And Gautama's teachings of discipline will all perish without exception!"
Such a vow the *māras* made, and thereby,
[The plant] later arose from the earth in Vaiśālī.
A *māra*-minister named Blood-Colored and a woman named
    Dharma-Confounder
Lay down in union near that [plant], overcome by desire.
At that time, Blood-Colored made a prediction, saying to
    Dharma-Confounder,
"If you offer this before the great king of the *māras*,
He will be pleased with you, because you will be offering him the very thing
To which the destruction of Gautama's teachings has been entrusted. Offer it
    to the *māra*-king."
The king of *māras* was extremely pleased and said,
"Aha! Wonderful! Amazing!
You have found this supreme substance, which will destroy
Gautama's teachings in the final five-hundred-year period [of the Dharma].
    How wonderful!
Blood-Colored, Dharma-Confounder, you two deserve praise for your
    devotion."
Saying so, he made the *māra*-minister and the woman the heads of
The armies of one hundred thousand *māras* and five hundred *rākṣasī*-demons,
Bestowing upon them the tobacco plant, and they gathered in the north of
    India.
At the gathering assembly, they were charged with this vow:
"May this fruit become known throughout Jambudvīpa [i.e., the known world],
And may the followers of Gautama and the young people, male and female,
Make use of it. Firstly, within their sense-faculties and minds,

May desire, hatred, and ignorance increase,
And may the entire host of afflictions greatly spread.
May this [tobacco] overcome all the power of the holy Dharma, without
    exception.
Then finally, may the teachings of Gautama be utterly destroyed,
And may the forces of Māra and the host of afflictions spread!"
So they vowed, and there to the assembly,
[Tobacco] was brought, and they all took it up and used it in their noses.
The host of afflictions spread, desire blazed up,
And gradually they spread it throughout India and Tibet.

This is the heaviest of evils.
All of my followers must refrain from using it.
If one simply encounters its scent, they will go to the Black Line Hell.[19]
Especially, if any person belonging to the noble Sangha makes use of it,
It will destroy [their practice of] Secret Mantra and serve as an anchor
    dragging them down to the hells.
If its scent simply wafts inside, outside, or in front of the mandala,
You will fall into the Black Line Hell, Crying Hell, or the Mire of Rotting
    Corpses.
Since whoever makes use of this poison that utterly increases the afflictions
Will be completely cut off from any recourse to the Conquerors of the three
    times,
You must abandon this substance, tobacco.
Everyone says that the scent of a plant harbors no evil.
As a novelty, they make use of this *māras'* food like they are playing a game.
Right now it seems nice, but in the future,
When you are in the Black Line Hell, Crying Hell, or the Mire of Rotting
    Corpses,
Where will you find happiness or novelty? Think about this!
Right now, in an age when the Buddha's teachings have been established,
You need to call on the Three Jewels for just a simple headache.
After using this *māras'* food in your nose, greatly increasing your afflictions,
And inflicting injury upon the teachings, there will be none to protect you.
    How pitiful!
Therefore, abandon this *māras'* food, and practice the holy Dharma.
If you abandon it, then virtuous qualities and prosperity will greatly
    increase.
Happy now, happy in the future, you will go from happiness to happiness.
Therefore, my followers, take this to heart!
I have spoken this on this occasion for the benefit of migrating beings.
Samaya.[20]
Now, for the pith instructions on forcefully eliminating this *māras'* food,
    tobacco:

Visualize yourself clearly as the teacher Vajrapāṇi.

Your right nostril is Mañjuśrī and your left is Avalokiteśvara.

[They emanate] rays of clear light that invite the entire host of the Conquerors' heirs,

Whose compassionate blessings overcome the entire host of sufferings,

And cause great compassion and primordial wisdom to blaze brilliantly.

The host of *māras* loses heart and is overcome, and negative thoughts are pacified.

Thinking thus, recite these secret mantras:

OṂ VAGIŚVARI MUṂ

OṂ MAṆI PADME HŪṂ

OṂ VAJRAPAṆI HŪṂ

DÜ SIN TAMAKHA MĀRAYA PHAṬ[21]

If you recite this a thousand times with devotion, planting the nails of the creation stage,[22]

Not even a recollection of the *māras'* food will arise in your mind.

It will become completely clear to you what is right and wrong to adopt.

In the future degenerate age, the time of the five corruptions,[23]

If there are still a few followers who maintain *samaya*,

Then, by persevering in this, they will overcome the hostility of the *māras* and *rakṣasī*-demons.

May these [teachings] be disseminated by my compassionate emanations.

Samaya. Sealed. Sealed. Sealed.

Revealed by the treasure-revealer Jikdrel Tutop Lingpa

2. "GUIDANCE FOR THE BLIND ON TURNING BACK FROM THE
PRECIPICE OF PERVERSE PATHS: A BRIEF SUMMARY OF
THE FAULTS OF THE TOXIC SUBSTANCE TOBACCO"[24]

OṂ SVASTI.

The embodiment of the primordial wisdom of the Conquerors and their heirs,

The great one from Oḍḍiyāna,[25] in whom all the families are subsumed—

Having bowed down to you with supreme devotion,

I will now explain the history of tobacco.

Formerly, when just one hundred years had passed since the Buddha passed into *parinirvāṇa*, in the land of China there was a woman belonging to the race of *māras* whose mind was intoxicated with desire. On the verge of death, she spoke these words:

By making this vow, may this physical body of mine have the power to lead many sentient beings from Jambudvīpa to unpleasant rebirths. Let my body be buried unharmed and left alone. Shortly after that, from my womb there will emerge a flower that is like no other. Simply encountering its scent will cause inconceivable joy and bliss to arise in both body and mind. This bliss will be even more intoxicating than the pleasure of intercourse between men and women. That [plant] will spread abundantly, and, finally, most of the beings in Jambudvīpa will be irresistibly compelled to use it.

Things came to pass just as she said, and nowadays there is the [plant] known as opium, as well as its counterpart, tobacco, which can be taken in the mouth or nose. These substances cannot eliminate hunger or thirst or provide satisfaction with their flavors, and they possess not even a single quality by which they are capable of benefiting one's physical strength or bodily constitution. Additionally, the fact that they give rise to disorders of wind, blood, and phlegm, lung disease, and so forth, is common knowledge that can be directly observed. Nevertheless, nowadays all people, high and low, have become irresistibly attracted to them and use them insatiably. Truly, the *māra*-woman's vow has finally come to fruition.

From the treasure-prophecies[26] of the Dharma-king Ratna Lingpa,[27] it is said,

When the great teacher (*acārya*) Padmasambhava
Bound the nine *damsi* brothers[28] under oath,
The youngest of the nine brothers said,
"Brothers, do not despair—listen to my words:
In the land of China, I will emanate as tobacco,
And will be known by the name of 'black poison.'[29]
It will come to grow at the borders of Tibet,
And the people from the borderlands will bring it to central Tibet.
The Tibetan people, who enjoy bliss and happiness,
Will, through its power, become afflicted with the five poisons, which will
   increase.
Abandoning the ten virtues, they will engage in the ten non-virtues.
The lifespans of the holders of the [Buddhist] teachings will become unstable.
The poisonous smoke will go down into the earth,
Destroying hundreds of thousands of great *nāga* cities.
Rain will cease to fall, and crops and animals will not thrive.
Infighting, virulent diseases, and all manner of unwanted circumstances will
   arise.
The poisonous smoke will go up into the expanse of space,
And through its power will destroy the cities of the gods.
The planets will become opposed, the seasons disrupted, and ominous stars
   will rise.
The channels of enlightened mind[30] will wither in people who smoke it,
And the 404 diseases will be stirred up.
Those who die from smoking will take birth in the three unpleasant realms.
Even to just contact the exhaled vapor, or to sense its scent,
Is equivalent to ripping the hearts out of six million people."

From the treasure-prophecies of Sangyé Lingpa,[31] it is said,

> Here in the degenerate age, people carry out all variety of evil conduct.
> Especially, instead of relying on delicious foods,
> People make use of poisonous, foul, foreign substances.
> Never satisfied, their craving greatly increases.
> They become distracted from their work, clinging passionately to poison.
> Their saliva and mucus flow uncontrollably and their complexions wane.

In the prophetic writings of [Rigdzin] Gödem,[32] it is said,

> In the evil end times, the food of *gandharvas*,[33]
> Exhaled as disgusting vomit, will be consumed as food.
> By simply sensing its scent, one will go to the Hell of Incessant Torment.
> Therefore, it is crucial that it be abandoned immediately.

From the treasure-prophecies of Düdul [Dorje],[34] it is said,

> When the smoke of that plant enters the mouth,
> Or its powdered form is stuffed in the nose,
> Monks and nuns, men and women, are brought under its sway,
> And hosts of *samaya*-breakers fill the land.
> As a sign that they have been deceived by *māras*,
> Thoughts of desire will arise again and again.
> As a sign that their merit will be exhausted,
> Their unbidden tears will fall uncontrollably.

From the prophetic writings of Longsal [Nyingpo],[35] it is said,

> When people take the smoke of toxic substances into their mouths,
> Trustworthy friends will become corrupted by that substance.

From the treasure-prophecies of Tukchok Dorje,[36] it is said,

> Because many living beings will become hardened by the power of the five
>   poisons,
> Suffering due to desire, hatred, and conflict will blaze like fire.
> The Dharma of the ten virtues will be discarded, and non-virtue will circu-
>   late like the wind.
> All virtuous conduct will be abandoned, and all sorts of perverse conduct will
>   spread.
> Guardian deities will become derelict as the *māras'* malevolent influence grows.
> In these evil times, people will inhale the smoke of the substance tobacco,

Blocking the wisdom channels and causing the karmic winds of the afflictions
   to spread,
And because the central channel is blocked, the radiance of self-awareness
   will fade.
Merit will decline, and all existence will be roiled by conflict.
Blessed objects will deteriorate, and perverse views and teachings will
   spread.
The gods and protectors will turn their gazes inward to the realms of
   Mt. Meru.
Foreigners will dominate the central lands, and central [Tibetans] will
   wander in foreign lands.
The teachings of the *māras* will spread, and Jambudvīpa will become like the
   hell-realms.

From the prophetic writings of Drodül Lingpa,[37] it is said,

The leaves of this plant [which grew from] a *rakṣasī*'s menstrual blood—
Just inhaling their scent will send one down to the Vajra Hell.

From the prophetic teachings of Machik Labdrön,[38] it is said,

In the end times, the age of strife,
A food that is replete with the five poisons
Will arise from China,
Spread to Mongolia,
And be consumed by beings in Tibet.
Under its power, here in this land of Jambudvīpa,
Rainfall will become unbalanced, and frost and hail will arise.
If those who practice meditation consume it,
They will not accomplish the deity, even in a hundred eons.
In future lives, they will wander constantly among the unpleasant realms.
The compassion of the Three Supreme [Jewels] will be powerless to protect
   them.

These and other statements appear among the infinite scriptural teachings, and
many similar proscriptions have been made by eminent scholars and accomplished individuals from both the Old and New schools. Thus, since the vajra
words of the Precious One from Oḍḍiyāna are never deceiving, it would be completely inappropriate to think with the perverse view that "how can there be
such fault in the smoke of a plant?" Considering that aconite also belongs to the
category of plants, but consuming just a small amount can still be life threatening, then how could this fruit of a *māra* woman's perverse vow not also be capable
of cutting off the life-span of liberation? Therefore, if knowledgeable people do

their best to abandon it, then they will truly be extending great kindness to themselves.

> May this please those who are devoted and knowledgeable,
> And lead them away from the precipice of perverse paths.
> In the joyous forest of the bliss of liberation,
> May they obtain relief and good fortune.
>> *This was written at the encouragement of Jikmé from Serthang in Golok,*[39]
>> *by the one called Vajrajñāna. Virtue!*

3. "THE FAULTS OF SMOKING TOBACCO"[40]

Homage to the root teacher, the Buddha Śākyamuni!
Homage to the wisdom warrior Mañjuśrī!
Homage to the gracious lineage gurus!

The unexcelled, profound, subtle Dharma
Is difficult to encounter in hundreds of millions of eons.
Now that I am able to see, hear, obtain, and uphold it,
May I understand the true import of the Tathāgata's teachings.

In order to liberate all sentient beings, I ask everyone to generate the unexcelled, extraordinary mind of enlightenment. Today's lecture focuses on the faults of smoking tobacco.

Many of my friends here from the Buddhist Academy are monastics, and after becoming monastics they most likely do not smoke tobacco anymore, so perhaps it is not entirely necessary to speak about this. Nevertheless, previously in many places, among Tibetan Buddhists there are some people who call themselves *māntrikas*,[41] as well as a very small number of Chinese Buddhists in Mongolia and other places, who smoke cigarettes. I have seen this before when we visited Mt. Wutai. Probably, these people are not particularly well versed in the Buddhist doctrines, so today, although I am mostly speaking to monastics, I still want to talk a bit about the faults of smoking. Ultimately, you monastics will also go out to spread the Buddhist Dharma, so if you yourselves do not understand these principles, it will be difficult to explain them to others.

Whenever I go out to give teachings, I find that, in some remote places, many people are not aware that the faults of tobacco smoking are extremely great. Actually, the faults of tobacco smoking, drinking alcohol, eating meat, and so forth, have been explained really clearly in the Buddhist discourses and treatises, as well as in the oral instructions of some eminent lamas. If we do not understand what to accept and reject, we will unknowingly bungle many situations. Khenpo Achö[42] said, "In the course of studying with a master, practicing is not important, but listening to and contemplating [their teachings] is very important." This statement resonates very deeply with me. When my lama, who is like a wish-fulfilling jewel, was still alive, his requirements that we listen and contemplate were very strict. Only now that our lama has passed into quiescence, have we come to deeply appreciate the importance of this advice. Now if we wish to consult the lama's oral instructions, we have only words on paper, on tape, or on DVD. Back in the day, my lama was not very willing to be recorded, so many precious instructions were not set down. Therefore, everyone, in studying with a master, it is very, very important to closely listen to their teachings on the true principles of Buddhism. There are some people who, when they are studying with a master, feel that listening and contemplating are not important and that practice should be most important. I have also had such thoughts before, but when I look at my present situation, I actually still have a great amount of doubt and will never be able to receive enough instructions on all the various principles directly in the presence of my lama.

For many of us, our study of the Buddha's scriptural teachings is not entirely complete, so as we go about our daily lives, we lack a fundamental understanding of what to accept and reject: which faults are the greatest, which merits are the greatest. Now, after having this opportunity to listen and contemplate, everyone should be in a position to weigh the various merits and faults and to choose for themselves. Otherwise, if you just don't understand any principles of the teachings, you will not know how to begin to engage in virtuous actions or how to abandon non-virtuous karma. This would be really sad!

Today, I am using this time to talk a bit to everyone about the faults of tobacco smoking. There are some Buddhist disciples who especially enjoyed smoking tobacco before and were strongly addicted to it. After encountering the Buddhadharma [i.e., Buddhism], they basically quit, and now all that remains is a memory. Of course, those who possess particularly strong habitual patterns may suddenly have dreams in which they are smoking cigarettes. Among non-Buddhists, the phenomenon of tobacco smoking is pretty serious. Actually, the harmful effects of smoking tobacco are quite significant. Not only will it deplete your health, waste your resources, disorder your mind, and lead to many illnesses in this lifetime, but the karmic consequences in future lifetimes are enough to really make you shudder in fear. All eminent monks and great worthies recognize that tobacco came into being as the result of the evil vow of *Māra*. Therefore, people who smoke are really scary, and practitioners all do not dare to get close to them. This includes me; when I encounter someone who smokes, I also get really nervous, as I am afraid that this kind of corrupting influence could cause my spiritual practice and blessings to deteriorate.

There are different histories of the origins of tobacco, of which there are a couple that are relatively well known. I will explain a few different ones to you all.

The first explanation is that, once during the Buddha's lifetime, he entered into a deep meditative state while in the *nāgas'* palace, and two *māra*-women from the desire realm Heaven of Enjoying Others' Creations[43] tried to use their magical arts to bewitch the Buddha, wanting to destroy his discipline. The Buddha had already cut off all craving, and any sexual desire had long ago vanished in him, so the *mara*-women's bewitchment had no way of succeeding. The two *mara*-women harbored a deep grudge, and each made an evil vow. The elder *mara*-woman took a clump of excrement and threw it into China, where it transformed into garlic. If you eat garlic, your body and mind will become uncomfortable, which is due to the *mara*'s bewitchment. Your desires will also greatly increase. All the instructions concerning discipline and cultivation state that consuming garlic is a great fault, so usually, when eating, it is best not to take food with onion or garlic. Garlic in particular should be avoided. The other *mara*-woman sprinkled some of her menstrual blood in India, where it transformed into the tobacco plant. Since tobacco is the fruition of the *mara*-woman's vow, those who smoke or consume it will deplete and destroy their compassionate minds, and anger, perverse views, ignorance, and the rest of the five poisons will naturally increase. It can also destroy all the merit accumulated from practice.

The second explanation is that, a long time ago, the *mara*-king Pāpīyān was on the verge of death yet was unable to take his last breath. His eldest daughter said, "I will kill a thousand sentient beings." Yet Pāpīyān was not able to die. His second daughter said, "I will kill a hundred million beings." Yet Pāpīyān was still not able to die. Finally, his youngest daughter said, "I will sprinkle my menstrual blood on the ground, and by all means make this vow: 'I vow that from this menstrual blood poisonous leaves will grow, so that ordinary men and women and especially Buddhist monastics will smoke this tobacco, and the fault of doing this will prevent their three generations of family members from attaining liberation. For a thousand eons, they will not be able to escape from the pitch-black smoking parlors. Wherever the tobacco plant spreads, there the gods, *nāgas*, earth spirits, and the rest of the eight classes of supernatural beings will be subdued. The people there will see their life-spans and blessings depleted, and their relatives and the common people will become weak. Because they will have short life-spans and many illnesses, they will be fearful and bitter, and many conflicts will arise. In future lifetimes they will fall into the eighteenth level of the hell-realms.'" Only after she made this evil vow was the *mara*-king Pāpīyān finally able to die in peace. Therefore, the mind of anyone who smokes tobacco will be overpowered and bewitched by the *maras*.

The third explanation is that when the Buddha Śākyamuni was turning the wheel of Dharma, there was a disciple who had broken the precepts and criticized the Three Jewels. She grew bitter in her heart and vowed that in the future, she would plant an evil seed within the human world that would prevent sentient beings from practicing the Buddhadharma. Because the power of her evil vow was especially great, after she died, she became a *mara* and entered into the human realm, plotting to destroy the Buddhist Dharma. She planned to take an egg conceived by a *mara* and *mara*-woman to India, where the Buddhadharma was flourishing the greatest. But when she got to India, because the buddha-light of the Buddha Śākyamuni was shining so broadly, she had no way to enter. For the five hundred years in which the true Dharma flourished, she had no opportunities. Five hundred years after the Buddha's parinirvāṇa, she again wanted to appear to stir up the wind and waves, but as soon as she emerged from the earth, she encountered the buddha-light of the great master Padmasambhava. The great master Padmasambhava was the foremost among the hundred mantra-masters, and he possessed extremely great power to subjugate *māra*s, so she still had no way to cause chaos. However, she did not give up at this. She crushed the *māra*-egg into powder and sprinkled it in space, where it was blown by the wind to a neighboring city in India. A year later, a strange plant grew there: tobacco.

Later, this plant was discovered by a Brahmin who was over five hundred years old. She thought that, although she had lived over five hundred years, she had never before seen such a strange plant. Feeling that it was very strange, she took it and brought it to an Indian town to sell. In that town, there was a *māra* who had transformed into a prostitute. As soon as she saw that plant, she developed a fierce craving for it and purchased it at a very high price. Afterward, she burned the plant and inhaled its smoke. This made her entire body feel blissful, so she began to cultivate it. Through her *māra*-powers, the next year she obtained a bountiful harvest. From this, one person spread it to ten people, ten spread it to a hundred, and they began to cultivate it in many different places. Gradually, it spread from India to Yunnan and other places in China. Tobacco first came to China during the Ming dynasty (1368–1644); prior to that, there is no historical record of tobacco.

Smoking tobacco presents extremely great dangers for our vows and cultivation; this is something that most people who have some understanding of Buddhism are aware of. After the great master Padmasambhava, many great treasure-revealing teachers gave instructions on how smoking tobacco can cause one to fall into negative rebirths. Not only do such writings exist within Buddhism, but even most worldly people have a fairly low opinion of the value of tobacco smoking. There was once a story about an American tobacco merchant who went to France to do business. One day, he was in the marketplace going on about the benefits of smoking tobacco, when suddenly an old man got on stage and said loudly, "Ladies and gentlemen, there are three great benefits of smoking tobacco: First, dogs are afraid of smokers; second, thieves do not dare to rob smokers' houses; and third, smokers will always be young." Off stage, the audience grew excited, and the businessman was even more elated. The old man waved his hands and continued, "Why is this? First, most smokers develop hunchbacks, so when dogs see them, they think that those people are hunched over collecting rocks to throw at the dogs. Second, smokers cough all night, so thieves assume that they are still awake. And third, smokers have short lives, so they are always young."

Of course, things cannot be so easily lumped together. There are smokers who live to see old age; they don't all necessarily have short lives. And not all people who cough are smokers. But no matter what, the dangers of tobacco smoking are extremely great. Those who have smoked cigarettes in the past should engage in the practice of Vajrasattva and other methods of repentance. If they do not clear away this defilement, then they will certainly experience suffering either at the moment of death or in the next lifetime.

Many lamas have said in their teachings that if the number of smokers increases over time, this will be especially dangerous for the Buddhist teachings. Recently, I heard that some lamas would bless cigarettes and then instruct the assembly to smoke them; this is a very bad phenomenon. Once there was one [lama] who, no matter which city he went to, would get a couple packs of cigarettes and empty them into a basin. No matter who came, whether lay or monastic, he would make each person smoke one cigarette. At the time, many laypeople found themselves in a difficult situation because they themselves did not smoke and would ask, "Is it OK if I don't smoke it?" Then some other laypeople would scold them, saying, "These were blessed by the lama! This is a rare opportunity; why would you not smoke them? If you don't smoke them, then you will break your karmic connection [with the lama]; you must smoke!" Those people were not very bright and could not refuse smoking as instructed. This is a very negative influence. I know a few of those people and have criticized them in person for this.

Of course, it is not for me to say whether or not these lamas had some secret intentions. But, according to the instructions of the great master Padmasambhava and other lamas throughout history, it is not permitted for ordinary people to smoke tobacco. The venerable Jikmé Lingpa[44] even said, "If you lamas smoke tobacco, then anyone with karmic connections to you will fall into negative rebirths." If lamas themselves smoke, then whoever makes karmic connections with them—for example, by listening to them teach the Dharma, or receiving empowerments from them—will all fall into negative rebirths. He then said, "If you high officials smoke tobacco, then all your subordinates will fall into negative rebirths." So, I am pretty worried for these people, because nowadays there are very few leaders who do not smoke. Will all their subordinates fall into negative rebirths? Ultimately, these admonishments were spoken by the venerable Jikmé Lingpa; if we look in the history of Tibetan Buddhism, eminent monks and great worthies such as Longchenpa,[45] Jikmé Lingpa, and Patrul Rinpoche[46] are difficult to encounter. Since [Jikmé Lingpa] has made this definitive statement as his vajra-speech, then I think that there are a few people who should be worrying about what will happen after their deaths.

Nowadays, there are some so-called lamas who say, "The Buddha never prohibited smoking tobacco within the Vinaya, so there should be no problems with smoking." This kind of statement is really stupid. The ultimate import of all the Buddha's teachings is to avoid committing all evil acts and to uphold all forms of virtuous conduct. Given that tobacco was produced by the magic power of the *māras*, it certainly falls within the scope of things that are obstacles. Moreover, all the eminent monks and great worthies, headed by the great master Padmasambhava, have proclaimed the harms of smoking. There are only a very small number of people who, to preserve their own interests, have proclaimed the merits of smoking tobacco, and most people generally recognize that they have done so as a deliberate attempt to destroy the Buddhadharma. If one deliberately attempts to destroy the Buddhadharma, it is said in the tantric scriptures that "those who are capable of harming Buddhism and defaming the lamas—the wise should eliminate these." For those who harm the Buddhadharma and slander the lamas, their speech is completely empowered by the *māras*, and so we should use the esoteric methods of subjugation to stop them.

Nowadays there are a rare few laypeople who, not understanding the Buddhadharma in the slightest, regularly expend great efforts to spread non-Dharmic practices. They do not understand that the Dharma taught by the Buddha Śākyamuni consists of the Dharma of transmission and the Dharma of realization. Apart from these, the scholar Vasubandhu has said that there is no other Dharma. The Dharma-king Jikmé Phuntsok often used to say that "when someone generates a virtuous mind, this is the Tathāgata's Dharma of realization; when someone speaks a scriptural verse, this is the Tathāgata's Dharma of transmission." To produce a mind of compassion for just an instant, or a mind of kindness or enlightenment—such kinds of virtuous mind represent the Dharma of realization. To recite a scriptural verse for another, or to listen to one yourself—this is what is called the Dharma of transmission. The Dharmas of transmission and realization are difficult to spread these days. Even if one has an opportunity to spread them, it is as though some people have been bewitched by the *māras*, so that their conduct is very inappropriate and troublesome. So, after this, if everyone is capable, whether you are monastic or lay, you should exert yourself toward spreading the Buddhadharma. Even if you don't have the power to do this, you should at least not be involved in getting others to do harmful things. Nowadays there are some people who are pretty good at creating negative karma, and there is a great deal of power behind the promotion of tobacco smoking. In fact, many ordinary people spend all their time engaged in illegal and non-virtuous activities; they do not need any so-called spiritual friends or lamas to exhort them to create negative karma. Therefore, if you know any smokers among your close friends, you should think of some way to get them to quit smoking.

Of course, when you talk to them about the karmic consequences of smoking in their future lifetimes, there will be some who will not necessarily accept such explanations. Instead, you can attempt to convince them from the standpoint of medicine or health. This way, it will be easier for them to accept your advice. Actually, the dangers of tobacco were already understood in premodern medicine. In the Ming-dynasty *Diannan Materia Medica*,[47] it says, "Tobacco is bitter and warm and greatly poisonous." The Qing-dynasty text on health maintenance, *Common Sayings for the Elderly*,[48] says, "Tobacco has a bitter flavor, and its nature is dry. When burned, its smoke will deplete the vital essence and cause people to become dull, as though drunk." Recently, studies have shown that 90 percent of lung cancer cases, 75 percent of emphysema cases, and 25 percent of heart disease cases are brought on by tobacco smoking. Every year throughout the entire world, there are 2.5 million people who die from various smoking-related illnesses. Many people think that smoking cigarettes can make your body feel happy and comfortable; they do not know that it is a chronic killer, and they unwittingly suffer great damage from it. Once in the United States, they did an experiment. They put a frog in a pot of boiling water, but as soon as the frog felt the heat, it used all its strength to jump out of the pot. Then, they put a frog in a pot of cold water and gradually heated it up. The frog did not notice and remained there contentedly, and when the water finally got so hot that the frog could not stand it anymore, it was already unable to move. Many people are like this. If they encounter strong suffering or pain, they will immediately avoid it. But when it comes to those things like drinking alcohol or smoking tobacco, which gradually weaken the body, they drop their defenses and invite calamity. So, without discussing Buddhist ideas of karmic cause and effect, just from the standpoint of caring for one's own health and longevity, we can still say that smoking tobacco is entirely harmful with no benefits.

Nowadays in our modern society, people especially like to smoke, puffing continuously on one cigarette after another, converting their monthly salaries into cigarettes and letting their money fly away through their noses. Although they know that tobacco smoking is bad for their health, they find it very difficult to break their addiction to tobacco. Actually, it is not that difficult to quit smoking. You only have to make a sincere vow in front of the Buddhas and bodhisattvas, or a lama capable of bestowing blessings, and you will obtain inconceivable assistance and protection from them. The great master Padmasambhava said, "When you make a vow before a spiritual friend, and genuinely refrain from tobacco, I will follow like your shadow to protect you." When a Buddhist disciple has faith, and then the blessings of the Buddha and the lama are added to that, they should have no problem quitting tobacco. I have encountered quite a few people who were originally greatly addicted to smoking but later made such a firm resolution and then no longer had any desire to smoke.

Even if you do not believe in Buddhism, you could still follow the examples of well-known worldly persons who quit smoking. For example, Emperor Qianlong of the Qing dynasty really liked smoking tobacco and would smoke whenever he had some free time. Later, he developed a chronic cough, and the imperial physician told him, "Your Majesty's cough is due to lung damage from smoking tobacco. If we are to cure the cough, you must first quit smoking." Emperor Qianlong heeded the imperial physician's advice well, and after he quit smoking his cough was cured.

Marx also went through a phase in which he was greatly addicted to tobacco. He would often smoke while working, and once said, "The amount that I was paid for writing *Capital* was not even enough to cover the money spent on cigars while I was writing it." Later he came down with tracheitis, and his doctor prohibited him from smoking, so he decided to quit.

The American president Ronald Reagan once hoped that by the year 2000, the U.S.A. would become a "smoke-free country," and so he himself decided to quit smoking in 1985. This vow has still not been realized; nowadays a fairly large number of American smoke.

The president of Singapore Lee Kuan Yew used to be a chain-smoker. Later, in order to create a smoke-free country, he quit smoking himself to set an example for the whole country, defeating this addiction of many years with a single blow.

Others such as De Gaulle, Lenin, and so forth also quit smoking for the sake of their personal health. By relying on worldly methods and pledges, they were able to defeat this habit.

Actually, there are no harmful effects whatsoever from not smoking. Among the thousands of people at our academy, you will not find one who smokes. The atmosphere of a Buddhist school is really great and very different from the outside. You won't see people drinking alcohol, smoking tobacco, or engaging in all sorts of illegal activities, and yet within this environment, everyone is living completely fulfilled and happy lives. There is also the country of Bhutan, which is famous throughout the world for being smoke free.[49] When the Dharma King Jikmé Phuntsok went there, he was very pleased and said, "It is already rare for there to be an entire country whose people follow the Buddhist teachings. The fact that they all have faith in the great master Padmasambhava and the Nyingma school, even to the point that not one of them smokes cigarettes—such a country as this is truly rare throughout history." We did not see anyone smoking when we were in Bhutan, and the histories also say that there are no smokers there, but I do not know if they really have any or not.

It's just as I said before: Solely from the standpoint of caring about your health, you should all make the greatest possible effort to not smoke. Tobacco and its smoke contain more than four thousand kinds of harmful substances (some say six hundred kinds). The amount of nicotine in one cigarette can kill a mouse, so the amount of nicotine that builds up in the body of long-time smokers will undoubtedly pose an extreme threat to their health. Nowadays doctors have discovered through experiments that smoking one cigarette will take eleven minutes off your life-span. So, if you want to live to a ripe old age and be free from illness, it is best not to smoke tobacco.

From the perspective of the Buddhist teachings on cause and effect, the faults of smoking tobacco are too innumerable to fully set down in writing. The great lama Tsongkhapa[50] once said, "As an evil thing that was produced by Māra's wicked vow, what need is there to speak of directly using it? Even if there is tobacco in a medicinal formulation, within seven days of using it, then both the patient and the doctor will be condemned to seven eons in the hell-realms with no chance of liberation." Abu Rinpoche [i.e., Patrul Rinpoche] also said, "If you inhale a tiny bit of tobacco from your fingernail, you will be unable to repent of this karmic transgression with even a hundred million recitations of the mantra of Avalokiteśvara." Of course, the perspective expressed in these admonishments is intended to show that the extent of the faults produced from smoking tobacco is extremely frightful; it is not necessarily the case that they are truly so severe. For example, the treasure-revealing lama Düdjom Dorje[51] said that "just smelling the scent of tobacco will cause even a great eighth-stage bodhisattva to fall into the Black Line Hell one time." But the Great Vehicle scriptures all agree that an eighth-stage bodhisattva will not fall into negative rebirths, so why would he speak this way? This is to show clearly the particular severity of the degree of harm caused by smoking tobacco. For example, if someone does an especially awful thing, you might warn them upon finding out that "you should not commit such an offense; even the president would be put in jail for that!" The severity of this statement may be exaggerated, but it will get that person's attention.

However, no matter what, when we encounter smokers, we should be particularly careful. Of course, some people, for work reasons, regularly encounter cigarette smoke. If you are in a work unit where everyone smokes, there is no way that you will not have contact with them, so what can you do? When you go home, you should practice repentance. Sometimes some non-Buddhist leaders will come to visit me at home, and it is difficult to avoid them smoking cigarettes there. However, it would not do to be inhospitable, so I have no choice but to allow it. Tibetan people all basically understand the rules: You do not smoke tobacco in a monastic's home or in a Buddha-hall. But there are some leaders who do not know a single thing about Buddhism, so as soon as they enter, they will light up a cigarette. It makes me uncomfortable, but I still act like I am comfortable. After they are gone, I will quickly open all the windows and light incense. The treasure-revealing lama Ratna Lingpa said, "If you smoke tobacco in front of the mandala, then the wisdom deities will not descend into it." This so-called mandala refers to our Buddha-hall or to a practitioner's residence. In such places, it is best not to smoke. If people go and smoke there, then your tutelary deity will depart, and no matter which rites you practice, it will be difficult to get a response from them. So, you should all take great care to avoid such people. However, I am also worried about some laywomen who practice Buddhism sincerely but whose husbands like to smoke. How could two such people live together? There is no other solution but to regularly recite the mantra of Vajrasattva and perform repentance.

Not only are the faults of smoking extremely great, the faults of selling tobacco are also quite significant. The lama Shabkar Tsokdruk Rangdrol[52] said, "Those who sell tobacco will be reborn as hungry ghosts for five hundred lifetimes." Since we have obtained this human body, we must understand what is and is not meritorious, and especially the fact that smoking, drinking, and other such types of conduct are the activities of inferior people. If we speak this way, then perhaps many people will be unhappy, thinking that they understand everything the best, and fundamentally lacking any awareness of the negative repercussions. Actually, the famous singer Wang Fei's child was born with a cleft lip, and there are some medical specialists who say that this was brought about because she smoked tobacco. Therefore, if you want to be really conscientious about this life and the next, you have to understand that the faults of smoking are really great and that smokers cannot even rely upon the Three Jewels and the guardian deities for protection. The ḍākinī Machik Labdrön said in a prophecy, "In the final age of strife, there will be people who will consume a substance that is replete with the five poisons of greed, hatred, ignorance, pride, and envy. This substance originates in China, was transmitted to Mongolia, and was then consumed by Tibetans. . . . If meditators consume poisonous tobacco, then even if they practice for a hundred eons, they will have no chance of accomplishing the practice of their tutelary deity, and in future lives they will wander among negative rebirths—even the Three Jewels will have no power to protect them." Therefore, you cannot smoke cigarettes on the one hand and pray to the Three Jewels for blessings on the other.

During this short human life, we should do things that have some significance for Buddhism. If we are always "swallowing clouds and spitting fog," then in the end it will just harm our health and contribute to the destruction of the Buddhadharma. Nowadays many civilized countries have established regulations prohibiting smoking in public places, and May 31 has been declared "World No-Tobacco Day." I think that such a holiday is great. If we often had such holidays during which people would stop smoking or engage in freeing lives so that these meritorious activities were promoted in all quarters, then people would naturally come to understand what to adopt and reject.

Once, I was in a hotel somewhere in Jilin Province, where an anti-smoking group and a tobacco organization were both meeting at the same time. At that time, the tobacco organization seemed to be the stronger—their posters and signs were all really large, whereas the anti-smoking organization seemed relatively weak and pathetic in most respects. This was some years ago, but it left an impression on me. So, in this age of the decline of Dharma, if you hoist high the flag of the Buddhadharma, its power will still be quite weak. However, as people who have produced the mind of enlightenment, even if you encounter a smoker on the bus, you should say a few words to them about the dangers of smoking. Sometimes, when I am on the bus and I see some drivers smoking, no matter how far away I am sitting, I will move closer and talk to them about the faults of smoking. Of course, if you talk to them about karmic cause and effect in the next lifetime, they will not listen, but if you discuss some medical information with them, then after a few kilometers, some will get the idea about quitting smoking. So, we should try to develop our usefulness and take different opportunities to talk to others about quitting smoking.

Nowadays there are some Buddhists who think, "Drinking alcohol has some small faults, eating meat has some small faults, but there is no fault in smoking tobacco because it is just a plant, and it can make one's body feel pleasant." People like this who create negative karma will say all sorts of reasonable-sounding things to protect themselves, but this false reasoning will not stand up in the face of karmic consequences. So, it is best not to spend all day singing the praises of actions that produce negative karma. This is like a thief spending all day talking about how great stealing is—ordinary people will not agree with them. It's best to gain some small amount of self-awareness, understand that one's own actions are very pitiful and frightful, and then apply the method of repentance to deal with them.

If we are speaking truthfully, then there are a lot of bad people in today's society. Among such a mass of bad people, it is truly as Sakya Pandita[53] said: "How can the wise be respected?" It is like a place where many poisonous snakes dwell; the brightest light will not be able to illuminate it. For example, if you go to attend a meeting, and all the leaders are drinking alcohol and smoking cigarettes, and not only are you the only one who does not drink or smoke, but you also do not eat meat, everyone will think that you have some mental problem and will take you for a crazy person. Of course, monastics have a slightly easier time facing society in this way, because everyone knows that shaven-headed people don't drink or smoke. If, after shaving your head, you go around drinking alcohol, then, unless you are the monk Jigong,[54] people will not necessarily respect your behavior. But if you are a lay Buddhist, then you have to be brave when facing the misunderstandings, opposition, and criticisms of the masses. Do not follow them in thinking that it is so glorious to create negative karma, and so shameful to avoid negative karma and uphold virtuous conduct, that not smoking or drinking causes you to hang your head in shame before worldly people.

The scholar Candrakīrti (from the seventh century) said that in a crazy world, a sane person will have difficulty facing society and in the end will have no choice but to be like the king who decided to go crazy.[55] However, Buddhist disciples who possess right understanding and right mindfulness should not care how they are treated by others and should persist in holding themselves to high standards of conduct. If you can follow the instructions of the lineage gurus and exert your mind and body in upholding meritorious and virtuous practices, and then promote Buddhism to whatever extent you are capable, then this will bring you unspeakable benefits!

NOTES

1.   Laufer 1924.

2.   Berounský 2013.

3.   Bell 1928: 242–45.

4.   Berounský 2013: 11–12.

5.   Daniel Berounský has surmised based on this fact that some Tibetans understood opium as a kind of tobacco; see Berounský 2013: 18–19.

6.   Treasure texts are believed to have been originally concealed in various locations around Tibet and later to have been revealed by individuals known as "treasure revealers" (gter ston) who possess special powers for discovering concealed texts. On this genre, see Doctor 2005.

7.   For a brief biography, see Nyoshul Khenpo 2005: 511–13.

8.   For a brief introduction to Düdjom Rinpoche's life and activities, see Düdjom Rinpoche 1991: xxv–xxvii.

9. It bears mentioning that, as Daniel Berounský (2013: 19–24) has pointed out, several of these texts are attributed to authors whose lives predated the introduction of tobacco to Tibet. Further research remains to be done on whether these prophetic texts, which are often quoted second- or third-hand, can actually be found among writings that can be reliably attributed to these authors. However, notions of authorship related to the genre of treasure literature are fluid and complex; on this subject, see Doctor 2005.

10. For a brief introduction to this teacher, see Holmes-Tagchungdarpa 2017.

11. On Māra and *māras* in general, see Boyd 1971. For a specific discussion of *māras* (*bdud*) in Tibetan Buddhism, see de Nebesky-Wojkowitz 1956: 273–77.

12. This is consistent with the form of Tibetan millenarianism particularly prominent in the treasure texts and prophecies of the Nyingma school, which focus on the danger that foreign invaders pose to the welfare of the Buddhist teachings in Tibet. On Tibetan millenarianism, see Brauen-Dolma 1985. On the relationship between millenarianism and the treasure genre, see Cuevas 2008: 55–57.

13. For more on *samaya*, see Dorje 1991.

14. By Tutop Lingpa (1858–1914). Translated from Mthu-stobs gling-pa 2013, vol. 9: 717–24. For an alternative translation of this text, see Avertin 2012.

15. That is, the five paths (*pañca-mārga*) and ten stages (*daśa-bhūmi*) of the bodhisattva's progress.

16. An epithet for the Buddha Śākyamuni.

17. Traditionally the Buddhist canon, known as the *Tripiṭaka*, consists of three divisions: *sūtra* (discourses), *śāstra* (treatises), and *vinaya* (ethics). The Vajrayana tradition adds a fourth division: *tantra* (esoterica).

18. Tib. *Dga' rab dbang phyug*, an epithet for the deity Kāmadeva.

19. *Thig nag* (*kālasūtra*), a hell so called because black lines are drawn on its inhabitants' bodies, which are then sliced up along those lines.

20. In a treasure text such as this one, the word *samaya* is often added at the end to indicate that the text is "sealed" by the sacred commitments of the treasure-revealer and guardian deities.

21. The first incantation invokes the bodhisattva Mañjuśrī, addressed as the "lord of speech" (*vāgīśvarī*). The second incantation is the well-known mantra of Avalokiteśvara, and the third invokes Vajrapāṇi. The final line, written in a combination of Tibetan and Sanskrit, asks these bodhisattvas to eliminate (*māraya*) the *māras* (*bdud*), *rakṣasīs* (*srin*), and tobacco (*tamakha*) itself. Note that I have transcribed these incantations as written in the original Tibetan text, without adding additional Sanskrit diacritics.

22. Tib. *bskyed rim gzer thebs*. This is a reference to the "four nails" (or "four stakes" [*gzer bzhi*]), four key points concerning the meditation and visualization of the creation stage (*bskyed rim*) of Tantric Buddhist practice, in which practitioners visualize themselves in the form of their tutelary deity. See Dharmachakra Translation Committee 2006: 81–96.

23. These are the five corrupted conditions that appeared in the final times of the Buddha's teachings: the corruptions of the age, wrong views, emotional afflictions, sentient beings, and diminishing life-span.

24. By Düdjom Rinpoche, Jikdrel Yeshe Dorje (1904–1987). Translated from Bdud-'joms' jigs-bral ye-shes rdo-rje 1979: 24.369–74.

25. This refers to Padmasambhava, also known as Guru Rinpoche, believed to have come to Tibet from the land of Oḍḍiyāna.

26. This refers to prophetic texts revealed as *termas*.

27. Ratna gling-pa (1403–1478). See Düdjom Rinpoche 1991: 793–95.

28. *Damsi* (*dam sri*) is a particular kind of demonic spirit found in Tibetan literature. See de Nebesky-Wojkowitz 1956: 300–303.

29. That is, opium.

30. *Byang chub sems rtsa*. This refers to energetic channels within the body believed to hold the essence of the enlightened mind.

31. Sangs-rgyas gling-pa (1340–1396). See Düdjom Rinpoche 1991: 784–88.

32. Rig-'dzin rgod-ldem-can (1337–1408). See Düdjom Rinpoche 1991: 780–83.

33. *Dri za*, a kind of supernatural being depicted in Indian mythology as consuming scents.

34. Bdud-'dul rdo-rje (1615–1672). See Düdjom Rinpoche 1991: 813–17.

35. Klong-gsal snying-po (1625–1682).

36. Thugs-mchog rdo-rje (fl. seventeenth to eighteenth century).

37. 'Gro-'dul gling-pa, possibly a reference to Orgyen Drodül Lingpa (O-rgyan 'gro-'dul gling-pa, b. 1757).

38. Ma-gcig lab-sgron (1055–1149). See Edou 1996.

39. Probably Khenpo Jikmé Phuntshok ('Jigs-med phun-tshogs, 1933–2004), who founded the Larung Gar monastery in western China.

40. Khenpo Sodargye 2008.

41. Tib. *ngakpa* (*sngags pa*). *Māntrika* (or *mantrin*) is a general name for a class of lay practitioners of Indo-Tibetan Tantric Buddhism. See Bogin 2008; Sihlé 2013.

42. Mkhan-po a-chos (1918–1998).

43. This is the sixth of the heavens in the desire realm, where Māra resides.

44. 'Jigs-med gling-pa (1730–1798). See Düdjom Rinpoche 1991: 835–40.

45. Klong-chen rab-'byams (1308–1364). See Düdjom Rinpoche 1991: 575–96.

46. Dpal-sprul o-rgyan chos-kyi dbang-po (1808–1887).

47. *Diannan bencao*.

48. *Laolao hengyan*.

49. The prohibition of tobacco in Bhutan dates to the eighteenth century. See Bell 1928: 242–43; Aris 1986: 141.

50. Tsong-kha-pa blo-bzang grags-pa (1357–1419).

51. Possibly Traktung Düdjom Dorje (Khrag-'thung bdud-'joms rdo-rje), also known as Lcags-khung sge'u-gter (1857–1921).

52. Zhabs-dkar tshogs-drug rang-grol (1781–1851).

53. Sa-skya paṇḍita (1182–1251).

54. Jigong (fl. late twelfth to early thirteen century) was a Chinese monk whose iconoclastic behavior, including eating meat and drinking alcohol, became the subject of popular folktales.

55. The story of the king who chose to become insane because everyone else in his kingdom was insane is paraphrased from Candrakīrti's commentary on Āryadeva's (second to third century) *Catuḥśataka*. See Lang 2003: 182.

9. Buddhism and Biomedicine in Republican China

Taixu's "Buddhism and Science" (1923) and Ding Fubao's *Essentials of Buddhist Studies* (1920)

GREGORY ADAM SCOTT

The Chinese publishing industry in Shanghai, established using foreign technology and local expertise in the late nineteenth century, grew explosively in the first two decades of the twentieth century,[1] and Buddhism played an important role. Monastics and laypeople from across the nation made use of print to engage in lively discourse, promoting new approaches to Buddhist thought and practice. Two prolific Chinese Buddhist authors of this period were the monk Taixu (1890–1947) and the lay physician and publisher Ding Fubao (1874–1952). Both embraced modernity and advocated for change among Buddhists, while also recognizing the authority of the Buddhist scriptures and their centrality to the Buddhist religion. Both were interested in science and Buddhism, but their understanding of the relationship between the two was vastly different. Taixu, a monk, viewed the Dharma as the ultimate truth and as the only system of thought that could fully comprehend existence; Ding, on the other hand, saw science and Buddhism as authorities in separate realms of human life, with neither having a monopoly on truth.

Taixu became caught up in the radical politics and philosophies that circulated in China during the crucial period around the time of the Xinhai Revolution, which ended the Qing dynasty and established the Republic of China in 1912. He first worked to transform Buddhism from within the structures of the powerful monasteries of the Jiangnan region and, when his plans were thwarted, turned to publishing as a means of circulating his ideas and promoting his program of education, reform, and modernization.[2] Taixu, like many others of the early twentieth century, believed that Buddhism contained knowledge that modern science was only now beginning to grasp. He held that the Buddha had, among other things, been among the first to see microscopic organisms, long before the invention of the microscope.[3] This view placed Buddhist authority above that of science, which was considered to be only a small portion of the complete field of knowledge and truth represented by the Dharma. The translation below is from his article "Buddhism and Science" (literally, "Buddhadharma and Science") published in the Buddhist periodical *Sound of the Sea Tide* (*Haichao yin*) on September 3, 1923. Taixu cites five examples of scientific phenomena that had already been described in the Buddhist scriptures. Two relate specifically to medicine: the discovery of microscopic organisms such as bacteria and the discovery of cellular bodies in animal tissue.

A physician by trade, Ding Fubao was a lifelong bibliophile and book collector (later in his life his personal library was said to include 150,000 titles), and he established two publishing companies: Civilization Press and Medical Studies Press. Ding also had an abiding interest in religion. He was something of a religious chimera, drifting through several religious traditions throughout his life without seeing the need to settle on a single religious identity. The book series that he published from 1918 to 1923, *The Buddhist Studies Collectanea*, consisting of thirty core titles, marks the high point of his involvement with Buddhism.[4] This series appeared precisely at a time when Buddhist publishing was beginning to take off in China, propelled by Buddhist periodicals, monographs, and scriptural works reprinted using woodblock printing. Many prominent monastics and laypeople in China were enthusiastic about the applicability of Buddhism to people's lives in the modern era and published eloquent discourses on the relationship between Buddhist traditions and different elements of modernity such as science, nationalism, and education, discourses spread through print to a wide public. Many others, however, viewed Buddhism and other religious traditions simply as superstitions, false beliefs that ought to be swept away by true— which in many cases was understood as scientific—knowledge.[5]

One title in Ding's series, *Essentials of Buddhist Studies*, addresses questions about the differing truth claims of Buddhism on the one hand, and science, a broad category of knowledge understood to include modern medicine, on the other. *Essentials* was first published in 1920, during the earliest stages of a raging debate among Chinese literati on whether modern science alone was a sufficient guide to human life or whether Chinese cultural heritage, including Buddhism, should continue to be valued as China began to modernize.[6] The second translation below is the first section of *Essentials of Buddhist Studies*, in which Ding converses with a friend who is eventually won over to the spiritual value of Buddhist studies. This text is one example of how Chinese Buddhists in the modern era worked to integrate the value of religious ideas into scientific frameworks of bodily health, and how Buddhism continued its historically close associations with health and healing during an era of biomedicine and the scientific method.

In the original text, the section translated below is followed by several sections of stories from classical literature dealing with the existence of spirits and the effectiveness of spiritual means in dealing with them; these are omitted here.

Although both Taixu and Ding are Buddhist apologists, there are important differences between the views expressed in the following translations, published only a few years apart. They exemplify two broad approaches to science and biomedicine among Buddhists during this era: (1) that science was belatedly proving insights that had been expressed in Buddhist scriptures for centuries; and (2) that Buddhism was applicable to matters of the spirit while science was applicable to matters of the body. What was at stake in these discourses was the continued relevance of Buddhism in a world in which science was daily producing new knowledge and where religion appeared to be rapidly losing ground.

FURTHER READING

Andrews, Bridie. 2014. *The Making of Modern Chinese Medicine, 1850–1960*. Vancouver: University of British Columbia Press.

Crozier, Ralph C. 1968. *Traditional Medicine in Modern China: Science, Nationalism, and the Tensions of Cultural Change*. Cambridge, Mass.: Harvard University Press.

Hammerstrom, Erik J. 2015. *The Science of Chinese Buddhism: Early Twentieth-Century Engagements*. New York: Columbia University Press.

Ritzinger, Justin. 2017. *Anarchy in the Pure Land: Reinventing the Cult of Maitreya in Modern Chinese Buddhism*. New York: Oxford University Press.

Rogaski, Ruth. 2004. *Hygienic Modernity: Meanings of Health and Disease in Treaty-Port China*. Berkeley: University of California Press.

Scott, Gregory A. 2015. "Navigating the Sea of Scriptures: *The Buddhist Studies Collectanea*, 1918–1923." In *Religious Publishing and Print Culture in Modern China, 1800–2012*, edited by Philip Clart and Gregory Adam Scott, 91–138. Boston: De Gruyter.

EXCERPT FROM "BUDDHISM AND SCIENCE"[7]

Scientific knowledge can provide verification and hypotheses for Buddhism but cannot comprehend the reality of Buddhism.

The discoveries of science have caused religion to lose influence. Common teachings such as that of *ātman*[8] and so on, at their core have little truth, and once a little wind blows against them, they can't help but be shaken. One only fears that if they are not disputed enough, they will continue to cause fear amongst people, force them toward incorrect conclusions, and make them lose their autonomy. These types of people are truly lamentable. Buddhism is unique in that it only fears that science is not vigorous, that science is not valorous and bold, that science does not determine a direction nor plumb the depths of truth, that science does not clearly discern all existence nor reach the most thorough awakening. If it were able to have these qualities, then science would be more advanced, but Buddhism would still be more elucidated. That which is illuminated by Buddhism is the true essential nature of the universe and all existence. If science were more vigorous, then it would be because it approaches nearer to Buddhism.

People of today and the past have spoken of astronomy. In the Eastern lands in former times, they knew only that Heaven was above (the sun, moon, stars, planets, and so on), Earth was below (the four Great Rivers, the plants and trees, and so on), and in the middle was humankind. In the West, Christians adopted the view of Greek philosophy, which said that the earth was the center of the universe, and they spread it throughout the world. Later on, after French philosophy discovered that the sun was the center of the universe, from then until now there have also been those who proclaim a theory of "no center." Overall, this has already progressed through several degrees of development. If we consider the knowledge that the stars in the sky are truly infinite in number, absorbing and repelling each other, without anything directing it all, then the theory that the stars are the center of the universe must also be discarded. Here, we start to prove what the Buddhist scriptures say: "Emptiness is without limits. Thus, worlds without number interact with and interpenetrate each other, like a net of many pearls." They also say, "The world is based upon a wind-wheel; the wind-wheel is based upon emptiness." These are all true views. This is the first way in which science approaches Buddhism.

Scientists hold that within water there are [microscopic] creatures. The Buddhist texts also say, "The Buddha perceives in one drop of water eighteen thousand [microscopic] creatures." As for this fact, more than ten years ago at the Nanjing residence of Mr. Yang Renshan, I used the highest-powered microscope and saw this for myself. This is the second way in which science approaches Buddhism.

Darwin holds that the origin of the human race stems from racial qualities being passed down, left aside, or gradually transformed. Although this shares with Buddhism an illumination of why there is a diversity of things in the world, they all achieve their differences as a result of the accumulation of karmic power, moral character, personal behavior, and so on. According to their karma, each rises or sinks, disappears or is strengthened. There is still much to be learned, but, compared to the old teaching that the gods created or the heavens gave birth to [humankind], it is certainly an improvement. This is the third way in which science approaches Buddhism.

Biologists believe that the human body is composed of circulatory organs and so on. But its blood and flesh are able to operate thanks to innumerable cells accumulating, living, and dying. Along with what the Buddhist scriptures call "viewing the body as an accumulation of creatures," these can be considered the first steps of incarnation. It is from these "root bodily creatures" that a body comes about. Clearly the two concepts match each other. This is the fourth way in which science approaches Buddhism.

Physicists believe that the three natures of solid, liquid, and gas are the basic qualities of all things. The Buddhist scriptures speak of the Four Great Elements: Earth is solid nature; Water is liquid nature; Wind and Fire are gaseous nature, since when the Wind moves, Fire heats up. All are forms of energy, like light, electricity, heat, and so on. This is the fifth way in which science approaches Buddhism. Additional ways I won't mention.

Two thousand years ago, these theories were already present in the Buddhist scriptures. There are no new discoveries of science that someone has not already described. Thus, the more vigorous that science becomes, the more that Buddhist studies will welcome it. That this is greatly sufficient as an initial step in verifying Buddhism should be abundantly clear.

EXCERPT FROM *ESSENTIALS OF BUDDHIST STUDIES*[9]

On the first of June, 1920, a fellow from my home region, Han Xuewen, came to Shanghai seeking medical treatment. I urged him to read Buddhist scriptures in addition to his treatment, and he respectfully agreed to do so. After a few days, his illness improved, and he again visited my home. He said to me [. . .], "In this sick world, there are those who rave wildly about the gods and spirits; they are all mentally ill. The Japanese have translated this illness as 'psychosis.'[10] Of course none of it is real: There are no gods or spirits, and thus the karma, rebirth in the past, present, and future, and other matters discussed in the Buddhist scriptures are all just absurd falsehoods! Recently, new teachings are being developed day by day, and science is daily thriving more and more. Looking at all the superstitions from ancient times, such as gods and spirits, karmic retribution, and so on, they have all crammed up the minds and spirits of the New Youth.[11] They are also the enemies of science. It would be good to sweep them all away at once! How is it that you, sir, can take on the task of promoting Buddhist studies, yet without verifying the truth of karma, rebirth, and so on described in the Buddhist scriptures, you constantly talk of the existence of spirits? How is that not equal to constantly going against the common sense of this new world? As for this sort of absurd false reasoning, those who now study new learning would not only cry out loudly and bitterly denounce it, but if you printed it and distributed it throughout the country, they would all rise up and attack your error. You, sir, are a physician. For you to be like this, I'm afraid that your good name will be sullied and have thus used these harsh words to give you advice." [. . .]

I answered him, saying, "If something does not exist and yet one believes that it does, that is called superstition. If something does exist and one believes in it, that is true belief and should not be termed superstition. Spirits, karmic retribution, Hell, and so on, these are all true things. They are not falsities expounded by people in the past. To expound them is not some kind of stratagem, and to believe in them is not superstitious. A blind person may, not seeing the sun, say that it does not exist, and a deaf person may, not hearing thunder, say that it does not exist. Yet the sun and thunder, they certainly do exist. For the blind and deaf to say that they don't, this is in fact them fooling themselves. Those today who do not believe in the existence of spirits, karmic retribution, and other such things, how are they different from this?"

Mr. Han said, "Spirits, karmic retribution, Hell, and so on, I believe that they do not exist, while you, sir, believe that they do. For these types of conundrum, there's never any conclusive evidence either way. If I may ask, sir, what means do you have of proving that they exist to refute my belief that they do not?"

I answered, saying, "I actually have a wondrous method of proving that they do exist and, thus proving that they do, to refute your belief that they do not. However, today I will first make an agreement with you, which will calm your mind and steady your *qi*. Take this book in which this wondrous method is inscribed, and read it from cover to cover. Don't stop in the middle before you've read to the final section, for this would be to fall prey to empty talk. If you encounter doubts, please consult the writings that others have made on their true investigations, in order to experimentally confirm their truth or falsity. In this way, your ring of doubt will be totally smashed apart."

Afterward, Mr. Han gradually read through each of the writings that are listed below in this very collection, and as he read and inquired, after a day's work he finished reading all of the evidence that I had mentioned regarding the existence and spirits and so on. Thereupon Mr. Han asked about the best way to start reading Buddhist scriptures, and I guided him through them one by one.

Mr. Han was overjoyed and said to me, "Today I have confirmed that there are indeed spirits, there is indeed karmic retribution, there is indeed rebirth and all the rest! All one needs to do is read the Buddhist scriptures. What I have gained in ten years of reading books is not equal to that gained by one evening of discussing them! Sir, first you used medicine to treat my body, then you used Buddhist studies to treat my soul! Once the body reaches its end, the soul continues forever without end. My gratitude is boundless; how could I repay you?"

NOTES

1. Masini 1993; Y. Lu 2004; Reed 2004.
2. Ritzinger 2017.
3. Hammerstrom 2012.
4. G. Scott 2015.
5. Hammerstrom 2015.
6. These debates exploded in print in 1923, with one of the earliest combative articles being the text of a speech by Zhang Junmai published in the weekly journal of Tsinghua University.
7. Reprinted in Huang 2006, vol. 157:12–17.
8. The "Great Soul" or "universal self" of Southern Asian Brahmanical teachings.

9. Ding 1920: 1a–3a. Portions of this discourse that have been omitted are marked with "[. . .]."

10. The term "psychosis" (*jingshen bing*) was originally coined in Japanese and later entered into modern Chinese. *Jingshen* can refer to the physical nervous system but also to a person's spirit or mental condition.

11. New Youth (*xin shaonian* or *xin qingnian*) is a generational term referring to students and others in the 1910s and 1920s who embraced progressive ideals such as science and democracy and who blamed traditional Chinese culture for China's national crises.

10. Reconciling Scripture and Surgery in Tibet

Khyenrap Norbu's *Arranging the Tree Trunks of Healing* (1952)

WILLIAM A. McGRATH

Khyenrap Norbu was perhaps the most influential Tibetan physician of the twentieth century.[1] Born in Tsetang in 1883,[2] Khyenrap Norbu enrolled in the Ngachö Monastic College in Tsetang at a young age, where he gained a reputation for kindness, patience, and diligence. In 1897, at the age of fourteen, Khyenrap Norbu was selected to study medicine at the illustrious Chakpori Medical College in Lhasa. While there, he mastered the *Four Tantras* and its associated commentarial literature and was appointed medical officer at Drepung monastery in 1912. This appointment marks the beginning of Khyenrap Norbu's long career as a both a physician and scholar, and from this point onward he is known to have written scores of commentaries, treatises, and instructional manuals on the theory and practice of medicine.[3]

From 1913 to 1914, Khyenrap Norbu traveled to India with the Tibetan representatives participating in the Simla Convention, and while there he impressed the British participants with his knowledge of and skill in medical practice.[4] As early as 1914, following his return to Lhasa, Khyenrap Norbu expressed an interest in securing smallpox vaccinations for the monks at Drepung monastery,[5] presumably inspired by the efficacy of inoculations that he had witnessed during his first visit abroad. By 1920, he had had extensive interactions with the British officers responsible for running the biomedical clinics in Lhasa, who were impressed by the curiosity of the so-called Men-tsiba Lama.[6] Lieutenant Colonel Robert Kennedy, for example, the medical officer accompanying Sir Charles Bell in Lhasa from 1920 to 1921, described how Khyenrap Norbu displayed "great interest in the work of the [British] Dispensary and came to see several operations [during which] he asked very pertinent questions and made copious notes."[7] Thus, the image of Khyenrap Norbu presented by his British acquaintances is that of the progressive physician, expert of the old tradition and scrutinizer of the new. As we shall see in his reflections translated below, however, in addition to his candid excitement and admiration for the efficacy of biomedicine, Khyenrap Norbu also held deep-seated reservations about the safety and long-term benefits of inoculations and invasive surgery, particularly when compared with the therapies of the Tibetan medical tradition.

As part of the reform program instituted in the 1910s,[8] the Thirteenth Dalai Lama ordered the establishment of a new medical college in Lhasa in 1916, which helped facilitate astrological and pediatric health care programs in Tibet.[9] Following his success at Drepung, Khyenrap Norbu was eventually appointed head of both the newly established Mentsikhang, as well as his alma mater, the Chakpori Medical College.[10] His fame as a scholar, educator, and practitioner of medicine attracted students from even the furthest reaches of the Tibetan plateau, and thousands of physicians in both modern China and Tibetan communities in exile currently represent his lineage.[11] Khyenrap Norbu contracted a bout of pneumonia and died on December 24, 1962, at the age of seventy-nine.[12] Following his death, his close disciple Jampa Trinlé (1928–2011) was appointed head of the Mentsikhang,[13] continuing Khyenrap Norbu's vision of Tibetan medical practice, scholarship, and education.

Three years before the death of Khyenrap Norbu, in the wake of the Tibetan uprising of 1959, the Mentsikhang was converted into a public hospital for biomedical treatment.[14] Although the practice of biomedicine in Central Tibet was nothing new—for the British had been operating small clinics in Gyantsé and throughout the Himalayas for most of the early twentieth century[15]—there is little evidence of Tibetan physicians offering inoculations, performing invasive surgeries, or engaging with biomedicine beyond the realm of observation prior to the forced political reforms of the 1950s and '60s.[16] Following the popularization of biomedical techniques and technology in Lhasa during the 1960s, however, despite the violence and tumult of the Cultural Revolution, the Mentsikhang became a site known for the integration of biomedicine and Tibetan medical traditions over the second half of the twentieth century.[17]

In 1951, the People's Liberation Army entered Lhasa, and, in an attempt to win over the Tibetan people, Chinese officers quickly established a free biomedical clinic there.[18] It was during this transitional period of the 1950s[19]—following the arrival of the Chinese army but before the flight of the Dalai Lama into exile in 1959—that Khyenrap Norbu concluded his scholastic exegesis of the *Four Tantras*. This work embodies what the historian Henry E. Sigerist called the "Janus head" of medical writing.[20] Looking back with the eyes of the monastic scholar, Khyenrap Norbu lauds the traditional physician who understands the anatomy of vulnerable points, humoral etiology, and orthodox treatments in accordance with the Buddhist tradition of medical scriptures. Indeed, such is the focus of his own work, *Arranging the Tree Trunks of Healing*, in which he summarizes and organizes the instructions of the *Four Tantras* using the image of a tree with trunks, branches, and leaves (a central explanatory metaphor for commentarial literature on the medical tantras). Looking forward with the eyes of the bodhisattva physician, however, he expresses admiration for the power and precision of biomedical techniques, as well as an admonition against their potential harms. In the end, he encourages practitioners to reconcile potential conflicts between the Tibetan and biomedical traditions by separately diagnosing diseases caused by internal factors (imbalances in the *tridoṣa*, which might be called "chronic diseases") and those caused by external conditions (wounds, tumors, poxes, and so forth). The physician who is able to effectively integrate new biomedical techniques and technologies with the theories and practices of the Buddhist medical tradition is rare indeed. If done safely and carefully, however, such a physician would be like a manifestation of Bhaiṣajyaguru in the flesh, capable of dispelling the sufferings of all sentient beings.

FURTHER READING

Adams, Vincanne. 2007. "Integrating Abstraction: Modernising Medicine at Lhasa's Mentsikhang." In *Soundings in Tibetan Medicine: Historical and Anthropological Perspectives*, edited by Mona Schrempf, 29–43. Leiden: Brill.

Hofer, Theresia, and Knud Larsen. 2014. "Pillars of Tibetan Medicine: The Chagpori and the Mentsikhang Institutes in Lhasa." In *Bodies in Balance: The Art of Tibetan Medicine*, edited by Theresia Hofer, 257–67. Seattle: University of Washington Press.

McKay, Alex. 2007. *Their Footprints Remain: Biomedical Beginnings Across the Indo-Tibetan Frontier*. Amsterdam: Amsterdam University Press.

Van Vleet, Stacey. 2010–2011. "Children's Healthcare and Astrology in the Nurturing of a Central Tibetan Nation-State, 1916–24." *Asian Medicine* 6: 348–86.

Yeshi Dönden. 1986. *Health Through Balance: An Introduction to Tibetan Medicine*, translated by Jeffrey Hopkins. Ithaca, N.Y.: Snow Lion.

AN EXCERPT FROM
ARRANGING THE TREE TRUNKS OF HEALING[21]

The physician who does not know the anatomy of the body is like a housekeeper in an unfamiliar place.

The physician who does not know the characteristics of the body is like one who does not know the secret centers of the *cakra*-wheels.

The physician who does not know the causes and conditions of disease is unable to differentiate between the classifications of diseases.

The physician who does not know the thermal properties of medicaments
   will bring both benefit and harm [to patients].
More specifically, the physician who does not know the strength
   [of medicaments] will come to be like the enemy of [the patient].
The physician who does not know the practical methods for healing is like
   one who tries to punch the darkness with his or her fists.
Thus, the physician who is not deluded in terms of anatomy, diagnosis,
   medicaments, or methods for healing—
The physician who practices according to the Word of the Victors
   [i.e., Buddhist scriptures]—such a physician is worthy of homage.
Regarding the "medical elixirs of quintessence" [i.e., vaccines] that have
   spread everywhere at the present time,[22]
As well as the methods for [the creation of these] medicines, their
   performance, and their equipment [i.e., syringes], beholding them fills
   one with wonder and rapture.
Regarding excisions, incisions, and other types of lacerations [i.e., invasive
   surgery],[23] although their precision is glorious and intriguing,
The physician who believes in the "vulnerable points" [of the body][24] should
   use his or her senses to discern both the long- and short-term benefits, as
   well as the long- and short-term dangers [of piercing the body in those
   locations].
Although dangerous types [of medical practice] involving the vulnerable
   points of the body and so forth are also clearly explained in the glorious
   [Four] Tantras,
As a result of various [historical] causes and conditions, their performance
   has decreased significantly since previous times.
Because the three roots of disease—Wind, Bile, and Phlegm—exist within
   [the body], they are induced by conditions [that cause disease].
External conditions are not limited to wounds, flesh and bone [disorders],
   repletion and depletion, tumors and poxes, [and so forth].
Although it is possible that approximately one hundred of the four hundred
   classes of disease are [caused by external conditions],[25]
One must not confuse the methods for diagnosis and healing for each of the
   classes of disease.
If one were to understand [diseases caused by external conditions] in
   accordance with the tradition of the Great Nation [of Tibet],
And if one were to definitively master this class of [biomedical] techniques,
   one would be the true manifestation of Bhaiṣajyaguru, dispelling suffering
   and disease.
Thus, one should cherish the descriptions of the object of healing [i.e., the
   patient], the classification of disease, and healing medicaments,
As well as the descriptions of anatomy that are essential for medical practice
   and the instructions for examination and diagnosis [as described according
   to the Tibetan medical tradition in Arranging the Tree Trunks of Healing].

NOTES

1.   The following biographical account and translation are primarily based on the writings of the late Jampa Trinlé (*byams pa 'phrin las*, 1928–2011), the former director the Mentsikhang in Lhasa, a celebrated scholar, and an intimate student of Khyenrap Norbu. For a biography of Khyenrap Norbu, see Byams pa 'phrin las 2000: 435–46; for a history of the Mentsikhang in Lhasa, see Byams pa 'phrin las 1996: 1–64.

2.   Rechung Rinpoche (1973: 22) lists the birth year of Khyenrap Norbu (*mkhyen rab nor bu*) as 1882, while Byams pa 'phrin las (2000: 435) provides both the Tibetan—the "water-sheep year of the fifteenth sexagenary cycle" (*rab byung bco lnga pa'i chu lug lo*)—and Gregorian calendar year cited here. The mistaken date of 1882 was possibly given owing to the established fact that Khyenrap Norbu died on December 24, 1962, at the age of eighty according to traditional Tibetan reckoning (in which an individual is considered to be one year old at the time of birth) but at the age of seventy-nine if one counts only the years after his birth in 1883.

3.   See, for example, A ru ra 2007. For a list of titles from specific works, see Byams pa 'phrin las 2000: 435–46.

4.   See, for example, the account of his disciple in Tenzin Choedrak and van Grasdorff 2000: 58. On the Simla Convention, see Goldstein 1989: 76–80, 300–303, 832–42.

5.   Khyenrap Norbu expressed this interest in a letter to David Macdonald (British Library Asia Pacific and Africa Collection, IOR Mss. F80/173, 1938), the British trade agent in Yatung (Yadong), a small town on the Sikkimese border. See Van Vleet 2011: 360–61n45.

6.   For a general description of the British clinics and inoculation programs in the Himalayas, see McKay 2007a, as well as McKay's other articles included in the references.

7.   Kennedy report from October 12, 1921, forwarded to the Government of India by Charles Bell on December 5, 1921 (OIOC, L/P&S/12/143–69). Cited in McKay 2007a: 156.

8.   Goldstein 1989: 78 passim. As noted by Van Vleet (2011: 350), Goldstein mentions Khyenrap Norbu briefly in his consummate history of modern Tibet but does not address the establishment of the Mentsikhang as part of the state-building program in early twentieth-century Lhasa.

9.   Van Vleet 2011.

10. For a brief history and analysis of these two medical colleges, see Hofer and Larsen 2014.

11. For a list of Khyenrap Norbu's most famous students, see Byams pa 'phrin las 2000: 445–46. On his most famous female student, Khandro Yangkar (1907–1973), see Hofer 2011. See also the works composed by some his students who eventually went into exile: Yeshi Dönden 1986, 2000; Tenzin Choedrak and van Grasdorff 2000; Lobsang Wangyal 2007.

12. Byams pa 'phrin las (2000: 444–45) states that Khyenrap Norbu died of a "throat cold" (*mgur cham*), which I interpret as pneumonia. For an English-language account of a meeting with Khyenrap Norbu in the early 1960s that is less than charitable, see Gelder and Gelder 1965: 87–88 passim (in which he is called "Chinrob Nobo").

13. Byams pa 'phrin las 1996: 44.

14. Byams pa 'phrin las 1996: 41.

15. See the description in McKay 2005–06: 125; for example, where he indicates that by the 1930s and 1940s, the British no longer reported resistance to smallpox inoculation among patients, as if the presence of British clinics had come to be accepted in Central Tibet.

16. As we have seen, Khyenrap Norbu received the most attention among his contemporaries for his curiosity about vaccines and surgeries, but he does not seem to have integrated such techniques into his own practice.

17. For an anthropological study of biomedicine at the Mentsikhang in Lhasa around the turn of the twenty-first century, as well as the complexities involved in integrating biomedical and Tibetan medical traditions, see Adams 2007. A more thorough analysis of this historical process, along with a detailed English-language history of the Mentsikhang in Lhasa, remains a major desideratum in the field of modern Tibetan medical history.

18. See the Lhasa Mission of the Government of India's report from 1951, cited in Goldstein 2007: 212: "A free medical dispensary, staffed by very courteous personnel, has been opened in Lhasa by the Chinese. In the first five days of operation, it deprived the Indian hospital of half of its patients" (copy in U. S. National Archives, 793B.00/1–2552). See also the Panchen Lama's formal request to Chairman Mao for medical clinics in Tibet in 1950, cited in Goldstein 2007: 279.

19. This commentary is called *Arranging the Tree Trunks of Healing* (*gso tshul gyi sdong 'grems*) and can be found in A ru ra 2007: 14–50. Byams pa 'phrin las (2000: 443) cites the year of composition as 1952.

20. See Sigerist 1932, vol. 1: 5; cited in Temkin 1977: 9: "But the history of medicine has a Janus-head. One face looks to the future with the eyes of the physician, and the other one is turned backward. With the eyes of the historian it tries to light up the darkness of the past."

21. This passage can be found in A ru ra 2007: 49–50 and is also cited in Byams pa 'phrin las 2000: 443–44. For an alternative translation and interpretation of parts of this passage, see Van Vleet 2011: 361 passim.

22. I interpret "medical elixirs of quintessence" (*sman bcud dwangs ma*) as referring to vaccines, and their "equipment" (*cha dpyad*) as syringes.

23. I interpret "excisions, incisions, and other types of lacerations" (*rma rigs 'dral gcod la sogs pa*) as referring to invasive surgery.

24. The "vulnerable points" (*gnad*) refer to points of the body the disturbance of which can result in severe injury or death. See, for example, Parfionovitch, Dorje, and Meyer 1992, vol. 1: 44–47; vol. 2: 199–202.

25. Here Khyenrap Norbu is referring to the traditional classification of all diseases by the *tridoṣa*: 101 that are primarily caused by Wind, 101 that are primarily caused by Bile, and 101 that are primarily caused by Phlegm. Typically, the remaining 101 are attributed to the combination of the three; however, he concedes that it might be possible for the remaining 101 diseases to be caused by what he calls "external conditions" (*phyi rkyen*).

11. Healing Wisdom

An Appreciation of a Twentieth-Century Japanese Scientist's Paintings of the *Heart Sūtra*

PAULA K. R. ARAI

I wasaki Tsuneo (1917–2002) was a Japanese biologist raised in a Pure Land family. He studied Zen Buddhist teachings[1] and took up the contemplative practice of calligraphic scripture copying in retirement. After brushing nearly two thousand rounds of the *Heart Sūtra*, he was motivated to make the wisdom of the scripture more accessible to the modern world.[2]

Iwasaki deftly harmonized Buddhism, science, and imagery to generate potent healing images that encourage experiences of interrelatedness,[3] shaping the Chinese characters of the pithy and popular *Heart Sūtra* into artistic imagery drawn from ephemeral beauties of nature, Buddhist cultural life, and microscopic and telescopic wonders.[4] His paintings were intended to function as healing talismans to make the wisdom of the *Heart Sūtra* visible and accessible. Iwasaki's genius was to bring into focus the role the senses play in perceiving different dimensions of reality.[5] An understanding of visual arts and science fundamentally relies on sensory experience, but Buddhist teachings caution that senses untrained in wisdom can misinform, leading to delusions that result in suffering. Perception is the fulcrum that funnels one either into the trenches of suffering or along the path of liberation. Experiencing one's interrelatedness is key to clearing away mental afflictions that derail one into suffering.[6] Iwasaki's paintings are like a visual dose of medicine that guides the viewer to see wisdom encoded in the objects he portrays and, by extension, in all things. Moreover, Iwasaki prayed, chanted, and offered incense to consecrate his paintings and instill them with healing energy. He died without knowing the fourteenth Dalai Lama[7] would one day bless his art for its power to illuminate resonances in Buddhist and scientific views of reality.[8]

Three of Iwasaki's paintings are reproduced below. The first is titled *DNA* (figure 11.1). The double helix is clearly recognizable and appears stable, but on closer examination the seemingly solid form dissolves into the shimmering gold characters of the *Heart Sūtra*. The midnight-blue background evokes deep space, placing DNA in the expanded context of the cosmos. The delicately porous pattern shaded by strokes of dark ink evoke volume but not solidity, making the golden DNA a visual metaphor for the insubstantiality and impermanence of the double helix image and, by extension, our conventional models of reality.

In choosing DNA, common to all living beings from bacteria to blue whales, the artist evokes all life. But, this "building block," as it were, is not a block at all. Whether one applies a Buddhist understanding of emptiness or a scientific understanding of biological processes, DNA is not a concrete, independent entity or object. Rather, it is interconnected with every condition that affects its activity. Iwasaki thus merges the ecological vision of a thoroughly interrelated biosphere and the Buddhist teaching of universal interrelatedness. DNA is the unifying template of life, revealing a profound commonality that, in Buddhist terms, underlies empathy and calls for compassion. Iwasaki points beyond socially constructed distinctions that justify neglect, exploitation, and harm by drawing attention to what living beings share.

Iwasaki makes the assertion that DNA—like meditation, study, ritual, and ethical activities—can be a vehicle to move from the shore of suffering to the shore of enlightenment. He symbolizes the shore of suffering in the lower right corner of the painting with a dark, horizontal stripe, and he depicts the shore of enlightenment in the upper left corner of the painting with a horizontal line of pure gold.

In the second painting, *Mizuko: Water Child* (figure 11.2), the power of art to ameliorate the pain of heartrending relationships is palpable. Iwasaki once visited a temple at which rituals for "water children" (*mizuko*; the Japanese term for unborn fetuses) were performed daily and was moved by how the poignant grief experienced there was shared in an environment of mutual respect and healing. Not delineating the cause of a fetus being unborn—whether by stillbirth, miscarriage, or abortion—the focus is on compassion for the child returning to the primordial waters to be reborn in auspicious circumstances.

Iwasaki found that the *Heart Sūtra* guided him to a deeper awareness of interdependence, leading to a stunning reversal of expectations in this painting. He draws on an iconic image of Avalokiteśvara (commonly known as the "Bodhisattva of Compassion") pouring an elixir of compassion out of a vase. Notice, however, that in Iwasaki's rendering, the *Heart Sūtra* is flowing back *in*, as indicated by the characters being upside down and reading from bottom to top. Iwasaki paints water children protected in womblike bubbles generating the elixir of compassion. Visually imparting wisdom into the interdependent nature of reality, this painting soothes hearts rent with the loss of innocents and inoculates against rigid thinking and harsh judgments. Iwasaki fuels compassion and healing by making invisible connections visible. This provocative and visually compelling painting evinces a love that transcends life and death, a compassion that knows no bounds.

In the third painting, *Mandala of Evolution* (figure 11.3), Iwasaki focuses on the causes and conditions of dependent co-arising and the nature of emptiness in his vision of enlightened reality. This mandala answers his question, "Who are my ancestors?" He begins with himself, or any viewer, represented as a seeker in the lower left quadrant of the painting. In concentric rings, each ancestral father is represented as a white buddha and each mother as a red buddha, making humans the progeny of buddhas. The sum of all ancestors reaches well more than a billion. Such a figure brings home the point that we are not just metaphorically one big family; we are also biologically interrelated. This sublime and expansive genealogical tree then spreads out to the perimeter of the circle in a continuous extension that includes asteroids, protein molecules, amoeba, paramecia, mollusks, star fish, amphibians, tree ferns, dinosaurs, marsupials, conifers, primates, and cherry blossoms.[9] He shows our sun swelling into a red giant, eventually becoming a planetary nebula and releasing energy for new forms, including hydrogen atoms that might one day form stars.[10]

To connote how energy does not necessarily flow in a linear and singular direction, he interlaces the text of the *Heart Sūtra*, streaming it both clockwise and counterclockwise. As a scientist, Iwasaki selects Amitābha, the Buddha of Infinite Light, for the center of his mandala of evolution. Light is energy. Enlisting the Greek Uroboros symbol of infinity and perfection, the dragon swallows its own tail to illustrate the *Heart Sūtra* teaching that there is no beginning or end. No birth, no death. Transformation keeps happening, weaving us all together in a cosmic egg, swirling in a womb of compassion. He reflects how it is hard to find a difference among people, animals, and plants, because we are all just various groupings of carbon, hydrogen, oxygen, calcium, iron, and nitrogen.

FURTHER READING

Abe, Ryuichi. 1999. *The Weaving of Mantra: Kūkai and the Construction of Esoteric Buddhist Discourse.* New York: Columbia University Press.

Arai, Paula. 2019. *Painting Enlightenment: Healing Visions of the Heart Sūtra—the Buddhist Art of Tsuneo Iwasaki.* Boulder, Colo.: Shambhala.

Bass, Jacquelynn. 2004. *Buddha Mind in Contemporary Art.* Berkeley: University of California Press.

O'Neal, Halle. 2018. *Word Embodied: The Jeweled Pagoda Mandalas in Japanese Buddhist Art.* Cambridge, Mass.: Harvard University Press.

Winfield, Pamela. 2013. *Icons and Iconoclasm in Japanese Buddhism: Kukai and Dogen on the Art of Enlightenment.* New York: Oxford University Press.

NOTES

1. For an introduction to Pure Land Buddhism, see Unno 2010. For an introduction to Japanese Zen Buddhism with a focus on art, see Suzuki and Jaffe 2018.

2. For an accessible English translation and commentary based on scholarly and experiential insights, see Thich Nhat Hanh 2017. On the origins of the sūtra, see Nattier 1992.

3. To understand Iwasaki's art in a deeper Japanese Buddhist context, see the discussion and insights in Winfield 2013. Other examples of contemporary Buddhist art are discussed in Bass 2004.

4. For further discussion of Japanese Buddhist art that uses Chinese characters to form Buddhist images, see O'Neal 2018.

5. For further discussion of theories and practices engaging religious visual culture, see Morgan 2005. Specifically on art and perception, see Langer 1957.

6. K'uei-chi 2001.

7. For His Holiness the Dalai Lama's insights into the *Heart Sutra*, see Tenzin Gyatso 2005.

8. For examples of research and insights that integrate scientific and Buddhist teachings, see Varela 1991; Matthieu 2001; B. Wallace 2003.

9. The evolutionary biologist Dominique Homberger provided information critical to understanding and identifying the biological aspects of this painting.

10. The astrophysicist Geoff Clayton helped with the astrophysical phenomenon represented in the painting. The quantum physicist Ravi Rai helped with the atomic activity represented in the painting.

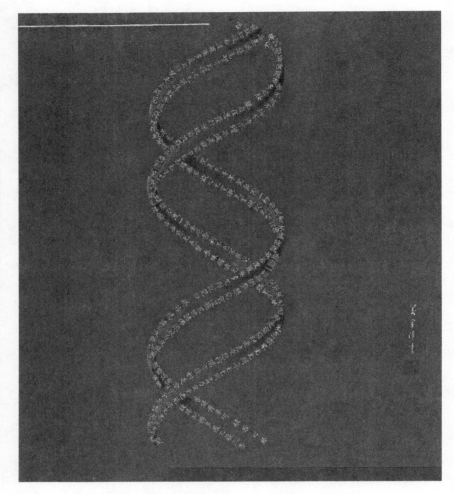

FIGURE 11.1 *DNA*. GOLD ON WASHI PAPER (30 × 27 CM).

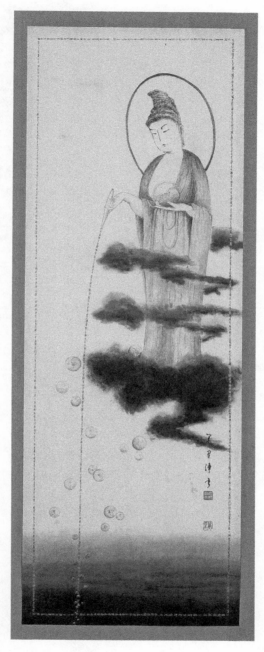

FIGURE 11.2 *MIZUKO: WATER CHILD* (120 × 35 CM, 1997).

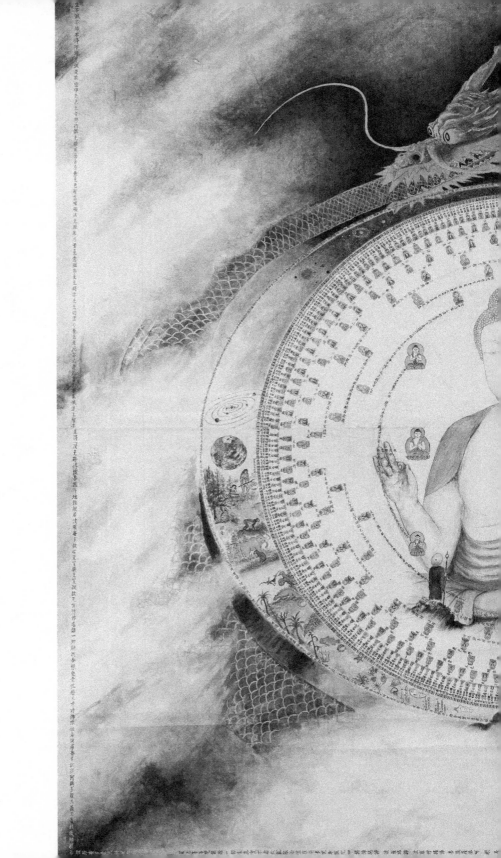

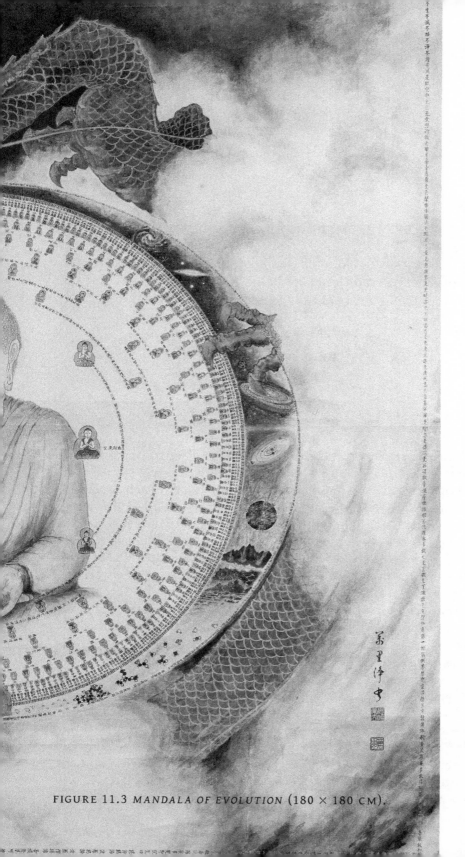

FIGURE 11.3 *MANDALA OF EVOLUTION* (180 × 180 CM).

12. Mantras for Modernity

Nida Chenagtsang's "Mantra Healing Is an Indispensable Branch of Tibetan Traditional Medicine" (2003) and "A Rough Explanation of How Mantras Work" (2015)

BEN P. JOFFE

This chapter presents translated excerpts from two Tibetan-language essays on mantra healing written by the Tibetan doctor and yogi (Tib. *ngakpa*),[1] Nida Chenagtsang (b. 1971). The first essay, "Mantra Healing Is an Indispensable Branch[2] of Tibetan Traditional Medicine," was originally published in a Tibetan literary journal in 2003, while the second, "A Rough Explanation of How Mantras Work," appears as a chapter in Nida's book *The Science of Interdependent Mantra Healing*, published in 2015.[3] Mantra healing refers to preventive and curative ritual healing practices that involve reciting and visualizing mantras. Derived from sacred scriptural languages like Sanskrit, Tibetan, and Shangshung, mantras are understood to possess unique transformative power. In these excerpts, Nida discusses the pedigree of mantra healing as a specifically Buddhist form of healing, while arguing at the same time for its compatibility with biomedicine, contemporary psychology, and science,[4] as well as other more secular modes of treatment in Tibetan traditional medicine.

Nida grew up in a nomad community in Mahlo county, Amdo, northeastern Tibet, during the latter part of the Cultural Revolution. In addition to a secular, Chinese-mandated education, he was exposed to Tantric Buddhist teachings from local religious experts at an early age. Following a brief stint working as a teacher at the middle school for "ethnic minorities" (Ch. *xiaoshu minzu*) in his home region, Nida apprenticed with doctors and lamas in the local area. He was subsequently accepted into the University of Traditional Tibetan Medicine in

Lhasa, where he studied from 1991 until 1997. During this period, he sought out extensive teachings and initiations connected with esoteric Tantric Buddhist practices from several Buddhist masters living in and around Central Tibet. He also engaged in a number of short, intensive retreats through which he had several transformative experiences and gained greater confidence in the profundity of Vajrayāna (Tantric) Buddhism and its compatibility with medicine and psychology.[5]

While mantra compilations and tantric grimoires (i.e., books of ritual formulas and sorcery) are well represented as genres within Tibetan Buddhist literary traditions, books in Tibetan *about* mantras are few and far between. Nida's 339-page mantra healing volume is thus groundbreaking, both for how it brings Buddhist scriptural material about tantric practice into conversation with the regional oral traditions of Tibetan yogis and for how it develops the genre of the mantra compilation by evaluating Tantric Buddhist ritual healing against alternative and competing epistemologies. Throughout the discussion translated below, Nida recognizes medicine and religion as separate, albeit overlapping, domains. He unambiguously situates mantra healing within the realm of religious practice and inspiration and is well aware of the caricature of mantra healing as fanciful folk superstition by "barking-dog" materialists. Nevertheless, framing mantra healing as simply a more spiritual or less material form of Tibetan medical treatment risks ignoring the distinctly embodied and material dimensions of mantra practice. Mantra healing may operate on more subtle or psychological levels than therapies like massage or bloodletting, but Nida makes it clear that to think of mantra healing as "nothing more than a psychological or psychosomatic cure" is to misunderstand or to deny the Buddhist truth of interdependence or contingency—the doctrine that guarantees that body, speech, and mind, inner and outer, subtle and gross, will overlap and influence one another and that ultimately accounts for why the skillful and careful alignment of such levels of being must necessarily produce tangible results. Rather than being innately spiritual or immaterial, then, mantra healing can be better thought of as an essentially integrative therapy that treats disease and adversity via perceived resonances across different levels of being.

While Nida highlights the convenience and accessibility of mantra healing for ordinary people, in stressing the practice's alignment with Buddhist principles and the activities of great Buddhist scholars and saints, he resists critics' relegation of it to mere folk superstition. In keeping with tradition, he admits that the ultimate extent of mantras' magical efficacy in the hands of realized adepts is "inconceivable"; yet, at the same time, he frames mantra healing as something more immediate and amenable to empirical, scientific investigation. In this way, Nida is able to strike a compromise between the view of mantra practice as difficult-to-quantify magic ultimately linked with the transformation and transcendence of conventional reality on the one hand, and as a kind of therapy linked to more habitual psychosomatic processes and worldly domains and dilemmas on the other.

Today, Nida teaches Tibetan medical and tantric practices to students in more than forty countries. His current work to preserve traditional Tibetan Buddhist healing practices like mantra healing involves revitalizing these practices in both their native, largely nomadic-agrarian, Tibetan contexts and transmitting them in new forms in non-Tibetan settings around the world.[6] Through these activities and in line with his discussion below, Nida advocates for a return to the early precedent of the founding figures of Tibetan medicine, who, as so-called yogi-doctors,[7] practiced tantric ritual healing and exoteric Tibetan medicine side by side in thoroughly integrated ways.

Yet Nida is hardly an antimodernist. While his efforts to preserve lapsed traditions and to promote earlier orientations pose a counterpoint to the formal secularization of Tibetan traditional medicine in Tibet since the Communist Chinese invasion in 1950,[8] his fusion of religion and medicine neither collapses nor firmly ranks these categories. Ritual healing is beneficial and relevant for particular conditions, at particular times. While its mechanisms may be associated with a higher order of Buddhist truth, this does not mean that ritual healing trumps other treatments in every instance. Ultimately, even as Nida gently suggests that religion (and specifically the subtle states of consciousness cultivated by virtuoso ascetics) may be the ultimate source of medical knowledge, we see that he nonetheless allows for a complex division of labor and jurisdiction when it comes to relations between medicine and religion and between traditional and modern knowledge systems.

FURTHER READING

Chenagtsang, Nida. 2015. *Mirror of Light: A Commentary on Yuthok's Ati Yoga*. Vol. 1. Portland, Ore.: Sky.

Cuevas, Bryan. 2009. "The 'Calf's Nipple' (*Be'u bum*) of Ju Mipam ('Ju Mi pham): A Handbook of Tibetan Ritual Magic." In *Tibetan Ritual*, edited by José Ignacio Cabezón, 165–86. Oxford: Oxford University Press.

Joffe, Ben. 2017. "Interview with Dr Nida Chenagtsang on Tibetan Tantra and Medicine." A Perfumed Skull. https://perfumedskull.com/2017/02/18/interview-with-dr-nida-chenagtsang -on-tibetan-tantra-and-medicine.

Schrempf, Mona. 2011. "Between Mantra and Syringe: Healing and Health-Seeking Behaviour in Contemporary Amdo." In *Medicine Between Science and Religion: Explorations on Tibetan Grounds*, edited by Vincanne Adams, Mona Schrempf, and Sienna Craig, 157–84. New York: Berghahn.

1. Excerpts from "Mantra Healing Is an Indispensable Branch of Tibetan Traditional Medicine"[9]

I prostrate, give offerings, and go for refuge to Yuthok, King of Physicians and Medicine![10]

Mantra healing was disseminated by sage-ascetics[11] from Dharma-countries like Shang Shung, Oḍḍiyāna, and India, right from the time of the earliest and original king of the world.[12] At a time when there was no vibrant culture and practice of medicine or of autonomous or self-sufficient rule, some people who feared the dangers of worldly karma and the laws of kings went alone without companions to stay in the mountains and dense forests. By isolating their minds and bodies, these so-called upright ones attained meditative absorption and, through the power of their clairvoyance and meditative stability, received [lit., "accomplished"] mantras, or "true words." By relying on the magical power of repeating mantras and speaking these words of truth, these sages offered beings tormented by sickness and demons extremely practical methods for treating illness and preventing infectious diseases. We can reasonably propose that such practices are the ultimate origin or "foundation-stone" of medical treatment.

These sages treated sickness either just with mantras or in some cases treated disease by using mantras in combination with compounded herbs; whole, dried, unprocessed medicines; and things like the flesh, blood, and bone of animals that they had discovered were appropriate [to use] through either their own efforts and experience or as a result of their clairvoyant vision. These saints originated these practices, and later, I suspect that what happened was that gradually, practitioners who solely treated with medicines, people who only did mantric rituals and ceremonies, and people who performed medical and mantra cures in combination became distinct [categories of practitioner]. Sages of the past, such as Ātreya and Dhanvantari, who held medical lineages together with religious ones thought to start treating problems with mantras in various ways: piercing or bursting different kinds of swellings and protuberances by saying mantras, staunching bleeding caused by weapons through mantras, extracting stones and pieces of wood from sores by blowing mantras, taking out cataracts with mantra water, healing by sucking out illnesses, and so on. So, saying that the traditional practices of Sowa Rigpa or Tibetan traditional medicine derive from ancient religious traditions is hardly just an arbitrary statement. [. . .][13]

From the eighth century onward, mantra healing became an important part of Tibetan medicine. As a result of this, there are several instructions on mantra healing taught in the sections of the *Four Tantras* that deal with children's diseases, diseases caused by astrological influences, and [those caused] by chthonic water spirits. One example among these deals with treating sickness caused by poison. By reciting the mantra taught in the text twenty-one times, one can cure and protect oneself from being afflicted by poison and can prevent [the possibility] of poisoning [as well]. If one recites the mantra one hundred or one thousand times, not only does it have the power to cure things like arsenic poisoning and poisoning from compounded poisons [i.e., the kind mixed in food, etc.], but it is taught that if one writes the letters of the mantra using cursive script[14] and gold ink as one recites them and then fastens this inscription to one's body, one will be able to cure and prevent [various] kinds of poisoning. We can see that research into mantra healing and mantra healing practice in the Tibetan medical system of that time were at a very high level. The number of recitations of a mantra, the benefits that these brought, the manner in which one should fasten the charm, and so on are all explained clearly and laid out with great confidence.

Given mantra healing's long history and its dissemination in earlier times, looking at the historical origins of specific mantras found within Tibetan traditional medicine, we can clearly see that there exist many mantras that derive from various non-Buddhist [religious] doctrines of unclear background, from Buddhism, and from the ancient Bön tradition. Mantra healing is taught in many of the translated texts from India that make up the *Kanjur* and *Tenjur*, the canonical collections of the Buddha's teachings and learned commentaries. Scholars of Tibetan traditional medicine, and awareness-holders,[15] great treasure-revealers,[16] and masters accomplished in deity and mantra practice from the Nyingma or Ancient Translation school of Tibetan Buddhism, in particular, also invented and collected together new mantras [which they received] through the inconceivable,[17] magical power of the true words of their aspiration prayers[18] and through their miraculous displays of clairvoyance. Such adepts revealed mantras through their treasure texts, preserving and spreading teachings that existed in earlier times without deterioration. [. . .] It goes without saying, and we can see as plainly as something right before our eyes, that the reading transmissions and oral instructions for these collections are wholly unbroken, that the potency of the current of their blessing-power has not at all vanished, and that these texts are a glowing, radiant jewel within the ocean of the Tibetan tradition of medicine.

When it comes to cases of sickness specifically, if the "three gatherings" [i.e., the *tridoṣa*] that make up the constituent Elements of the ordinary human body increase, are depleted, or are disturbed as a result of various causes and conditions, one's basic Elements become imbalanced. This is then remedied through the four approaches of diet, lifestyle, medicines, and [external or surgical] treatments. Mantras as a therapy fit with all of these approaches: things like "mantra water," "mantra butter" [i.e., in which one recites mantras, then blows onto water or butter, and the power of the mantras enters into these], "edible letters" [see chapter 33 of this anthology], and just generally making use of food and drinks that have been blessed by mantras fit with diet-based therapy. Reciting mantras and carrying things like mantra syllables or mantra-containing protective "magic circle" amulets around one's neck, shoulders, or upper arms while traveling, staying put, or sleeping goes with treatment through lifestyle. Reciting mantras during moxibustion, hot cupping, and bloodletting increases the efficacy of these and can also be used to stop bleeding and prevent treatments from going awry— this is an indispensable tool in surgical and external treatments.

Not only does mantra healing align with all four of the remedies or healing approaches [for those who are sick], but things like mantra-containing talismans, mantra inscriptions, and protective amulets fastened to the body are able to ward off epidemic and contagious diseases, the pollution and harm caused by demonic sickness, and wounding by weapons, as well. As such, mantra healing is inestimably valuable for keeping people who are not sick safe, too. Also, if one looks at the cures for sicknesses affecting types of livestock collected throughout some of the revealed "treasure-text" (terma) teachings, it is easy to see as well that mantra healing is extremely broad in scope and not just for humans who are chief among the six classes of beings. Beyond this, in some cases mantra healing has many distinct qualities, superior even to those of the usual four remedies. These are listed below as I myself understand them:

1. Mantra healing is convenient and only minimally difficult: Any individual who has received tantric empowerment, reading transmission, and oral instructions,[19] and who has properly accomplished the "approach and accomplishing" practices of visualizing the form and reciting the mantras of their meditational deity[20] [hundreds and thousands of times] who then recites these or any sort of healing mantra three, seven, twenty-on, or one hundred times can cure sites of illness.
2. Mantras work quickly and keenly. [. . .]
3. Mantras are emergency cures: Mantras can stop blood loss from things like cuts, wounds, and bloodletting.
4. They are inexpensive: Merely reciting mantras and blowing or saying mantras over everyday objects like butter, water, and salt can be a treatment or make these [substances] into medicine.
5. A single mantra possesses special capacities for a hundred illnesses: Using various methods such as fierce, wild mantras like the Dorje Gotrab or the "Vajra Armor" and "Four BAT" mantra of Padampa [Sangye] can cure many different kinds of illness through just one mantra.
6. One can treat some difficult-to-treat illnesses using mantra-healing procedures: Most kinds of illness caused by demonic spiritual forces have to be treated with mantra-healing rituals. In addition, other types of illness that are difficult to treat can be treated with mantras. For example, Ra Lo[tsawa] Dorje Drakpa joined together torn lips and ears to their original condition just by using mantras.
7. Mantras can protect against contagious diseases and being wounded by weapons.
8. Mantras possess inconceivably good or "spiritual" qualities [the kind that cannot be explained by current science]: When one gives edible mantra letters and uses mantra butter for difficult childbirth, the baby comes quickly, and the butter and other ritual substances can directly be seen stuck to the baby's head. Broken bones can also be joined together through the blowing of mantras. Current science cannot explain these sorts of thing.
9. Mantras cure illnesses solely through mantras. [. . .]
10. Illnesses are cured through the combination of blessed substances and medicine. [. . .]

Now, when it comes to [all of] this, materialists claim, like so many wretched barking dogs, that, since mantra healing is [just] some myth in the minds of superstitious religious people, it is useless or has no value. If mantra healing is even a little efficacious, such people say that it was no more than a psychological cure. But, once one examines things like [mantra] butter sticking to babies' heads and the benefits that come from reciting mantras for cattle and livestock, it is easy to see that mantra healing is not just a psychological remedy.

The profound and special qualities of mantra healing show up in the hagiographies of the great Tibetan saints of previous generations. For example, in *The Secret Path of Ten Million Ḍākinīs*, the first section of the holy woman Machik Labdrön's biography of complete liberation says, "Moreover, she thoroughly restored 427 people with advanced leprosy, returning their flesh to its former condition, and helped with the demonic afflictions and diseases of countless beings." [. . .] The elder and younger Yuthoks, the Kings of Physicians, and all of the early great and titled physicians who were the primary expounders of Sowa Rigpa, being thoroughly trained in the teachings of both the Buddhist sutras and tantras were all exclusively "yogi-doctors" who practiced [exoteric] medicine and tantra/mantra healing inseparably in a thoroughly integrated way. Likewise, this approach has not gone extinct today—there are currently powerful yogis and respected reincarnated lamas who dispel the suffering of many patients through mantra healing rituals.

By using mantras to incite the "three roots,"[21] along with the principal deities of the mandala and their retinue, one obtains both common and uncommon *siddhis* [i.e., spiritual powers and blessings]—having gained control over the outer and inner elements, one manifests unimaginable magical power. While the ways this is accomplished may be beyond the domain of [scientific] investigation, it is clear nonetheless how very important it is for us to investigate and move forward in our understanding as much we can by doing research on things like the difference between water and salt before and after they have had mantras recited over them and on how exactly the elements making up sick people's bodies are transformed or counteracted. [. . .]

2. Excerpt from "A Rough Explanation of How Mantras Work"[22]

The learned authority Ju Mipam Namgyal Gyatso stated, "Thus, since the magical efficacy of mantras is unimaginable, if one exerts oneself properly [in their use], all sorts of sicknesses will surely be pacified." He taught with great confidence that the power or efficacy of mantras is unimaginable and that, if one authentically accomplishes their practice, one will have the power to pacify any illness whatsoever. We can see, too, that great qualified physicians and powerful yogis of the past achieved visible and tangible results[23] through mantra practice and the stages of mantra-healing training. For example, when uttering the necessary specific recitations and [doing the] visualizations for the joining of broken bones, they would speak mantras over pieces of [broken] slate to see whether or not they could join the pieces [of slate] together. If they could, their mantra-power was authentic, and they would say mantras for patients. They would also utter mantras over quicksilver and would drink it directly without any harm. They could lick metal that had turned red hot with their tongues, and, having actualized their tongue mantra-power, they would [then] lick patients. [. . .] When saying mantras for poisoning, initially when the poisons reached the liver, [the urine] would go black. If they said mantras over it and it turned red, this was a sign that the mantras had worked and that they would be able to perform mantra healing. Thus, when we investigate phenomena such as these, we can see that the power or efficacy of mantras is difficult to fathom with the [conceptual] mind, is beneficial, and is of a scientific nature. For this reason, mantra healing is something more than just mere mental imputation devoid of benefit, and no one can say that it is just fruitless superstition or blind faith.

When it comes to putting mantra healing into practice, one absolutely has to understand the reasons why or the basic mechanisms through which mantras produce results. However, explanations about how mantras function have only rarely appeared in any of the books that have been written from ancient times until the present in either the New or Old translation schools [of Tibetan Buddhism], nor is it particularly easy to express the many subtle key points relating to interdependent origination in a way that accords with either our vocabulary or with [ordinary] human understanding. Nevertheless, I think that, if you are someone who uses mantras, it is important to at least understand a little about how mantras work, or at least to put some thought and investigation into the subject. If one does not do any research into the way that mantras are efficacious, one will never be able to become someone who understands the essence or ultimate meaning of the tradition.

NOTES

1. Tib. *sngags pa/ma*, male and female nonmonastic, noncelibate practitioners of tantric Buddhist yoga (literally, "mantra wielders"). Buddhism in Tibetan and Himalayan societies is upheld by two distinct communities (Tib. *sde gnyis*) of professional religious vow-holders: the shaved-headed community of "saffron-robed monastics" and "the white-robed, dreadlocked" (Tib. *gos dkar lcang lo*) community of *ngakpa/ma*. Ngakpa/ma raise families and engage in worldly work in addition to spending considerable time in retreat and as ritual specialists (e.g., weather controllers, healers, funerary experts, exorcists) for hire.

2. Tib. *Yan lag*. Here, this term suggests both "branch" or "limb" and the additional sense of "supplement" or "supporting practice."

3. Since its publication in 2003, however, the first of these essays has also appeared in various forms on a number of websites. My translation is based on the three-part version of the essay that appears on the website of Sorig Khang International: http://bod.sorig .net/?p=32, last accessed February 2, 2018.

4. Despite Nida's overtures toward Western biomedical categories, scientific findings, and various other etic categories, his account remains rooted within indigenous Tibetan cosmological understandings. Concepts like *rlung* (Wind or vital energy), *rtsa* (channels of the subtle yogic body), and the Five Elements—all of which are central to Tibetan traditional medicine and tantric yoga's theories of body and mind—appear as irreducible, ontological givens and are discussed unapologetically.

5. Nida Chenagtsang, personal communication, May 2017; cf. Joffe 2017.

6. Nida is the director of Sorig Khang International and a cofounder of the International Ngakmang Institute for the preservation and promotion of the Rebkong *ngakpa* tradition. More information about these organizations and Nida's activities can be found at www .sorig.net/.

7. Tib. *Sngags sman.*

8. For more information on transnational developments around the intersection of religion and science in Sowa Rigpa or Tibetan traditional medicine, cf., for example, Adams, Schrempf, and Craig 2011; Craig 2012.

9. Chenagtsang 2014a.

10. Yuthok Yönten Gonpo. Two figures bear this name in Tibetan tradition. Yuthok the Younger of the twelfth century and his more mythic forebear, Yuthok the Elder, postulated to have existed in the eighth century, are both considered to be the founders of Sowa Rigpa.

11. The term used here is *drang srong*, the Tibetan translation of the Sanskrit *ṛṣi*. The Tibetan translation literally means "truthful, upright ones" or "straightened-out ones."

12. Tib. *Mang bkur rgyal po*, the first primordial king of this world system.

13. Sections of the text that have not been translated are marked by "[. . .]." Nida offers further qualifying information regarding the ultimately religious and not necessarily Buddhist origins of Sowa Rigpa in Chenagtsang 2014b.

14. Tib. *Tsheg med*, a kind of Tibetan cursive writing that lacks the *tsheg* (point) that divides syllables in other scripts.

15. Tib. *Rig 'dzin*, the Tibetan for the Sanskrit *vidyādhara*, a "keeper or holder of knowledge or awareness" and esoteric knowledge or gnosis, in particular. In *Vajrayāna*, the term denotes accomplished practitioners of tantric Buddhism, especially those whose realization has granted them miraculous abilities. Its Tibetan gloss (*rig 'dzin/ma*) suggests someone who recognizes the ultimate nature of mind and sustains natural, uncontrived, pristine awareness (Tib. *rig pa*).

16. For more information on treasure revelation and revealers, see the glossary and c.f. J. Gyatso 1999; Jacoby 2015; Gayley 2017.

17. Nida uses terms meaning "inconceivable," "unimaginable," and "beyond imagining" (*bsam gyis mi khyab pa, bsam yul las 'das pa*) to describe the magical power of mantra practice throughout his writing. Such terms suggest not only that the extent of mantras' efficacy is difficult to imagine but also that they operate at or through a level of awareness or perception that literally "goes beyond" or "cannot be encompassed" (*las 'das pa, mi khyab pa*) by ordinary imagination, thought, or conceptual mind (*bsam*).

18. The implication is that using prayers that already contain powerful "true words" (*bden tshig*) received by previous religious virtuosi can enable the further revelation of new words of truth or power.

19. The triad of initiation or "empowerment" (Tib. *dbang*), reading transmission (*lung*), and direct, personalized instruction (*khrid*) involves the key transmissions one must receive from a qualified lama before one can undertake advanced tantric Buddhist practices. Empowerment transforms and ripens the student, revealing the nature of the practice and the student's ultimately realized body, speech, and mind. Through empowerment, students are initiated into the mandala (see glossary) of a particular set of tutelary tantric Buddhas on whom they will meditate. With reading "transmission," the student listens to the teacher read the words of the practice text aloud, thereby connecting to the practice lineage, while "instruction" involves specific technical advice about the practice given to the student by the lama or guru.

20. That is, *yidam*, the tutelary Buddha form(s) into whose practice or cosmology tantric Buddhists are initiated and whom they imagine themselves as, as part of "deity yoga" practices for achieving spiritual powers and buddhahood.

21. The "three roots" (*rtsa gsum*) in Vajrayāna or Tibetan tantric Buddhism are the lama (*bla ma*; one's personal teacher who reveals and models the path to enlightenment), the *yidam*, and the *khandro* or *ḍākinī* (*mkha' 'gro ma*; specific female buddha forms with which the practitioner engages in meditation and ritual). These three roots are the esoteric or tantric expression of the Three Jewels and are the focus of various contemplative, devotional practices in Tibetan Buddhism.

22. Heruka and Drolma 2015: 36–37. Chenagtsang is Nida's family or clan name and the one he uses most often as a surname in English contexts. In both Tibetan and English texts, however, he prefers simply to go by "Dr Nida" (*sman pa nyi zla*). When writing specifically about tantric as opposed to more exoteric medical subjects, Nida tends to use his *sngags pa* name, Nyida Heruka (*nyi zla he ru ka*). Nida's sister-in-law, Yeshe Drolma, assisted with the preparation of his book on mantra healing and is listed as its coauthor, although the book's contents were written by Nida.

23. Tib. *Mig mthong lag zin gyi 'bras bu*, literally "results [that can be] seen by the eyes and held by the hands."

13. Science and Authority in Tibetan Medicine

Gönpokyap's "Extraordinarily Special Features of the Human Body" (2008)

JENNY BRIGHT

The translation below is an excerpt from one of twenty essays written by Gönpokyap (b. 1970) included in his self-edited volume, *Moonbeam of Delightful Jasmine: Collected Essays on Tibetan Medicine*, published in 2008 in Beijing.[1] The essay makes explicit an underlying assumption shared by many of his generation of Tibetan medical writers working in China. This is the argument that Buddhist philosophy is "scientific" by today's modern standards, making Buddhist knowledge about the body not only compatible with medical thought but also constituting a vital resource for new research and development of the Tibetan medical tradition. Gönpokyap's works about medicine and the body are also often philosophical, speaking directly or implicitly to the contemporary social and political climate in Chinese Tibet. In this translated essay, he quotes from the likes of Friedrich Engels, Sun Yat-sen, and several other Chinese intellectuals to support his argument about the scientific nature of Buddhist philosophy.

According to his brief biography outlining his medical credentials, Gönpokyap has studied and practiced medicine throughout Tibet's Central and Eastern regions, including the Luqu Prefecture Medical Hospital, the Qinghai Tibetan Medical University, the Central Tibetan Chakpori Medical University, the Lhasa Medical-Astro University, as well as the medical centers in Sog County, Nagchu Province, and Langzhou. He has a robust academic portfolio, having published his research in more than thirty domestic and international journals. A colleague from the Central Tibetan Medical Hospital writes in the preface to the work

discussed here that Gönpokyap is a "modern intellectual"[2] and a great proponent and disseminator of knowledge about Tibetan medicine. He is believed to
merge tradition with innovation, resulting in the further development of Tibetan
medical science.

As is customary in Tibetan medical publications from China, both Gönpokyap's
biography and the preface to the volume clearly state the three criteria for
demonstrating medical authority in contemporary Tibetan medicine. First, medical authority rests upon knowledge of the texts of the Tibetan medical tradition.
Gönpokyap's biography tells us that he was a top student at his medical school,
having studied the texts of the Tibetan medical system in depth. Second, modern
Tibetan medical authority requires that one know the theories and clinical practices of biomedicine, which Gönpokyap has demonstrated by engaging with international medical journals and relating the Tibetan system to biomedicine in his
own published writings. Third, and crucially, Gönpokyap has ample medical
experience throughout Tibet. On the first page of the volume—even before the
table of contents—Gönpokyap's medical authority is established, and we are told
that the book is the result of his expertise in these three areas.

His essay "A Short Discussion on Why We Need to Continually Develop and
Advance Our Unique Insights Into the Extraordinarily Special Features of the
Human Body" argues that Tibetan medicine, coupled with Buddhist knowledge
of the body, is as empirical and scientific as modern biomedicine. The key
strength of Tibetan medicine, according to Gönpokyap, is its close relation to
Buddhism, which provides both an epistemological and materialist blueprint for
knowledge-building, as well as a soteriological map of the workings of the
universe, human life, and death.

The essay is composed of two parts. The first section, "On Extraordinarily
Special Insights," maintains that the unique features of Buddhist knowledge,
such as the notion of the *bardo* (the liminal space between one lifetime and the
next), make the Tibetan system "extraordinary."[3] Yet, because a notion such as
this is not currently considered scientific by modern standards, Gönpokyap
argues that Tibetan researchers must innovate ways to show that Buddhist
knowledge is not superstitious, but indeed scientific. The second section, "Why
We Must Do Critical Research to Clarify the Meanings of the Root Texts" emphasizes that, despite the remarkable achievements of Tibetans throughout history
in understanding and mending the body, there is a current need to synthesize
and standardize the interpretation of authoritative medical texts and, based on
this, produce a standard textbook for all Tibetan medical students.

A key element of Gönpokyap's argument for understanding Buddhism as
containing scientific elements is that this notion is also supported by socialist
intellectuals, writers, and officials of the highest social and political echelons of
the People's Republic of China. By stating this, he signals to his fellow Tibetans
that they can openly embrace Buddhism as an aspect of modern Tibetan
medicine and confidently refer to Buddhist texts about the body as authoritative
medical sources. Gönpokyap also walks the fine line of merging politically safe

elements of Tibet's past with the official history of modern China. Hence, while he explicitly narrates Tibet's "liberation" and development under the Chinese state, and presents Tibetan Buddhism and medicine as aligning with the ideals of modern socialism, Gönpokyap makes several implicit nods to Tibetan medicine's Indian Buddhist origins.

For Gönpokyap and many of his peers, research into Tibet's authoritative medical texts and Buddhist tantras is a central way to establish and bolster the legitimacy of Tibetan medicine, while at the same time integrating, or at least accounting for, biomedicine. In much of contemporary Tibetan medical literature, these authoritative texts are often treated as resources for innovative ways of interpreting biomedical thought and, in the process, for developing and expanding upon the already rich knowledge of the Tibetan medical system. Significantly, in his essay, Gönpokyap explicitly signals to other Tibetan medical writers that Buddhism, science, and communist ideals can co-exist in a way that benefits the Tibetan medical system, making it viable and relevant in the contemporary age.

FURTHER READING

Adams, Vincanne, Renqing Dongzhu, and Phuoc V. Le. 2010. "Translating Science: The Arura Medical Group at the Frontiers of Medical Research." In *Studies of Medical Pluralism in Tibetan History and Society*, edited by Sienna R. Craig et al., 111–36. Andiast, Switzerland: International Institute for Tibetan and Buddhist Studies.

Craig, Sienna R. 2012. *Healing Elements: Efficacy and Social Ecologies of Tibetan Medicine*. Berkeley: University of California Press.

Cuomu, Mingji. 2010. "Qualitative and Quantitative Research Methodology in Tibetan Medicine: The History, Background and Development of Research in Sowa Rigpa." In *Medicine Between Science and Religion: Explorations on Tibetan Grounds*, edited by Vincanne Adams, Mona Schrempf, and Sienna R. Craig, 245–63. New York: Berghahn.

Garrett, Frances, and Vincanne Adams. 2008. "The Three Channels in Tibetan Medicine with a Translation of Tsultrim Gyaltsen's 'A Clear Explanation of the Principle Structure and Location of the Circulatory Channels as Illustrated in the Medical Paintings.'" *Traditional South Asian Medicine* 8: 86–114.

EXCERPT FROM "A SHORT DISCUSSION ON WHY WE NEED TO CONTINUALLY DEVELOP AND ADVANCE OUR UNIQUE INSIGHTS INTO THE EXTRAORDINARILY SPECIAL FEATURES OF THE HUMAN BODY"[4]

The current trend in biomedicine is the idea that if we are able to thoroughly understand the physical nature of human beings, then we will be able to treat illnesses and imbalances of the body when they arise. Furthermore, biomedicine prescribes preventive measures to enable longer and healthier lives. Tibetan medical thought is no different. According to the *Root Tantra*, "If one desires to be healthy, to cure sickness, and live a long life, they should learn the oral instructions of the Tibetan medical tradition." And, according to the *Explanatory Tantra*, "The ultimate purpose of medicine is to treat people when they are sick and to help them achieve a healthy, long life." As clearly stated in the above quotations from the *Four Tantras*, biomedicine and Tibetan medicine have the same aim.

During Tibetan medicine's 3,900-year history,[5] it has been able to gain an understanding into the nature of human bodies. Some of us claim that it is inconceivable that our medical system arose from ordinary individuals, making it very different from modern medicine.[6] Some assert that the practical teachings of the classical texts are not well understood, and, because there is not a single, common rendering of them, errors exist. Focusing on these two [interrelated] points, this essay explores the current study of the extraordinary knowledge of Tibetan medicine through an examination of instances wherein what appears as backward or unintelligible can be made clear.

On Extraordinarily Special Insights

It is explained in the literature of modern medicine that the human body is created exclusively by the flawless reproductive fluids of the parents. In the Land of Snows, according to the texts of our Tibetan medical tradition, the father's semen, the mother's red element,[7] and the migrating consciousness of a *bardo* being[8] are necessary to conceive a child. At the time of [Tibet's] "liberation,"[9] this idea of a migrating consciousness was considered irrational. Up until the late 1980s, all of the wisdom of the Buddha's teachings was labeled as superstitious [by the Chinese authorities]. Near the end of the 1980s and [at] the beginning of the 1990s, Buddhist teachings began to be thought of as containing genuine scientific elements. And, in the twenty-first century, Buddhist insight is being taught in universities. This situation gives us reason to be happy. It is also a sign that in order to move away from [the belief that the Buddha's teachings are] superstitious, we need to begin to confirm everything empirically.

According to the early *sūtras*, the founder of our religion, the Buddha, taught that the world is spherical in shape and that the [circumference of] the earth or globe is three hundred thousand *yojanas*.[10] It is said that the Buddha claimed that the elevation of Mount Meru is twenty thousand *yojanas* and that the distance between the earth and the moon is forty-two thousand *yojanas*. These days, according to scientific reasoning and through the use of new technologies such as satellites, it has been calculated that the distance between the earth and the moon is approximately 537,000 kilometers. Therefore, when the distance of forty-two thousand *yojanas* is converted, it shows that the Buddhist texts are actually correct.

Sun Yat-sen[11] writes, "The Buddha's religion is the mother of philosophy. Other sciences are not able to grasp a thousandth of what Buddhism does." Similarly, Zhao Puchu[12] writes, "Buddhist philosophy is pregnant with exceedingly deep and profound knowledge that allows humans to understand the world rationally and examine their own personal faults through inferring from the whole human species. Having examined Buddhism's defining characteristics closely, it is evident that it is a scientific path that possesses features that are deep, profound, and unique."

[As these statements by Chinese political and religious leaders indicate,] just because something is not yet measurable by science does not mean that it should necessarily be considered superstitious. The knowledge contained in our Buddhist teachings comes from the times of ancient society. In present times, people are unable to interpret these and say that according to Buddhism, a deity created the world, or they even go as far as to say that our karma is a matter of fate [rather than of cause and effect]. But this is nothing but foolish chatter, and even Chinese revolutionaries and intellectuals who think from sophisticated scientific viewpoints have confidence in the material origins [of the Buddha's teachings]. The great writer Lu Xun,[13] after having read many Buddhist texts, told his friend Xu Shoutang,[14] "The Buddha Shakyamuni is all-knowing and a great discerner of the way things really are. Because we humans continuously have countless difficult points in our lives that are hard to overcome, his teachings from ancient times have remained constant." One would need to be utterly crazy not to agree that [what Lu Xun] says is the truth.

Likewise, Engels,[15] giving an explanation of dialectical reasoning, writes, "What makes the Buddhist religion unique is that it has reached a very high level of dialectical reasoning. The Buddhist world view does not accept a wondrous or unrivaled deity, but rather that all phenomena, from beginning to end, are based on the web of cause and effect." When it is put like this, it is easy to see that the teachings that make up our Buddhist knowledge do fulfill our [modern] wishes, having been born of scientific and materialist foundations.

I am making a similar argument in regard to our Tibetan medical texts, which state that for pregnancy to occur, the joining of the semen, the blood, and a consciousness is necessary. It is precisely because the consciousness is an extremely hidden phenomenon that it can not be easily pointed to, and, because of that, from the materialistic point of view, the notion of the consciousness is not accepted. But, in reality, sometimes when we see someone laughing, we also involuntarily laugh, and, similarly, when we see people cry, we cannot help but feel like crying.[16] During the thirty-eight weeks that our body is in the process of being created, the consciousness, together with the function of thirty-two different Winds,[17] forms the support for the growth and development of the body. [For a Buddhist account of gestation, see Anthology, vol. 1, ch. 5.] It is precisely this knowledge that modern science is not able to accept as scientific. Even if you circle the globe three times, it would be difficult to find [a scientific system that would accept this], and, because of that, we need to zealously pursue [research confirming the validity of] the unique and extraordinary features of our [Tibetan medical tradition].

Why We Must Do Critical Research to Clarify the Meanings of the Root Texts

Overall, the Tibetan medical system is founded on a thorough examination of the parts of the human body. During the reign of the tenth Tibetan king, Esho Leg, flawed bone could be removed, and damaged flesh could be sewn back together. Knowledge on sewing up skin is clearly expanded upon in Shentön Yeshé Lodrö[18] of Darding's text, *The Instructional Water That Revives the Dying Through the Treatment of Wounds*. And especially, during the time of the eighth century, His Eminence Yuthok the Senior[19] composed the text *Essence of Nectar* [i.e., the *Four Tantras*] and surgically replaced a skull fragment for the Kashmiri king's minister, Sengé Bépa, which today is difficult to imagine. Other texts from that century include *Measurements of Living and Dead Bodies, Combining the Nine Anatomical Threads*, and *Magic Mirror of Anatomy*.[20] Having researched the human body empirically, [I have found that] basic principles [of medicine] were discovered [by our early forbearers].

After visiting many cremation grounds, one of the ten great Tibetan thinkers, Machik Labdrön,[21] was gradually able to clearly understand in fine detail the basic nature of the body's constituent parts, leading to the composition of the text *Machik's Complete Explanation: Casting the Body Out as Food*. Likewise, Drangti Palden Tsoché[22] wrote *Clear Illumination of the Fabric of Knots of the Upper Body*. In the seventeenth century, the famous Buddhist virtuoso[23] Desi Sangyé Gyatso,[24] having consulted the earlier medical drawings of the human body, commissioned seventy-nine new medical paintings to illustrate the inner meanings of the authoritative medical texts and commentaries. Some other essential details were established by Lhodrak Tendzin Norbu,[25] who made empirical illustrations of the human body, having dissected actual human corpses.

Similar to these accomplishments recorded in our history books, our ancestors created and gifted us, their descendants, a wondrous and unsurpassable tradition, which, like the precious lapis lazuli stone [of the Buddha Bhaiṣajyaguru],[26] is our unique cultural treasure. However, because there is not yet a common way of understanding the words and meanings of the authoritative texts, those of the younger generation interpret them in many different ways. And, many of these interpretations are not in keeping with the original meaning [of the authoritative treatises] and remain doubtful. For example, there are currently several different interpretations surrounding the [problem that] some authoritative texts and illustrations of the body posit seventy-seven blood channels, which, compared alongside a [dissected] body, cannot be identified. This is a very serious situation, which, if continued, threatens the very existence of the *Four Tantras*. Therefore, in regard to the body's anatomy, we need to be able to definitively label each of the body's constituent parts so that we can refer to any specific part of the body [and understand which part of the body is being spoken of].

This method, however, is hard rather than easy. Nonetheless, at first, [we must] synthesize the [works of] the great scholars on how the body is constituted, and, based on that, [we must produce] colored medical diagrams that label the specific classifications of the 364 different bones, the white and black channels, and [all the other constituent parts of the body]. In short, we need to be able to identify all the parts of the body according to the authoritative texts of the Tibetan medical tradition. And from that, a book should be composed, published, and taught to all the Tibetan medical students. [In addition to authoritative medical texts,] such a book would need to be composed considering the fundamental works of [Buddhist] tantra, as well as the writings belonging to the "writing from experience" [genre].[27]

NOTES

1. Some parts of this translation were published in my dissertation, "Women and Hormones in Tibetan Medical Literature" (University of Toronto 2017). Some minor revisions appear in the present translation. I would like to express my appreciation to Pierce Salguero for his generous assistance and careful edits and to Jia Luo, Khenpo Kunga Sherab, Tsering Samdrup, Lauran Hartley, Gerald Roche, and Remy Landau for their helpful suggestions and unique insights.

2. Tib. *Da lam tshe rig pa*.

3. Tib. *Thun mong ma yin pa*. Mgon po skyabs 2008: 127.

4. Mgon po skyabs 2008: 126–35.

5. This 3,900-year history dates Tibetan medicine as emerging at the same time as the earliest recorded histories of the Tibetan civilization—long before the advent of Buddhism.

6. This is an implicit nod to the narrative that Tibetan medicine, and its foundational text, the *Four Tantras*, originated from the omniscient mind of Bhaiṣajyaguru and is therefore perfect and unerring, unlike the medical systems arising from the minds of ordinary individuals.

7. The "white and red elements" (*khams dkar dmar*) are the reproductive fluids, the white semen of the male and the red menstrual blood of the female.

8. Bardo (*bar do*) literally means to be "in the middle" or "in between"; thus, a "*bardo* being" (*bar do ba*) is a consciousness migrating between lifetimes. See glossary.

9. A common epithet, Tibet's "liberation" refers to the decade of the 1950s during which time China's military took administrative control over Tibet. For a detailed history of this period, see Shakya 2000.

10. A *yojana* (Tib. *dpag tshad*) is a Sanskrit term referring to a measure of distance of about seven to nine miles.

11. Sun Yat-sen (1866–1925), known as the father of the Chinese nation, was a physician, writer, intellectual, and revolutionary, who in 1912 became the first president of the Republic of China (see Schoppa 2000: 186–87).

12. Zhao Puchu (1907–2000), who had close ties to the Chinese Communist Party, was the leading voice of official Chinese Buddhism for most of the twentieth century. Especially in the 1980s, during the so-called period of opening up and reform in China, and until his death, Zhao Puchu promoted the legitimacy of Buddhism within Chinese culture, aiming to counter the dominant view of the Chinese government and the public that religion is superstitious and dangerous (see Zhe 2016: 312–48).

13. Lu Xun (1881–1936) is considered by many to be modern China's preeminent essayist, poet, writer of short stories, historian of Chinese literature, and translator of Japanese and German (see Davies 2013: 1–7).

14. Xu Shoutang (1883–1948) was a close friend of Lu Xun. A couple stories of their friendship can be found in Gu 2013: 68–69; Khempo Sodargye 2013: 10.

15. Friedrich Engels (1820–1895), the German socialist philosopher and writer who worked collaboratively with Karl Marx (1818–1883) to write a number of influential works, including *The Communist Manifesto*.

16. That is, we know that laughter is contagious based on our own experience; therefore, we cannot say that it is untrue or does not exist just because we do not have the technology to know the mechanism by which such a phenomenon occurs.

17. The "thirty-two Winds" allude to the subtle energy channels of tantric anatomy (see I. Baker 2017).

18. Shentön Yeshé Lodrö (Gshen ston ye shes blo gros) was a physician dating from the pre-imperial Yarlung dynasty (second to sixth centuries). He is mentioned briefly in a list of early "Renowned Tibetan Physicians" in D. Gyatso 2010: 271.

19. "Yuthok the Senior" refers to Yuthok Yönten Gönpo (G.yu thog yon tan mgon po; 708–833), a central founding figure in Tibetan medicine accredited with composing an early version of its premier text, the *Four Tantras*, to which Gönpokyap refers by its alternative and abbreviated title, *Essence of Nectar*.

20. *Söntik dang Rotik* (*Gson thig dang ro thig*), *Rotra Tugu Gujor* (*Ro bkra thu gu dgu sbyor*), and *Rotra Pülgyi Melong* (*Ro bkra 'phul gyi me long*) are three of many works attributed to Biji Tsenpashilaha. All are listed in D. Gyatso 2010: 623. The contemporary medical historian Jampa Thinley (see 'Byams pa 'phrin las 1996: 370–71) describes these three texts as including illustrations, descriptive measurements, and grids of the body (see J. Gyatso 2015: 46, 415fn64).

21. Machik Labdrön (Ma gcig labs sgron, 1055–1149) is one of the few preeminent female Tibetan religious teachers; she is known primarily for propagating the practice of *chöd* (*gcod*). A significant element of this practice is that it ideally takes place in cremation grounds or places that contain corpses on which to contemplate. Hence, Machik Labdrön is presumed to have had considerable knowledge of the empirical body, in addition to her insights into its "true" nature as taught in Buddhism. For more on this figure and the work mentioned by Gönpokyap, see Ma gcig lab sgron 2003.

22. Drangti Pelden Tsoché (Brang ti dpal ldan 'tsho byed; c. thirteenth to fourteenth centuries) was a famous Tibetan medical historian and teacher of the Drangti (*brang ti*) lineage of Tibetan medicine. The work Gönpokyap refers to here, *Byang khog yul gyi thig 'grems gsal ba'i sgron me*, is discussed in Taube 1981: 58. The works of Pelden Tsoché are among the few Tibetan sources of medical illustrations from which Desi Sangyé Gyatso looked to in the creation of his own seventy-nine medical paintings (see J. Gyatso 2015: 46).

23. A *paṇḍita* is a scholar virtuoso who has mastered the five sciences of Buddhist learning: religious philosophy, dialectics and logic, grammar, medicine, and applied arts and crafts.

24. Desi Sangyé Gyatso (Sde srid sangs rgyas rgya mtsho; 1653–1705) was an enormously influential political and religious figure of the seventeenth century, as well as a monk, scholar, and medical historian. His *Mirror of Beryl* is considered a definitive, authoritative source of Tibetan medical history (see J. Gyatso 2015: 23–80).

25. Lhodrak Tenzin Norbu (Lho brag bstan 'dzin nor bu; seventeenth century) was one of the artists commissioned by Desi Sangyé Gyatso for his seventy-nine paintings. For more on "illustrating the real," see J. Gyatso 2015: 54–57.

26. Lapis lazuli is highly significant in Tibetan medicine. For example, Bhaiṣajyaguru is always depicted and described as being a radiant bright blue, and one of his common titles is "King of Lapis Lazuli Light." For a detailed study of this term in its Tibetan, Indian, Chinese, East Asian, and Greco-Roman contexts, see Winder 2001. By calling Tibetan medicine a unique national treasure like a lapis lazuli stone, Gönpokyap is again pointing to Tibet's Buddhist heritage. On the Master of Medicines Buddha, see also *Anthology*, vol. 1, ch. 25.

27. For more on the medical genre "writing from experience" (*nyams yig*), see J. Gyatso 2004.

14. "We Will Live Long Lives and Attain Great Health"

Monk Changlyu's *The Book of Diagnosis and Natural Foods* (2014)

EMILY S. WU

Morality books, usually published in the form of small booklets and pamphlets, are often found free to take in local Buddhist and folk temples in Taiwan.[1] Besides the extremely popular stories about good deeds leading to an accumulation of karmic merit and bad deeds leading to horrific outcomes, books promoting healthful living are also common. *The Book of Diagnosis and Natural Foods* (*Tianran shiwu zhenduan shu*), published in 2014, is a contemporary example. The author, the Taiwanese Dharma master Changlyu (addressed simply as "Monk" by his followers and in his own writings), cites *sūtras*, as well as health tips based on contemporary hearsay, to support his central argument that a dharmically and scientifically informed vegetarian lifestyle can prevent and cure cancer.

The significance of *The Book of Diagnosis and Natural Foods*, at least from a religious perspective, lies in the integration of three important discourses in contemporary Taiwanese Buddhism, each of which is based in Mahāyāna Buddhist ideals of compassion and the bodhisattva vow. The first of these discourses is a justification of vegetarianism. Although a vegetarian diet is not a requirement in all strands of Buddhism, it is a signature practice in contemporary Chinese and Taiwanese Buddhism, not only among the monastics but also among lay followers. Historical interactions with Daoist and traditional Chinese medical thought led to the common perception that vegetarianism was desirable for spiritual development.[2] Prohibited foods include not only animal flesh and animal products but also pungent vegetables such as onions, scallions, chives, garlic, and shallots. These vegetables, commonly called the "five pungents" (*wuxin* or *wuhun*), are deemed detrimental for spiritual cultivation because the strong smells and tastes supposedly arouse physical desires and are therefore distractions to one's concentration on the spiritual path. Changlyu additionally argues that improper vegetarianism can also be harmful. He offers explanations of why certain vegetables and fruits are better than others to consume and how to best prepare those foods for consumption.

Second, Changlyu engages with long-standing notions of karmic retribution, or the belief that negative actions (such as killing animals) lead to negative outcomes. In Taiwanese Buddhism, the popular interpretation of karma takes on the form of daily practices designed to accumulate merit (Ch. *gongde*; Skt. *puṇya*). People who mindfully practice to earn merit are rewarded with prosperity, advancements, and good health; the opposite leads to obstacles, troubles, illnesses, and violent deaths. To Changlyu, cancer is a prominent category of karmic retribution. As such, it can be prevented and possibly reversed through proper lifestyle. For a full reversal of karmic retribution, one must practice sincere repentance, hold an intention to do good, and practice cultivation through traditional Buddhist means. One example of beneficial practice that he gives is to financially support his medical services, which in turn alleviate the suffering of fellow human beings.

The third discourse is that of Humanistic Buddhism, a socially engaged mode of Mahāyāna Buddhism popular in Taiwan that emphasizes one's social responsibility to elevate the conditions of oneself and all sentient beings. The creation of Humanistic Buddhism is usually attributed to the Chinese Dharma master Taixu (1890–1947), who actively participated in the social revolution led by Sun Yat-Sen. Taixu's disciple Yinshun (1906–2005) migrated from China to Taiwan in 1952 and deeply influenced the founders of several of the largest Buddhist followings in Taiwan.[3] Specifically, Changlyu's discussion of a vegetarian diet touches upon the question of a Buddhist's social responsibility. He points to the necessity for Buddhists to prove that a vegetarian diet can sustain strong, healthy bodies that allow one to fulfill social responsibilities such as caring for one's family. According to Changlyu, as a vegetarian diet also reduces the killing of animals, it can thus also prevent collective karmic retribution in the form of large-scale warfare. Not included in the excerpts here are his additional arguments that with a vegetarian diet, one also contributes to the preservation of natural habitats and the environment.

With this vernacular Buddhist articulation of health and medicine as a foundation, Changlyu has established a number of charity kitchens, free clinics, and hospices in Taiwan. Besides promoting a vegetarian diet, Changlyu also speaks strongly against biomedical treatments for cancer; for example, claiming that chemotherapy does more harm than good. While his community hospices have doctors and nurses with biomedical training, he states that traditional Chinese medicine is more beneficial for patients. His free clinics have only traditional

Chinese medicine doctors, who offer mostly herbal remedies. Changlyu had also planned to establish an oncology hospital based on his approach, and building commenced in 2017. However, the focus of the plan changed shortly thereafter, shifting from curing cancer to providing Buddhist hospice care for terminally ill patients.

FURTHER READINGS

Chandler, Stuart. 2004. *Establishing a Pure Land on Earth: The Fo Guang Buddhist Perspective on Modernization and Globalization*. Honolulu: University of Hawai'i Press.

Clart, Philip, and Gregory Adam Scott, eds. 2014. *Religious Publishing and Print Culture in Modern China: 1800–2012*. Boston: De Gruyter.

Eppsteiner, Fred, ed. 1988. *The Path of Compassion: Writing Socially Engaged Buddhism*. Berkeley, Calif.: Parallax.

Pittman, Don A. 2001. *Toward a Modern Chinese Buddhism: Taixu's Reforms*. Honolulu: University of Hawai'i Press.

Weller, Robert P., C. Julia Huang, Keping Wu, and Fan Lizhu. 2018. *Religion and Charity: The Social Life of Goodness in Chinese Societies*. Cambridge: Cambridge University Press.

EXCERPTS FROM
THE BOOK OF DIAGNOSIS AND NATURAL FOODS[4]

Each person only has one body. If the body is not treasured, when it gets seriously ill, not only does the person himself suffer, the whole family also suffers incredibly. It is a very simple logic: One person gets cancer, but the whole family is affected. The one person gets cancer physically, but the whole family gets the cancer of mental anguish, which is no less painful than for the actual cancer sufferer. In order to prevent family members from undergoing suffering, one must watch out for cancer. Everyone should condition the body daily with a healthful diet. Otherwise, cancer will ruthlessly come and take happiness away from your entire family.

Why Do Ordained People Eat Vegetarian Food but Still Get Cancer?

In Buddhism, there are two layers of understanding: this-worldly and other-worldly. In the this-worldly [understanding of things], the physical body is the most important. There is first the physical body, then there is the Dharma body; without the physical body, how could one cultivate? How would you spread the Dharma to benefit other sentient beings? The Dharma is vast like the ocean, and, even with lifelong devotion, one can still never achieve complete comprehension of it. One must cultivate both the this-worldly and other-worldly and remain unbiased—that would be a harmonious [state of mind]. Monk believes that one must first cultivate the this-worldly to reach perfection. Our vegetarian diet should lead to a strong, healthy physical body, and then we can give other people more confidence [in following the Dharma]. However, many Buddhists ignore their own [physical] health. Without a healthy body, how do you study Buddhism? How do you cultivate? How do you take care of your family? And how can you sustain the most basic survival in your life?

Many long-term vegetarians, because of their erroneous conceptions about their diets, end up with cancer! The blind spots of vegetarianism are in the overuse of cooking oil and over-consumption of bean products. Soybeans especially contain high levels of proteins and oils and can lead to high blood cholesterol, causing strokes, or having fatty liver, leading to liver fibrosis.

Also, after eating a full meal, it is not appropriate to eat soup, have fruits, or drink tea. This is because after food enters the stomach, the stomach needs to secrete stomach acid to digest. If you eat soup or fruits, the fruit acids will neutralize the stomach acid and easily cause ulcers. Drinking tea can dilute the acids and enzymes and cause gastroptosis, stomach ulcers, and other problems.

In addition, one must eat consistent amounts during consistent times of the day for the stomach and intestines to be healthy. The stomach secretes stomach acid during specific times. If one skips regular eating times, because there is no food in the stomach, the stomach acid will start to erode the stomach wall. Eventually, there will be problems in the digestive system. The coldness, hotness,[5] and thickness of the stomach wall vary from one person to the next. How to eat consistently—whether it is to eat a little but frequently or eat more but less frequently—depends on the conditions of each individual person.

In the old days, meat was a rarity in people's daily diets. However, people were physically healthy, calm tempered, and full of kindness. In contrast, modern people eat too much meat, fast food, and processed food. They lack mineral nutrients, and that causes weakness and myriad illnesses. In fact, many children have a hard time concentrating, have a bad temper, and are impulsive because they lack mineral nutrients. Physicality affects psychology, so we must trace the root causes.

Minerals are also one set of effective tools in the fight against cancer. If one wishes to get sufficient minerals, then one must eat properly to get a healthy body. When the immunity is strengthened, one does not get cancer so easily, and longevity comes naturally. How could anyone enjoy a beautiful life if there is no health?

The Healthiest Ways to Wash and Cook Vegetables

The safest and healthiest method is to boil the vegetables. Boil a full kettle of hot water. Put all the vegetables to be eaten in a meal in the boiling water to blanch for one minute. For vegetables with thick leaves, blanch for two minutes. This way, all the pesticide residues are eliminated, because pesticides are diluted once they are heated. After blanching, strain the vegetables and put into a wok to then stir-fry, or place onto a plate, and drizzle cooking oil on the vegetable leaves. For saltier flavor, drizzle some soy sauce and mix to blend in the flavor.

For fruits that are consumed with skin still on, we can also blanch them for one minute before eating. Fruits are more nutritious when eaten with their skins on, because the skins have more than double the nutritional value of the flesh of the fruits. Therefore, try to eat fruits with their skins if at all possible, so that you can absorb all the nutrients from the fruits.

Use one thousand cubic centimeters of clean water. Add two tablespoons of baking soda and the juice of one lime. Soak fruits and vegetables in the soda water and stir by hand for approximately three minutes. This should get rid of the pesticides.

For leafy vegetables, such as Napa cabbage, Savoy cabbage, bok choy, white cabbage, lettuce, and so forth, remove the outer leaves. Blanch the inner leaves with boiling hot water, or wash each leaf individually under running water.

If possible, do not consume vegetables raw. There are many pests and pesticides on raw vegetables, and they are difficult to wash clean. Pesticides are difficult to wash off completely with water. Especially water-soluble pesticides—those are absorbed by the plants from their roots, enter into the inside of the vegetables, and are impossible to wash off. Therefore, eat salads less frequently; if pesticides are consumed, that could cause meningitis.

As the Modern Diet Becomes Luxurious, Our Bodies Become Odorous

When Monk was going to school thirty years ago, whether I took the train or the bus, I felt that few passengers had body odor. Now when Monk takes the airplane or train, the strong odors from human bodies are overwhelming. After many years of a very light-flavored vegetarian diet, smelling body odor suffocates me and makes breathing difficult. As a result, now Monk habitually wears a mask before boarding any flight or train.

Our diets have become more and more rich and abundant, but our bodies have also become more stinky. When you are inside a very crowded bus in the summer, you can smell the terrible odor coming from the underarms of young men and women. The indescribable odor is especially dizzying coming from women with body odor who try to cover it with perfume.

Among the undesirable human body odors, the most problematic is the underarm odor. This odor comes from the secretions of underarm sweat glands—it is pungent sweat! And the reason why underarm sweat carries such pungent smell has to do with food.

The sweat glands located in the underarms are especially sensitive to metabolic responses. When the blood is not alkaline enough to neutralize the harmful acidic substances within it, these acidic substances will, in turn, be secreted by the underarm sweat glands. This secretion contains compounds of amino acids, cholesterol, and iron, as well as other acidic substances that have not been neutralized. [All these substances] accumulate under the arms and exude a strong, pungent odor. Therefore, we know that the only way to prevent underarm odor is to maintain ideal alkalinity in the blood.

Therefore, the underarm sweat glands can most concretely reflect the state of metabolism within the human body. From the underarm odor, we can tell that there is unhealthy blood in the body containing a lot of harmful acidic substances. Switching to a vegetarian diet can make the blood turn alkaline, neutralize these harmful acidic substances in the blood, and finally get rid of them and eliminate the terrible smell. Therefore, people who eat vegetarian diets do not have bad body odor.

Eat Less Meat to Save the World

The global population currently numbers six billion, and everyone has such hungry appetites! So whenever a new day dawns, countless butchers hold up their cleavers, and instantly countless sentient beings lose their lives. Their corpses pile up higher than Mount Tai, their blood pooled together overflows Lake Dongting,[6] and their calls for help roar like thunder. All that killing is truly very cruel.

Currently, it is very popular to eat meat in Taiwan. Every year, we consume more than two hundred million chickens. In addition to those, the consumption of cows and sheep, ducks and geese, fish and shrimp, increases the number to billions of lives. Taiwan has indeed become a fearsome killing field for animals.

With several billion animal lives eaten in Taiwan annually, in ten years we will be responsible for killing tens of billions of animal lives. The resentful spirits of these animals hover over Taiwan, and that hatred is hard to resolve. When all that hatred accumulates to a point of saturation, there will befall a huge negative karmic force that will naturally come back to the people, and our nation will suffer terrible warfare. This is the unchanging principle of karmic retribution. [. . .][7]

All the people in Taiwan should stop eating meat now, so that we can avoid the misfortune of warfare, and our relatives can all avoid the suffering of lost lives. Furthermore, meat products now contain many chemical toxins, and consuming them can lead to the unspeakable sufferings of serious illnesses like cancer, strokes, and high blood pressure.

Therefore, to save our nation from the disaster of war, the general public should have the self-redemptive spirit to save the nation by eating less meat. This is the urgent duty of all Taiwanese people—we must not procrastinate.

Therefore, promoting vegetarianism as a movement is far more meaningful than any other action. It is also more functional and practical than any preservation effort. Therefore, Monk calls on everyone to join hands in promoting vegetarianism. It will not only make you healthier but also make people more compassionate and the world more peaceful and kind.

Hopefully, after you read this article, even if you cannot immediately start on a vegetarian diet, at least please treasure your own health, and reduce your consumption of meat. It is limitless merit not to contribute to the karmic cycle of killing. Even if you cannot reduce the meat you eat, please at least do not hinder the determination of family members or others to go vegetarian.

The Karma of Many Diseases and Few Diseases
Among All Sentient Beings

According to the Buddha in the *Sūtra of the Buddha's Explanation of Distinctions in Karmic Retribution for the Layman Śuka*,[8] frequent donations of medicine or persuading others to donate medicine to treat the ill can lead to better health and fewer illnesses. Chengte[9] Charity Chinese Hospital permanently provides free medicine to members of the sangha and people in poverty. As for regular people, whether you have money or not, when you come to Chengte Hospital, you can donate at will for the medical services you receive. There is absolutely no set fee table, and we never charge fees for registration or services. There are many members of the Chengte Medical Charitable Foundation around the nation who donate NT $100 [USD $3.50] each month. They support the funding of the Medical Charitable Foundation so that we can regularly purchase beneficial medicine to give to the members of the sangha and sentient beings in poverty.

Monk truly appreciates the Medical Foundation members around the nation making monthly donations over the long term in support of the compassionate medical fund. Volunteers are also always fundraising tirelessly, so that Chengte Hospital can always purchase beneficial medicine to treat all sentient beings, so that they can be liberated from suffering. Monk is touched and comforted by the limitless merit everyone accumulates!

You see, when the general public come to Chengte's Chinese medicine clinic, because they are given five to seven servings of herbal tonics, and we do not charge fees for registration or services, every patient can save at least NT $1,500 [USD $50] each visit. In the twenty-five years since we started Chengte's clinic, we have donated countless medicines to sentient beings in poverty, as well as to the general public. We have helped many who suffered from pain and diseases and treated illnesses that big hospitals could not treat. We completely depend on the nationwide members of the Chengte Medical Charitable Foundation. Every month, everybody donates NT $100 here and NT $100 there. In twenty-five years, we have given out the equivalent of NT $50 million [USD $1.75 million] in medication and treatments.

So, as the Buddha would say, all the Chengte members and fundraising volunteers often offer beneficial medicine to people and raise medical funds to save lives. Since everyone accumulates limitless and boundless merit, we will live long lives and attain great health!

NOTES

1. For more discussion of Chinese morality books, see Clart and Scott 2014.

2. For examples of confluences between Chinese Buddhist and Daoist views on vegetarianism, see H. Lu 2002 and chapter 1 in Mollier 2008. Chinese medical classics, such as *The Yellow Emperor's Inner Classic (Huangdi neijing)*, typically encourage a diet that includes grains, fruits, meats, and vegetables and consider consuming meat to be nourishing, especially when it is the appropriate amount and suitable for the individual's disposition and condition (Unschuld 2003: 300).

3. Cheng Yen, who founded Tzu-Chi Compassionate Relief, was his disciple. Sheng Yen, who founded Dharma Drum Mountain (*Fagu shan*), and Hsing Yun, who founded Buddha Light Mountain (*Foguang shan*), also trace their interpretations of Humanistic Buddhism directly to Taixu and Taixu's disciples.

4. Excerpts from Changlyu 2014: 12, 17–20, 204–207, 232–35.

5. "Coldness" and "hotness" here do not refer to temperature but rather to traditional Chinese categories of the natural constitution of each person's individual physical state.

6. Mount Tai is a mountain in Shandong Province, China, and Lake Dongting is located in Hunan Province, China. In vernacular Chinese speech, they are referenced generically to signify enormous height and volume, respectively.

7. A portion of this chapter discussing the morality of vegetarianism has been omitted.

8. MN.135. *Culakam-sūtra.*

9. Chengte is the official English name of Changlyu's organization.

Hybridities and Innovations

15. Taiwanese Tantra

Guru Wuguang's *Art of Yogic Nourishment and the Esoteric Path* (1966)

CODY R. BAHIR

The excerpts translated below are from a Chinese-language treatise on the relationship among yoga, Esoteric Buddhism, and Daoist internal alchemy first published in 1966. Its author, Guru Wuguang (1918–2000), was a Taiwanese Chan monk, Shingon Buddhist priest, folk healer, and advanced practitioner of Kundalini yoga. He is famous throughout the Chinese-speaking Buddhist world for resurrecting Zhenyan (mantra; literally, "True Word"), an extinct form of Esoteric Buddhism that many believe flourished during the Tang dynasty. The Buddhist community he founded, the Mantra School Bright Lineage (*Zhenyan-zong guangmingliu*), is headquartered in a large complex in the rural mountains of Kaohsiung in Southern Taiwan and has branches throughout Taiwan and Hong Kong, as well as an offshoot in Malaysia. Before becoming a monk, Wuguang worked as a bamboo furniture maker, merchant sailor, and construction worker. He also performed exorcisms of both homes and people, and created medicinal herbal concoctions, which he sold out of his personal laboratory.

Wuguang's yogic treatise, *The Art of Yogic Nourishment and the Esoteric Path*, is his earliest published book. He wrote it while serving as a member of Taiwan's oldest Buddhist monastery, Zhuxi temple, in Tainan. The treatise was first published in 1966 as a two-volume set. The first volume links the practice of yoga to specific Buddhist concepts and Daoist alchemical techniques while outlining the fundamental components of Kundalini practice. The second volume is a

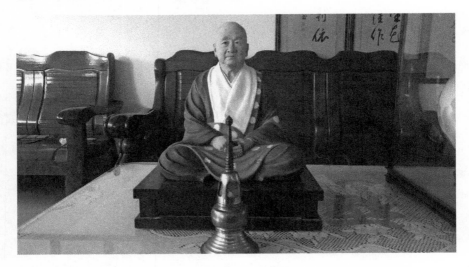

FIGURE 15.1 STATUE OF WUGUANG AT THE TEMPLE OF UNIVERSAL
BRIGHTNESS IN KAOHSIUNG, TAIWAN.
Source: Cody R. Bahir.

self-study course with instructions on how to perform various yogic exercises
and tantric practices. Wuguang's intended audience consisted of fellow Buddhist
monastics. He desired to convince his Dharma-kin that physical exercise was a
vital component of monastic life and that, although foreign, Indian yoga has
much to offer Chinese religionists.

In exploring Wuguang's writings, this chapter showcases the impact globalization has had on modern East Asian Buddhism in general and Taiwanese
religious practice in particular. In addition to the Chinese Chan and Daoist
traditions to which Wuguang belonged, passages in this chapter reference
Japanese martial arts, Shintō, and Tibetan as well as Indian forms of yoga. The
presence of each of these elements is rooted in the Japanese colonization of
Taiwan and the influx of Tibetan Buddhist masters after the Chinese Civil War.
In addition, the introductory section translated below explicitly states that
Western academia provided the inspiration for the work's composition. The
following section harmonizes Mahāyāna ontological doctrines concerning
Emptiness with Chinese concept of *qi*. Wuguang then outlines the key components of correct yogic breathing. From there, he concludes by contrasting Daoist
and Buddhist mantra recitation.

Wuguang firmly believed in the unity between mind and body, as well as
humanity's potential to perform feats that some would label as "magical" or
"supernatural." Thus, he was greatly troubled by the modernist tendency to
separate mind from matter and to label the miraculous as "superstitious."
Wuguang's displeasure was exacerbated by the fact that many influential
twentieth-century East Asian Buddhist reformers, attempting to make

Buddhism suitable for the modern world, had adopted a dualistic distinction between mind and matter and had attempted to purge Buddhism of its more esoteric side. The passages below represent Wuguang's response to such pressures. However, Wuguang was not a fundamentalist who rejected science and empirical thinking. Rather, he was a modernist who thought that science was the key to understanding the spiritual. His passionate belief in the underlying harmony between classic and modern, as well as the constituent parts of the human experience, reverberates throughout his work.

The excerpts below were chosen for their utility in understanding Wuguang's thoughts and his place within modern Buddhist discourse. Additionally, they clearly outline the underlying mechanics of his hybrid Buddho-Daoist yoga, describe how to perform a number of preliminary exercises, and explain how to put the core principles into practice while engaged in mundane activities.

FURTHER READING

Bahir, Cody R. 2013. "Buddhist Master Wuguang's (1918–2000) Taiwanese Web of the Colonial, Exilic and Han." *Electronic Journal of East and Central Asian Religions* 1 (1): 81–93.

Bianchi, Ester. 2004. "The Tantric Rebirth Movement in Modern China: Esoteric Buddhism Revivified by the Japanese and Tibetan Traditions." *Acta Orientalia Academiae Scientiarum Hungarica* 57 (1): 31–54.

Kohn, Livia. 2006. "Yoga and Daoyin." In *Daoist Body Cultivation*, edited by Livia Kohn. Magdalena, N. Mex.: Three Pines.

Liu, Xun. 2012. "Scientizing the Body for the Nation: Chen Yingning and the Reinvention of Daoist Inner Alchemy in 1930s Shanghai." In *Daoism in the Twentieth Century: Between Eternity and Modernity*, edited by David A. Palmer. Berkeley: University of California Press.

Excerpts from *The Art of Yogic Nourishment and the Esoteric Path*

Introduction[1]

For five thousand years, humans have been tirelessly investigating the secrets of the universe. Each investigator obtained a single piece of the mystery, which was then studied by later generations. This has made it impossible to glimpse a complete picture. As time passed and civilization advanced, more people penned their doctrines in order to promote them. The result is that there are hundreds of schools of thought, each with its own merits. It is a shame that the topics of which they spoke remain murky, without any clear exposition. When we read this type of literature, even if we expend a great deal of mental energy, it feels as though we cannot understand it.

The literature of which I speak concerns prolonging life, managing illness, and Daoist cultivation. Originally, Daoism was the philosophical school of purity and nonaction. Later, it became concerned with the elixir of eternal life, practical alchemy, male and female, *yin-yang*, sexual intercourse, the harvesting and collection of pharmaceuticals, religious offerings of fire and water, and practices related to pregnancy.[2] However, it has never been clearly explained how to use these practices in one's daily life. Furthermore, the massive number of Daoist texts and Buddhist *sūtras* can make people sigh in awe. They do not know where to begin studying, and beginners with a shallow understanding do not even dare to ask. Consequently, classic literary works from the past have become obsolete and nothing more than material for scholars to leisurely discuss.

Even though there are Eastern people who have both researched and practiced techniques aimed at achieving long life and health, they are reticent and do not publicly acknowledge it. Their accomplishments are remarkable, but they are increasingly secretive. It is as though they fear being disturbed if the world discovers them. Even if one such individual occasionally publishes a work to popularize their ideas, the book itself will include statements such as "one must have oral instruction from a master to understand the details." As a result, we have no sources to gain insight, and, as time has passed, people of later generations have no interest in these subjects. This style is an Eastern shortcoming. Westerners are not like this. Western academics spare no effort in their investigations of and research into Asia. They then make the results of their experiments public. Now, they have already turned Daoism, yoga, and Buddhism into practical, everyday topics.

While our Chinese scholars of Daoist longevity practices have been secretive, there has been an increasing interest in Indian yoga. The East and West have simultaneously become interested in this valuable method for achieving physical health and longevity. Recently, a great number of yoga studios have been established, enabling anyone to go and practice on site. We [Taiwanese] have only the opportunity to study the physically strengthening martial art of *taijiquan*, as there are still are not many people promoting breathing techniques[3] or yoga.

It is said that yoga was invented in India five thousand years ago. There are multiple aspects within Buddhism that come from yoga, and the most yogic-like form of Buddhism is Esoteric Buddhism [i.e., Tibetan Vajrayāna and Japanese Shingon].[4] In addition to prolonging life, Esoteric Buddhism can bring out one's supernatural abilities, *prajñā* [literally "wisdom," but here referring to powers that come with wisdom], and enable one to achieve salvation.

In this book, I introduce the universal principles that connect humans and all living things, discuss yogic techniques, and [discuss] the Esoteric Buddhist path of salvation. I have united the underlying key theories and practices to write this book. It is my hope that readers will achieve long life and obtain great supernatural abilities, *prajñā*, and escape *saṃsāra*. To this end, I have chosen not to use the encoded language of old, for it is too convoluted and complicated. Rather, I have synthesized and adapted the ancient teachings in accordance with the aim of modern people, that aim being verifiable evidence. It is a blessing if fellow lovers of the path find mistakes herein.

Buddhist Doctrine

Buddhism is an empty matter. *Emptiness* (*śūnyatā*) means that the characteristics of all things in the universe are produced by causes and conditions.[5] Some people think that *Emptiness* means that nothing is real, but this is a mistaken understanding. All phenomena within the universe are ceaselessly alive. They absorb material from the air, which replaces old matter while being turned into new forms of matter. Thus, the new is ceaselessly superseding the old. This demonstrates how everything rises from causes and conditions. From a mundane perspective, the short-term aspects of this process are invisible. However, we can observe that the appearances of phenomena change after a few days or years. For example, our bodies completely regenerate every seven years.

The myriad phenomena absorb the great *qi* of the universe. Each arises and disappears according to causes and conditions. This is an irrefutable fact. Each nonvirtuous action a person performs produces negative karma. This negatively impacts the body, causing dramatic changes and early death. All Buddhist teachings regarding karma are concerned with human thoughts, which is the function of one's spirit—and spirit can control matter. Therefore, Buddhism's main concerns are to bring about a mental transformation, to revert our consciousness to its original state through self-introspection, to cultivate our minds, nourish our nature, and thus avert negative physical repercussions. This is the practical application of *prajñā*. This enables one to reach the great path of enlightenment while making the body healthy. However, most of us mistake the false for the real and constantly misapply our mental faculties without ever stopping. This sort of mentality is called delusion.[6]

People with seriously deluded minds age quickly and are sickly. Their mentality causes their *qi* and blood to stagnate, making them susceptible to catching colds and more serious ailments.[7] Anger not only puts one in a bad mood but can also make one lose consciousness or even lead to high blood pressure. All sights, sounds, smells, tastes, and feelings influence the circulation of bodily *qi* and blood. The human desire to satisfy one's appetites is so inexhaustible that we are willing to wholeheartedly sacrifice ourselves. Some people say that this is natural, but that is gravely incorrect. People's desires should be rational. Their exaggeration is the product of mental attitudes. Naturally, we are able to live for a very long time, but violating the natural order brings about early death. Buddhism teaches that we must "illuminate our minds and see our original nature."[8] First, we must understand that our minds contain ideas that go against the natural order; then we can make sure we do not deviate therefrom by inspecting our original nature. If people can control their desires, then they can achieve peace of mind. Peace of mind will allow our *qi* and blood to circulate harmoniously, which will lead to a healthy body and joyous life.

The Method of Yogic Breathing

Breathing is the most important element for human survival. As the inability to breathe would equal death, controlling one's breath means controlling one's life. The longer one's breath, the longer one's life. Thus, long breath and long life are one and the same. This principle not only applies to humans, as any living creature that stops breathing dies after just a few minutes. There are some people who can add years to their life by fasting for months while only consuming small amounts of clean water.[9] However, if someone were to quit breathing for just a few minutes, their life would be forfeited—like drowning under water. People depend on breath, for it gives them life.

This is explained in terms of physiology. The bodily organs absorb oxygen from the air and their nutritious materials are transformed into blood. This replenishes the body and dispels fatigue. However, if a person's breath is unhealthy, their fatigue cannot be dispelled, as it is impossible for nutrients to reach the bloodstream. It is a physiological fact that this leads to poor health and a short life. This principle is not limited to physiology, as it can also be understood in spiritual terms. The ancients often spoke about the interdependent relationship between the mind and body, as well as the single substance within the air from which all activity and life spring. In yogic terms, this substance is referred to as *prāṇa*, and, in [Chinese terms,] it is known as *qi*. Know that this universal *prāṇa* or *qi* exists within all living beings and permeates the entire Dharma realm. Therefore, the universe is not composed of matter and air, but of *prāṇa/qi*. Even modern physical sciences teach that there is an ethereal substance, a great spiritual force, that exists in the universe. However, it is immaterial and has yet to be conclusively identified. From a yogic perspective, it is as necessary for one's life force as oxygen is to the blood because it performs the same vitalizing function. Like oxygen, *prāṇa/qi* from the air enters the blood, is absorbed by the nervous system, then travels through the veins, circulating throughout the whole body. Consuming *prāṇa/qi* is also indispensable for mental functions and the production of emotions, which is why it must be continuously replenished.

Ancient Daoist masters spoke of a deep-breathing method referred to as "breathing through one's heels."[10] This entails breathing through the backbone and down to the heels of the feet. They discovered that there is an intimate connection between the spirit and the breath and that the oscillation of the breath determines the length of one's life. Similarly, yogic practitioners invented various breath techniques to regulate one's life-span. Every person wishes for a long, healthy life devoid of sickness. However, people who understand the fundamental principles of *qi* are very rare, which is why so many of us live short lives plagued by illness. People's desire for fame, wealth, and beauty lead them to sacrifice their lives without hesitation. It is truly the greatest of shames that they are so reckless when it comes to preserving their lives. Yogic practitioners, on the other hand, place great importance on the fundamentals of life. Thus, they use various philosophical, biological, and intellectual principles to achieve levels of health and longevity that surpass those of the average person.

Since *prāṇa* functions as the fundamental element of human life, it is found throughout the universe, and there is nowhere that it is not present. People's physical and mental activity is made possible by absorbing various amounts of it from the air, food, water, earth, and the sun's rays. There is nothing that *prāṇa/qi* does not bestow. People who wish to live a long life and nurture their life force must know how to absorb and metabolize *prāṇa*.

There are multiple methods for metabolizing *prāṇa*, all of which boil down to exhaling and inhaling—nothing more than how to bring the breath in and keep it inside. The yogic breathing method is known as "treasure-vase breathing."[11] This entails "filling the vase" by filling the lungs with air like filling a vase with clean water, "assembling the vase" by exhaling in a manner akin to pouring the water out of a vase, and "resting the vase" by momentarily holding the breath and retaining it within the body without allowing any to leak out.

Prāṇa is the primordial element of life because it is the fundamental force underlying the universe. If there was no *prāṇa* in the air we breathe and the food we eat, then these would not sustain our lives, since they would be devoid of nourishment for us to metabolize. On the other hand, one can create a physical reservoir of *prāṇa* by consuming and metabolizing a surplus thereof. If you were to physically touch someone whose body had such a surplus of *prāṇa* energy, all your illnesses could be cured by receiving the magnetic influence of their *qi*.

There are a great many daily activities that correspond to yogic breathing. High-ranking monks often live for a very long time. When they perform *sūtra* recitation according to the prescribed chanting methods, they naturally breathe gently and prolongedly with power from the abdomen. This is in accordance with yogic breathing methods. People of old said, "The blessed are always at the gates of laughter," for when people laugh, they naturally exhale forcefully, pushing their diaphragm down with force from their abdomen. This, too, resembles yogic breathing. Moreover, since their mind and spirit are peaceful, their health improves, and their life is blessed. Other activities such as reciting poetry or singing out loud also entail forceful, deep, and prolonged breathing and are in accordance with yogic breathing. People who are unaware of these principles but breathe in a yogic manner can also attain good health and longevity.

There are people in every country all over the world who are unfamiliar with these breathing techniques and who recognize that smoking cigarettes is an unhealthy habit. Despite the fact that [cigarettes] contain nicotine—which causes physical harm—when people smoke, their breath is gentle and prolonged in accordance with the breathing methods of metabolizing *prāṇa*. This is why taking a few inhalations of cigarette smoke when one is uncomfortable can arouse the mind and dispel fatigue. If one can thoroughly grasp this underlying principle and breathe gently and prolongedly from the abdomen as though they were smoking—without inhaling toxic substances—then it would be in accordance with yogic breathing. One's body, mind, and self would then be peaceful and joyful. When a person's mind is groggy, they should speak in a loud voice. Doing so expels the stale *qi* inside the body that is lacking in life force. The mind will then naturally clear, and both mind and body will become peaceful. Japanese Shintō priests also have a chanting method that elongates the breath. When they perform the funerary rite,[12] they exhale prolongedly while singing the prayers in accordance with yogic breathing. This is why many Shintō priests are very healthy and live a long time.

To "assemble the vase," focus your mental energy while momentarily holding in a breath. Then, exhale as though a very heavy thing is rising out of your lungs, while *qi* enters your *dantian* [i.e., the area below one's navel]. All of your mental and physical energy should be concentrated at your waist and lower abdomen, making the *dantian* the focus of your attention. Naturally relax your shoulders and contract your anus. Creating the *qi*-vase is a sublime method to bring about mind–body unity.

You can use the above breathing method to influence others through spiritual means. If you are facing a physical confrontation, you can use the above breathing method, since victory depends on who has the strongest breath. In Japanese martial arts, this is called *kiai-jutsu*.[13] Nourishing your health and religious achievement requires metabolizing the universe's *prāṇa*. Those who have delved deeply into this method have more powerful breath. Therefore, people with peaceful bodies and minds certainly have a lot of power in their abdomens, as this is the power of their *qi*-vase. In the art of yoga, it is known that that the *qi*-vase can awaken our body's internal life force. This is why the *qi*-vase is especially emphasized in *prāṇa* metabolism. This topic is referred to as "the power of *qi*," meaning that there is power when exhaling *qi*. Every action is made manifest upon exhaling *qi*. Fighting, fencing, judo, and playing ball are all connected to exhaling *qi*. Take fencing for example. First, you inhale *qi*. It then resides in your body. When you exhale 20 percent, you strike. If you do not regulate your *qi*, your exhalations will be erratic.

The Function of Mantra Recitation

Talisman writing and mantra recitation are performed by [members of] a certain stream of Daoism.[14] Since ancient times, very few people have known its origins. It is said that Zhang Daoling [34–156 CE] founded this form of Daoism [the Celestial Masters] based on the teachings of Laozi.[15] Truthfully, however, Laozi's teachings and talismanic Daoism have little in common. Furthermore, mantras already existed during the time of the Yellow Emperor, rendering this origination myth a case of false attribution. Nevertheless, mantra recitation influences one's faith.

Mantra recitation has three primary aspects: vocalization, hearing, and mental feeling. The sound emitted by the reciter is similar to hypnosis, as it has the power to influence his own faith, as well as that of others who hear it. This is especially efficacious with devout individuals. Mantric forms of Daoism [involve reciting] mantras for every occasion and every action, including sleeping, waking in the morning, using the restroom, washing one's hands, showering, eating, traveling, breathing, swallowing saliva, changing clothes, treating illness, exorcism, writing talismans, etc. They have countless mantras, all of which draw from the power of external deities.[16] People whose mantra recitation is spiritually potent do not know wherefrom that potency stems.

Esoteric Buddhism can be called the "Mantra Vehicle," "*Dhāraṇī* Vehicle," or "True-Word Vehicle." Most people incorrectly believe that its form of mantra recitation is the same as [that of] Daoism and draws upon the power of external deities. However, after investigation, it becomes clear that it uses a form of yogic power drawn from both the individual self and external deities. As the sound one emits while vocalizing mantras comes from inside the body, it stimulates the channels [i.e., meridians] through vibration, arousing the concealed force of one's life-*qi*. Yogic practitioners can awaken this incomparable force that lies sleeping within their channels by refining *qi* and reciting mantras. This results in a mutual correspondence with the great force of the universe.[17] Sitting in *chan* is one meditation method that can arouse the mind. But by combining meditation with *qi*-refinement and mantra recitation as taught by yoga, it is possible to arouse one's life force much quicker—which is a unique characteristic of Esoteric Buddhism.

The contents of mantras are very mysterious, although scholars who research India do in fact clearly understand them. However, one need not translate or understand their meanings, as simply chanting them is adequate. Even though Daoist and yogic mantras have similarities, as time has passed, Daoism has accumulated many different mantras, making this practice more mysterious and increasingly difficult to transmit to others.

NOTES

1. The translator has been asked to state that, while I have sought to do justice to Wuguang's writings and make them accessible to Western audiences, the original Chinese text remains authoritative for understanding his teachings. The passages translated here are taken from the 1996 reprint (Wuguang 1996: 1–4, 16–18, 43–49, 57–58).

2. Here, Wuguang is using the distinction between "philosophical" and "religious" Daoism. The former—which never existed as an independent philosophical tradition—is based upon teachings found in the Chinese classical texts known as the *Daode jing* and the *Zhuangzi*. The latter denotes religious, magical, and alchemical practices incorporated by the Daoist religious tradition. See Komjathy 2013: 4–10.

3. *Tuna* is short for *tugu naxin*, "exhaling old and breathing in new [breath]," which is a general term for breathing techniques aimed at replenishing old or stagnant *qi* with fresh *qi*.

4.   For more information on Esoteric Buddhism, see Orzech, Payne, and Sørensen 2011: 3–18.

5.   For an explanation of the link between Buddhist beliefs concerning "emptiness" and doctrines concerning "causes and conditions," see Lopez 2001: 24–33.

6.   According to Buddhism, delusion is one of three cardinal negative virtues, the other two being greed and hate.

7.   According to traditional Chinese medicine, the stagnation of one's *qi* is the root cause of many serious physical and psychological ailments.

8.   The "nature" spoken of here refers to an individual's "original nature" and is synonymous with "Buddha nature," which represents a sentient being's potential to become a buddha.

9.   In his autohagiography, Wuguang (1999) claims to have done this for long periods of time during the years before he wrote his yoga treatise.

10. For information regarding heel breathing and related Daoist practices, see Komjathy 2013: 192–95.

11. The breathing method described by Wuguang here is a form of "vase breathing" common in many Tibetan yogic practices. For more examples, see Germano 1997: 296.

12. The *chinkon* rite is a funerary rite aimed at pacifying and aiding the spirit of a deceased person.

13. *Kiai-jutsu* is the art of using shouts during combat. This is primarily a facet of Japanese, rather than Chinese, martial arts.

14. The use of talismanic magic for protection, curing illness, and soteriological benefits is widespread in many forms of Daoism. In fact, the main topic of many sacred Daoist scriptures concerns the creation and use of talismans. See Bokenkamp 2008: 35–38.

15. Laozi is traditionally attributed with writing the Chinese work *Daodejing*. Zhang Daoiling is credited with founding the Celestial Masters school of Daoism (*Tianshi dao*) during the Han dynasty, based upon a vision of Laozi. Zhang's Celestial Masters Daoism was the first form of Daoism to resemble an organized religion. See Poceski 2009: 65–67.

16. Here, Wuguang references the "self–other" distinction used to distinguish different forms of Buddhist practice. Practices that rely on the aid of external deities, such as being reborn into the Western Paradise of Amitāyus through the recitation of his name, are said to draw upon "other-power," whereas those that function solely on the efforts of the individual practitioner, such as silent meditation, are fueled by "self-power." For more information, see Ford 2002.

17. "Mutual correspondence" (*ganying*) is an ancient Chinese metaphysical belief that geographically distant, categorically similar phenomena can influence each other. For more information, see Sharf 2002: 119.

16. Making a Modern Image of Jīvaka

"First Encounters with Jīvaka Komārabhacca, the High Guru of Healers and the Inspiration for Sculpting His Image" (1969)

ANTHONY LOVENHEIM IRWIN

Jīvaka[1] is a medical hero of the Buddhist world. He was the Buddha Gautama's physician, famously curing the Buddha's constipation with a special laxative and also attending to the health of the Buddha's early disciples (see *Anthology*, vol. 1, chs. 1, 20).[2] Throughout South, East, and Southeast Asia, Jīvaka is known by many names, including "Father Doctor," "King of Physicians," and "High Guru of Healers." He is a medical symbol that has been transmitted through Buddhist space and time, and examples of Jīvaka worship are present in Pāli, Sanskrit, Tibetan, and Chinese scriptures.[3] Jīvaka is highly revered in present-day Thailand, where he is honored as the principle guru of Thai Traditional Medicine (TTM) practitioners, including healers, massage therapists, and herbal doctors, but this was not always the case.[4] This chapter is about the recreation or reinvention of Jīvaka in mid-twentieth-century Thailand.

Since the 1940s, images and amulets of Jīvaka have proliferated throughout Thailand, where they are worshiped on the shrines of TTM practitioners and called upon for their healing properties. Most of the images of Jīvaka in Thailand are modeled after the one found on the grounds of Wat Somananam Borihan, a Vietnamese temple in Bangkok also commonly known as Wat Yuan Saphan Khao (figures 16.1 and 16.2). This highly realistic image was sculpted in 1954 by Khun Choti Samosot under the instruction of Wat Yuan Saphan Khao's abbot, Master (*luang pho*) Bao Oeng (1906–1964). The selection translated below, "First Encounters

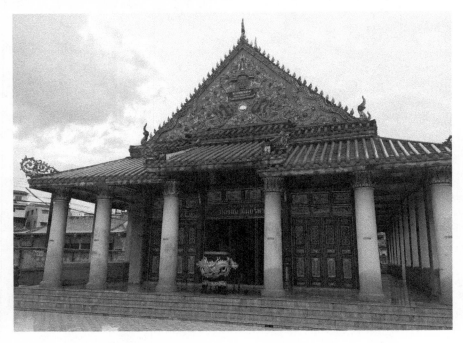

FIGURE 16.1 GROUNDS OF WAT SOMANANAM BORIHAN (WAT YUAN
SAPHAN KHAO), WITH A VIEW OF THE SHRINE HALL IN WHICH THE
STATUE OF JĪVAKA STANDS.
Source: C. Pierce Salguero

with Jīvaka Komārabhacca, the High Guru of Healers and the Inspiration for
Sculpting His Image," is an account of that image's inception and creation, as
well as the miraculous occurrences that brought it into the world.

Master Bao Oeng was a high-ranking member of the Annam Nikaya, a small sect
of Vietnamese monks officially recognized by the Thai state.[5] The Annam Nikaya
is a Mahāyāna sect, which differentiates it from Thailand's Theravada Buddhist
majority. While propitiating statues of deities related to healing is routine in
Mahāyāna and may have influenced Master Bao Oeng's reverence for Jīvaka, tradition holds that this innovation was not related to his Vietnamese background.
Instead, it stemmed from his role as a celebrated spirit medium and his direct contact with the world of spirits. We usually talk about the transmission of religious
ideas, symbols, and traditions as being the work of human actors—the people who
teach, translate, and carry religious forms and texts through time and space. In
the account translated below, however, Jīvaka's spirit seeks out Master Bao Oeng as
his disciple and then manifests in physical form to serve as a model for the sculpting of this now-famous image at Wat Yuan Saphan Khao.

This short account is about the work of art in the realm of miraculous repro-
duction. From ancient chronicles to contemporary rumors, accounts of Buddhist
material and spatial production, such as the one provided by this story of the

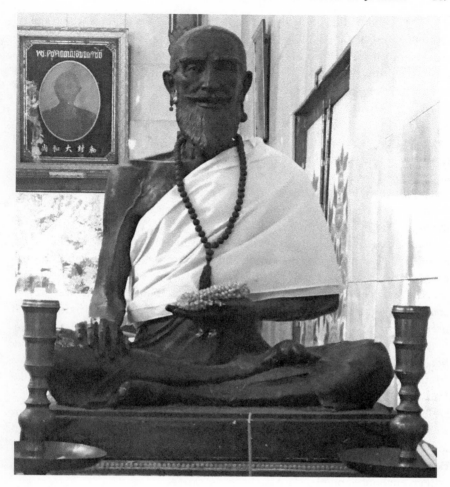

FIGURE 16.2 THE STATUE SCULPTED IN 1954 BY KHUN CHOTI SAMOSOT,
AFTER JĪVAKA'S REVELATION.
Source: C. Pierce Salguero

Jīvaka statue, are imbued with miraculous events, divine interventions, and
numinous powers.[6] Of course, however, these objects and spaces, and the stories
of their creation, are always framed by the historical and cultural contexts in
which they unfold. The story of the production of the Jīvaka image at Wat Yuan
Saphan Khao shows that spirits can play an integral role in the shape Buddhism
takes as it intersects with modernity. The image came into the world at a time
when Buddhism in Thailand (and Bangkok more specifically) had been experiencing the forces of modernization for at least one hundred years.

One of the more important elements of modern Buddhism in Thailand is a
concern for historical accuracy. The account below describes that when Khun
Choti presented Master Bao Oeng with his first attempt at sculpting Jīvaka in a
"Chinese style," the monk rejected it. Since Jīvaka was a man who lived during

the time of the Buddha, Master Bao Oeng insists that his facial features should resemble those of an Indian Brahmin. Master Bao Oeng's modern concern for the ethnic and historical accuracy of the image is actually the impetus for the account's primary miracle. To achieve the historical and ethnic accuracy that Master Bao Oeng requires, the monk calls Jīvaka's spirit to manifest on the tip of his thumb, which Khun Choti then uses as his first model to sculpt the image now enshrined at the temple. Other details in the accounts, such as the precise dates and times, the named university professors and officials who witnessed the miracle, and so forth, serve to further bolster the account's aura of accuracy and authoritativeness.

Finally, to understand this account as a reflection of modern Thai Buddhism, we must also consider how it is presented to the general public, and in what medium. The Jīvaka image was made in 1954, but the earliest printing of this account I have been able to find is in a 1969 cremation volume for a Thai royal, Mom Thongkham Singhara.[7] Printing and distributing collections of literature, religious writings, and poetry to mark funerary ceremonies emerged as a specific form of merit-making that followed the introduction of printing to the country.[8] Cremation volumes, then, are a particularly modern Thai Buddhist literary genre.

The translation below is from a cremation volume titled *Are Spirits Real or Not? and The History of Jīvaka Komārabhacca, High Guru of Healers*. It takes its name from the two main essays it contains. The story of the production of the Jīvaka image at Wat Saphan Khao, translated below, comes from the latter essay, which offers a resounding yes in answer to the question raised by the former: Are spirits real or not? This story about Jīvaka is notably bereft of the miraculous healings that Thai accounts often associated with the "High Guru of Healers." Nevertheless, it reminds us that the modern world is, for many people, still an enchanted one.

FURTHER READING

Horner, I. B. 2000. *The Book of the Discipline (Vinaya-Piṭaka)*. Volume 4, *Mahāvagga*. Oxford: Pali Text Society, 379–97.

Irwin, Anthony Lovenheim. 2017. "Partners in Power and Perfection: *Khrubas*, Construction, and *Khu Barami* in Chiang Rai, Thailand." In *Charismatic Monks of Lanna Buddhism*, edited by Paul T. Cohen. Copenhagen: Nordic Institute of Asian Studies, 87–114.

Salguero, C. Pierce. 2017. "Honoring the Teachers, Constructing the Lineage: A *Wai Khru* Ritual Among Healers in Chiang Mai, Thailand." In *Translating the Body: Medical Education in Southeast Asia*, edited by Hans Pols, C. Michele Thompson, and John Harley Warner, 295–318. Singapore: NUS.

Zysk, Kenneth G. 1998. *Asceticism and Healing in Ancient India: Medicine in the Buddhist Monastery*. Delhi: Motilal Banarsidass, 52–61.

"First Encounters with Jīvaka Komārabhacca, the High Guru of Healers and the Inspiration for Sculpting His Image"[9]

Master Bao Oeng's Testimony

On March 18, 1954, when I had the monastic rank of Ong Phochon Sunthon, I had contact with the spirit of Khun Phun Phen Chamrunchan, the deceased wife of Police Captain Thawi Chamrunchan. Her spirit came to me while I was in my residence, in the presence of two or three of my followers. When Khun Phun Phen was alive, she was a serious and devout Buddhist. Not long before she passed away, she came to me to fully devote herself as my student. I wholeheartedly accepted her devotion. After her funeral, Police Captain Thawi Chamrunchan, following his wife's wishes, had her remains installed in a small reliquary (chedi) built on a tiered finial on the top of my residence. Since then, Khun Phun Phen's spirit has stayed close to me.

During Thawi Chamrunchan's visit, the spirit of Khun Phun Phen entered him at 9:30 PM and said to me, "I [Khun Phun Phen] have come. I told you during a previous visit, Master Bao Oeng, that you are a healer who can cure many ailments, but I forgot to tell you that you should perform a ceremony requesting Venerable Jīvaka to come and assist you in your healing. You should offer yourself to Jīvaka as his disciple."

I then asked, "Who is Venerable Jīvaka?" Khun Phun Phen's spirit explained to me that when he was alive, Venerable Jīvaka was a physician who dedicated himself to the care of the Buddha and the original sangha donating medicine for their care. Intrigued, I asked, "On what day should I perform the ceremony to call his spirit, and what types of offering would be appropriate?"

Khun Phun Phen's spirit responded, "Perform the ceremony on the next full moon. As for the offerings, prepare a five-tray offering (khan ha) to donate to Venerable Jīvaka.[10] On Saturday, April 17, 1954, at 10:10 PM, I placed a five-tray offering prepared by Khun Wit Siwadit on a table that I set up on the porch of my residence. Then I offered prayers of obedience and called the spirit of Jīvaka, the High Guru of Healers, and requested that he accept me as his disciple. I asked to enter his lineage of healing, offering the khan ha donation as a way to introduce myself to him, so that he would know who I was.

Then, on Sunday, May 2, 1954, at 12:15 PM, I announced that I wanted to find a craftsperson to sculpt an image of the High Guru of Healers, Jīvaka. I therefore called on his spirit to appear on the tip of my thumb so that it could be used as a model for the image. This image would then be kept as a shrine for offerings to Jīvaka. Not long after, I was visited by the skilled sculptor Khun Choti Samosot (who has since passed away). I invited Khun Choti to my residence so that I could produce the image of Jīvaka for him to use as a model for the image. Khun Choti did not believe that I could produce an image for him through calling a spirit, but I told him that he would soon be convinced.

I then performed a ceremony to call the spirit of Jīvaka, the High Guru of Healers, to manifest a figure of his face so that Khun Choti could use it as a model for the image. When the figure appeared on the tip of my thumb, Khun Choti was so amazed that he exclaimed, "If I wasn't seeing this with my own eyes, I wouldn't believe it!"

Khun Choti then sculpted the image according to the form he saw on the tip of my thumb. It took two hours of sculpting until Khun Choti was done copying the face of Jīvaka. All in all, Khun Choti and his group of friends were thoroughly amazed by everything that had happened. Khun Choti gave his own account of the events to one of my other disciples.

Khun Choti Samosot's Testimony

This was the first time I ever came to Wat Yuan Saphan Khao, and, really, I just sort of wandered in here, following Master Chum Chai Khiri (a well-known Buddhist craftsperson) with whom I was working at the time. When I first entered the temple, I went to the merit-making pavilion, and I saw Master Bao Oeng perform a healing ceremony on a sick temple-goer. I instantly had faith in him and politely asked, "Master Bao Oeng, may I just sit here for a while as you care for this ailing person?" At that, Master Bao Oeng asked me, "You are a sculptor, aren't you?"

"Yes, I am," I answered. "Do you have something you would like me to make? If you have a sketch or model, please show it to me."

Master Bao Oeng said, "I want you to sculpt an image of Venerable Jīvaka."

When I heard Master Bao Oeng say that, I felt confused and a bit stupid because I didn't know who this Venerable Jīvaka was. When Master Bao Oeng saw the look of consternation on my face, he kindly explained, "Venerable Jīvaka was the Buddha's physician. I will call his figure to appear on the tip of my thumb as a model for you to work from."

When I heard these words from Master Bao Oeng, I felt like this was something I once knew but had forgotten. I also felt a bit skeptical and slightly amused because I didn't believe for a second that this monk was going to cause a figure to appear somehow on the tip of his thumb.

Just then, my friend who was with me, Professor Prasan Praempricha, who had lots of experience with spirit mediums, saw the look of doubt on my face. He quickly interjected, "This is the man for the job!" When I heard my friend volunteer me for the job, I was less than enthusiastic and utterly skeptical. We then prostrated before the monk, and I left the temple without any real interest in the monk's plan. That was on April 30, 1954.

The next day, I returned to the temple and met Master Bao Oeng at about 4 PM. He said to me, "Are you free tomorrow? I will call Venerable Jīvaka to appear on the tip of my thumb for you to use as a model for your sculpture."

"I am free," I quickly answered, accepting the job. I then left the temple to do some errands and returned to my house at around midnight. I sat down to rest for only a moment, and then a very strange feeling stirred in my hands. I immediately went and got some modeling clay. I figured that since Master Bao Oeng was in the Chinese monastic lineage,[11] the Jīvaka image that he wanted me to sculpt should be in the Chinese style and that Jīvaka should have the features of a Chinese deity. It rained all night, and I finished the image around 1 AM.

The next morning, I went to find two professors from Silpakorn University, Khun Chaloem and Khun Churairat, to accompany me to the temple and witness whatever was to unfold that day. We arrived at the temple around noon, and I presented Master Bao Oeng with the image I had sculpted the night before. When the monk saw that it was done in a very Chinese style, he said, "No! Jīvaka had Indian features, like a Brahmin, not Chinese!" He then told us to follow him to his residence.

As we sat there, Master Bao Oeng began the ceremony to call Jīvaka, which was simpler than I had expected. I watched his every move closely. He lit incense and placed some other offerings on his shrine. Then he said a prayer in Vietnamese and then in Pāli, so I had no idea what he was saying. At that time, I just wanted to see the image so I could make the sculpture.

Still holding the lit incense in his hand, Master Bao Oeng took his seat on his raised preaching platform. He then pointed the thumb of the hand that held the incense up in the air. My eyes fixed on the tip of that finger, which I saw transform into a white cloth that quickly expanded into a figure. I saw an image, but it was not very clear. I felt so amazed; this was unlike anything I had ever seen before.

Master Bao Oeng then shifted his position a bit, and, as a shimmering aura appeared, a figure came into focus on the tip of his thumb. I began molding my clay to resemble Master Bao Oeng's transformed thumb. I could hardly believe what was happening. As I was sculpting, I felt this elation, almost like I was going a bit mad. I just sat there and sculpted for about two hours without any plan or direction, as if I were in a type of trance.

Khun Chaloem and Khun Churairat, the professors from Silpakorn who were with me, can both attest that the image that I sculpted was similar to the figure we saw on Master Bao Oeng's thumb in every respect. When I finished sculpting, the three of us paid obeisance to Master Bao Oeng. I dared not take the image I had sculpted back to my house when I left the temple.

The next morning, I went to visit Khun Phraphichan Chorikit, the head of the Harbor Department. As we sat chatting, I began stroking the tip of my thumb, and, as I looked down, I saw an incredible miracle appear on the tip of my thumb. I began to see the same figure of Venerable Jīvaka that I had seen the day before on the tip of Master Bao Oeng's thumb. When my visit with Khun Phraphichan was over, I went directly to Wat Somananam Borihan. I met Master Bao Oeng in the ordination hall and lifted up my thumb to his guest, Khun In Thewaḍa (Sublieutenant of the Harbor Police). I asked him, with my thumb in his face,

"Do you see something here or not?" Khun In Thewada looked quickly and said, "Yes, I clearly see the face of a man with a beard." The figure was there for about two minutes, and I knew that it was Venerable Jīvaka.

Master Bao Oeng just sat there and laughed when he heard Khun In Thewada's response and then invited us both up to his residence. There, in his residence, Master Bao Oeng brought down the image that I had sculpted the day before. When Khun In saw the image, he cried "Yes! That's it!" He then quickly lowered himself and prostrated before the image. Upon seeing that, I came out of my stupor and began to believe that all of this was actually happening, that he had really seen the figure on my thumb, and that the image I had sculpted the day before was genuine. I then lowered myself and prostrated with sincere veneration before this image that I myself had sculpted.

Upon experiencing this miraculous and magical event, Khun In Thewada became a disciple of Master Bao Oeng. While requesting Master Bao Oeng as his master, he proclaimed, "I do not know what forces have brought me to this temple, I didn't really have a plan when I came here, but with this experience, having seen what I have seen, I am convinced [that these powers are real]."

The next day, another miracle occurred. At around noon, I came to the temple with one of my students at Silpakorn University, Khun Amphai, to assist with the production of the image. I told him the he should look at the tip of my thumb. He said that I was absolutely crazy, but when he sat and looked, the figure of Venerable Jīvaka appeared on the tip of my thumb after about five minutes. Not only did he reject what I told him, but he refused to even believe his own eyes. His doubt was insulting, so I told him to grab ahold of his own thumb and gaze at it. By the power of all that is sacred, he began to see a figure appear on the tip of his own thumb, but he saw it from the side. I asked him to describe and sketch what he was seeing. At the same time, I took a random piece of paper that was lying around the temple and sketched the figure on his thumb myself. While I was sitting there sketching, a group of police officers who were sitting around the temple ridiculed me, saying that I must have gone crazy. I took no notice of them and continued to sketch for about ten minutes.

That night, I took our drawings to Master Bao Oeng. Our sketches were identical to the image I had sculpted a couple of days before. I was then convinced that the image of Jīvaka was beyond what any artist could have thought up on their own and vowed to continue working on the image. When I looked again at my sketch, I saw that the English words "Medical Service" were printed on the back. When I went home, I opened my English dictionary and found that the words "Medical Service" refer to a place where people can receive medical attention. I then cried out, "This is either a crazy coincidence or due to some other powers!"

I now fully believe that spirits are real. Certain forces remain in the world according to one's merit or demerit and are the result of people's actions. I believe this because I have seen it with my own eyes, which is the most valuable type of evidence in the world.

Master Bao Oeng's Testimony

On the evening of Thursday, May 4, 1954, I had a large group of followers in my residence. At about 10 PM, Khun Soman Phongsuwan requested that I call on the bodhisattva Cintāmaṇicakra Avalokiteśvara[12] so he and his retinue could make offerings. We all went to the merit-making pavilion, and I identified Khun Chaum Watanachaeng, the nephew of the head of their group, to be the vessel for the bodhisattva. I began the ceremony, and Avalokiteśvara quickly entered the body of Khun Chaum, but not completely. His body just went limp right there. At that, one of my disciples, Prathum Chamsombun, was worried that Khun Chaum would not be able to handle it and offered herself as the vessel for Avalokiteśvara. Khun Prathum's intervention came just in time, because there was a possibility that the boy would not ever have come out of that state if it had gone on any longer. Avalokiteśvara left the boy's body and entered Khun Prathum completely. At that, Khun Chaum returned to normal.

After the group had made their offerings and requests of Avalokiteśvara, I said, "I have called Venerable Jīvaka here recently and want to ask what the proper type of comportment and offering he requires. Also, what does he require when entering someone's body as a vessel?"

The High Goddess answered, "You may call upon Jīvaka, but whatever vessel he enters must sit upon clean white cloth, as he is a very holy spirit."

Just then, Khun Prathum's hand pointed at Police Captain Thawi Chamrunchan, indicating that he should be the vessel for Jīvaka because he was such a pure person. Police Captain Thawi Chamrunchan then ran out from the merit-making pavilion, not wanting to be a vessel for the spirit. In his stead, I indicated Khun Chaum Watanachaeng, Khun Kasaem Sawawasu, and Colonel Aram Menakhongkha (of the First Artillery Battalion) as the ones who could care for the spirit. I then began the ceremony to call Venerable Jīvaka.

Once I began the ceremony, Police Captain Thawi Chamrunchan came back into the merit-making pavilion and sat among the other congregants. After a short while, though, Police Captain Thawi began acting strange. He started slapping his cushion with his hands, and the loud sound caught the attention of everyone in the pavilion. Right when we all turned our heads to look at him, Venerable Jīvaka entered his body. He was unable to escape, and, just as Avalokiteśvara had indicated, Police Captain Thawi was Jīvaka's chosen vessel.

When Venerable Jīvaka was fully in his body, I invited him to sit on a white-cloth-covered platform that had been prepared earlier. I then offered myself to him as his disciple and asked that I may study the healing arts with him. He fully accepted me, and I asked him about his personal history and [asked] some other questions. After answering my questions, the spirit left the police captain's body. I count that as the first time I ever met Venerable Jīvaka and had the opportunity to speak with him.

On Sunday, May 23, 1954, at 11:30 PM, I again invited Venerable Jīvaka to enter the body of Police Captain Thawi, but this time in the temple's ordination hall. During this session, I requested permission to cast images of him that could be used in offering shrines. I asked if we could make one large image and 108 smaller images measuring three inches from knee to knee.[13] I then showed the image that Khun Choti had sculpted, which would serve as the model for the bronze images.

Venerable Jīvaka responded, "This isn't going to get out of hand, is it? If the images are only for yourself and your disciples, then I grant permission." At that, Venerable Jīvaka gave the following prayer for curing diseases: NA A NA VA ROGĀ BYĀDHI VINĀSSANTI.

After receiving approval from Venerable Jīvaka, I had Nai Chin Chuemprasit sculpt the bodies for the images. I requested that the bodies be lifelike, so they would resemble what Jīvaka actually looked like when he was alive. My attention to detail in this regard slowed down production significantly. Nai Chin sculpted the images for two years before they were finished and ready to be cast in bronze.

A big miracle occurred during this time. Once Nai Chin was finished with his sculpting, I went to his foundry with Khun Prathum Chansombun. While at the foundry, I performed a ceremony to call Avalokiteśvara to enter the body of the most experienced sculptor there to check that the work Nai Chin had done was up to par. Avalokiteśvara entered his body and checked the right, left, back, and front sides of the image and said that the image was not exactly symmetrical. No one had noticed this before, and it took Avalokiteśvara to recognize it.

There were many other small matters that Avalokiteśvara noticed as well. For some of them, Avalokiteśvara directed the hand of the craftsperson right there and then to smooth them over. All the while, the eyes of the possessed craftsperson were closed as small details of the model were changed here and there. I held my breath the entire time, afraid that the image that had taken two years to perfect would be completely ruined. But in the end, I was delighted because the image turned out to be beautiful and lifelike in every respect. The image was not crafted from someone's imagination, or some design or plan, but from the image that appeared on the tip of my thumb. Nai Chin, the craftsperson who had made the image, accepted all the changes and said that the image now looked extremely lifelike.

When the entire image was ready to be cast, I performed a consecration ceremony for the casting of the large and small Jīvaka images. The ceremony was held on Thursday, April 24, 1956, at 5 AM. When the casting was finished, the craftspeople finished the images with black patina. I then invited Venerable Jīvaka to come to spiritually charge the life-size image and the 108 small images. This was on April 28, 1957, at 9 PM. This fulfilled my wish to have a life-size image of Jīvaka to make offerings to. I then named the image Jīvaka Komaraphat, High Guru of Healers. This image is installed on the left-hand side of the principle image of the ordination hall of Wat Somananam Borihan (Wat Yuan Saphan Khao).

Ong Soraphanamathurot (Master Bao Oeng)
Abbot of Wat Somananam Borihan
December 25, 1958

NOTES

1. Jīvaka's full name in the Pāli scriptures is Jīvaka Komārabhacca (Skt. Jīvaka Kumārabhṛta). For morphological reasons, his name is rendered in Thai as Chiwaka Komaraphat, often accompanied by the honorific *than* ("venerable") and the epithet *boroma khuru phet* ("High Guru of Healers"). For style and consistency, I refer to him simply as Jīvaka throughout this introductory essay. In my translation below, I have transcribed the Thai spelling of his name into Pāli, dropping "Komārabbhacca" but preserving the honorifics and epithets found in the piece. For ease of use and reading, this essay uses the Royal Thai General System of Transcription.

2. For biographies of Jīvaka, see von Schiefner 1906; Horner 2000; Schopen 2017; cf Zysk 1998.

3. Salguero 2009.

4. Salguero 2017.

5. For more information on the makeup and history of the Annam Nikay, see Tran Duy Hieu 2008. Thanks to Thomas Borchert for this source.

6. See Swearer 2004; Tosa 2014; Chiu 2017; Irwin 2017.

7. Ong Saraphanmathurot 1969. This was published as a cremation volume for Mom Thongkham Singhara, the wife of a disciple of Rama I.

8. Olson 1992.

9. Ong Saraphanmathurot 1969.

10. A *khan ha* offering is the typical offering given by disciples to their principle gurus during *wai khru* ceremonies. It includes white flowers, incense sticks, candles, white cloth, and decoratively folded banana leaves.

11. Vietnamese Buddhism is closely affiliated with Chinese Buddhism. Before Chinese temples were widely found throughout Bangkok, the Chinese population of the city frequented Vietnamese temples.

12. In Thai, this bodhisattva is referred to as Thepachao Thao Chai Phak. Thanks to Venerable Tran Duy Hieu (Thich Nhuan An) for help with the identity of this deity.

13. Thai Buddhist images are measured from knee to knee, a measurement known as *natak*.

17. Gross National Happiness

Buddhist Principles and Bhutanese National Health Policy

CHARLES JAMYANG OLIPHANT OF ROSSIE

The well-being of the individual citizen has most often been equated with the material improvement and higher living standards considered fitting for an economically developed nation. This assumption that a nation's gross domestic product (GDP) is a pivotal indicator of the citizens' subjective well-being both in material and social terms has, however, been proven somewhat flawed by various studies.[1] Recently, different conceptual models and analytical frameworks for measuring well-being have been devised. The United Nations has been encouraging such collective efforts. For example, on July 19, 2011, its assembly encouraged member nations "to pursue the elaboration of additional measures that better capture the importance of the pursuit of happiness and well-being in development with a view to guiding their public policies."[2] The resolution also stated that "the pursuit of happiness is a fundamental human goal."

Yet, with regard to institutionalizing the pursuit of happiness for their citizens, few governments have been as committed and rigorous as that of Bhutan. This small Himalayan country is nestled between two global superpowers, China and India, and thus has been concerned about the survival of its identity. Perhaps alarmed by neighboring Nepal's social and economic failures, Bhutan has devised its own unique development model. The term "gross national happiness" (GNH) is said to have been coined by Jigme Singye Wangchuck (b. 1955), the fourth king of Bhutan, in 1972. The GNH developmental philosophy and its related policies were envisioned by the king in the late 1970s. The GNH Index itself was developed at the Centre for Bhutan Studies and first deployed in 2010.

There are earlier examples of governments trying to translate principles into practice by promoting equality in health care and curbing the acquisitive impulse in society. The Labour government of the United Kingdom from 1945 to 1951 is perhaps the foremost example.[3] The GNH Index of Bhutan is, however, the first-ever attempt by a national government to statistically measure well-being via a systematic analysis of material and cultural indicators. The index measures the well-being of individuals across nine domains, as measured by 124 variables, and is based on survey data specific to different regions.[4]

The GNH model does not blindly emulate standard global models of production, trade, and economic growth. Instead it claims to focus on prioritizing the well-being of citizens, social harmony, and environmental protection in a system in which spiritual and material progress go hand in hand. These spiritual goals largely stem from Buddhist understandings, although opinions differ on how closely GNH is connected with Buddhist doctrine. Bhutan's prime minister from 2013 to 2018, Tshering Tobgay, connected GNH to Bhutan's Buddhist heritage in a general way: "Since we are largely Buddhist, everything we do has a basis in Buddhism, so in that respect, you can say GNH has its roots in Buddhism."[5] However, Khenpo Phuntsok Tashi, the director of the National Museum of Bhutan, has more explicitly stated that GNH "cannot be achieved unless Buddhist philosophy is fully incorporated and practiced by each and every citizen of Bhutan."[6] The GNH commission itself defines the concept of happiness in a way that is consonant with Buddhist ideas:

We have now clearly distinguished [the GNH concept of "happiness"] . . . from the fleeting, pleasurable "feel-good" moods so often associated with that term. We know that true abiding happiness cannot exist while others suffer and comes only from serving others, living in harmony with nature, and realizing our innate wisdom and the true and brilliant nature of our own minds.[7]

Thus, Buddhism's ultimate goal of a permanent state of mental balance, awareness, and happiness appears to form the backbone of the GNH Index and its indicators. More directly, in its quest for the optimal condition for society, the concept of GNH has taken inspiration from the Four Noble Truths, karma, and the Six Perfections (*pāramitā*).[8] The Bhutanese government, aware that everything starts with the single individual, also monitors individual human emotions through a systematic assessment of symptoms of psychological distress and socially destructive attitudes. States of mental happiness are also studied and fostered, since an individual's moods and emotions will have an enormous range of effects on their well-being.

It is not within the scope of this short contribution to evaluate the achievements or shortcomings of the GNH. Rather, its purpose is to briefly illustrate how Buddhist principles have impacted the national health policy of Bhutan. With this in mind, I have included below two excerpts from official Bhutanese documents. The first is a 2000 report on human development from the Planning Commission Secretariat of the Royal Government of Bhutan, which discusses the constituents of happiness and their connections with Buddhism. The second is an excerpt of the National Health Policy from the Bhutanese Ministry of Health that succinctly express the kingdom's perspectives and aspirations regarding the role of health care in GNH.

FURTHER READING

Costanza, Robert, et al. 2007. "Quality of Life: An Approach Integrating Opportunities, Human Needs, and Subjective Well-Being." *Ecological Economics* 61 (2–3): 267–76.

England, Richard W. 1998. "Measurement of Social Well-Being: Alternatives to Gross Domestic Product." *Ecological Economics* 25 (1): 89–103.

Givel, Michael 2015. "Mahayana Buddhism and Gross National Happiness in Bhutan." *International Journal of Wellbeing* 5 (2): 14–27.

Khenpo Phuntsok Tashi. 2004. "The Role of Buddhism in Achieving Gross National Happiness." In *Gross National Happiness and Development: Proceedings of the First International Conference on Operationalization of Gross National Happiness*, edited by Karma Ura and Karma Galay, 483–95. Thimphu, Bhutan: Centre for Bhutan Studies.

1. EXCERPT FROM *BHUTAN NATIONAL HUMAN DEVELOPMENT REPORT, 2000: THE CONSTITUENTS OF HAPPINESS*[9]

A great deal of consistency exists between the Bhutanese concept of Gross National Happiness (GNH) and human development. Commodity ownership may contribute to standard of living, but it is not a constituent part of that standard. Amartya Sen points out, for instance, that a grumbling rich man may well be less happy than a contented farmer, but he does have a higher standard of living than the farmer. It is the sense of discontentment or emptiness that the rich man experiences that constitutes unhappiness. Happiness may be subjective, but this subjectiveness is shared by all, regardless of levels of income, class, gender or race.

The pursuit of GNH calls for a multi-dimensional approach to development that seeks to maintain harmony and balance between economic forces, environmental preservation, cultural and spiritual values, and good governance. The articulation of happiness as the goal of development has strong roots in Bhutan's Buddhist traditions. Rather than talk of happiness per se, Buddhism talks about avoiding dissatisfaction through adequate provisioning of four necessities—food, shelter, clothing, and medicine. Significantly, however, it holds that meeting this hierarchy of wants is only the first step in avoiding human suffering which ultimately depends upon cultivating a sense of detachment and spiritual fulfillment.

Apart from the religious influences, the concept of GNH as it has evolved over the years has also been a reaction to the experiences of other developing nations. Bhutan's late start in development has had one major advantage: it allowed the country to learn from the experiences of other countries. The pursuit of growth in GNH rather than in GDP, reflects Bhutan's anxiety to avoid some of the more glaring failures of the blind pursuit of economic growth. By seeking to promote human happiness, the focus is on what matters most to people: their security, peace, and comfort. Consequently, Bhutan has identified four essential constituents of happiness: economic development, environmental preservation, cultural preservation and promotion, and good governance.

If happiness is among the cherished goals of development, then it does matter how this happiness is generated, what causes it, what goes with it, and how it is distributed—whether it is enjoyed by a few or shared by all. Human happiness may not automatically flow from economic growth. Conscious policies are needed to establish a link between economic progress and human happiness. Part of this will require improvements in socioeconomic conditions and the satisfaction of basic needs. But a growing income and better provisioning of basic social services are not sufficient by themselves; these have to be supplemented by appropriate employment opportunities, social security and adequate leisure time.

Bhutan seeks to establish a happy society, where people are safe, where everyone is guaranteed a decent livelihood, and where people enjoy universal access to good education and health care. It is a society where there is no pollution or violation of the environment, where there is no aggression and war, where inequalities do not exist, and where cultural values get strengthened everyday. A happy society is not a fatalistic society, but is built on hope and aspirations. It is also a more equal and compassionate society, where sharing and contentment come out of a positive sense of community feeling. A happy society is one where people enjoy freedoms, where there is no oppression, where art, music, dance, drama, and culture flourish.

Ultimately, a happy society is a caring society, caring for the past and future, caring for the environment, and caring for those who need protection. Establishing such a society will require a long-term rather than a short-term perspective of development. Much will depend upon how well the country's environmental resources are harnessed and managed. Happiness in the future will also depend upon mitigating the foreseeable conflict between traditional cultural values and the modern lifestyles that inevitably follow in the wake of development.

2. Excerpts from the Bhutanese Ministry of Health's *National Health Policy* (Sections 2 and 13)[10]

While Bhutan has overcome many obstacles in the past, it now confronts new and varied challenges such as 1) rising health care expenditure, 2) changing life style and disease pattern, 3) inadequate human resources, 4) changing political environment, 5) increasingly evolving health care needs of the population, 6) international health obligations, and 7) new health technologies.

Despite numerous challenges, it is envisioned that the National Health Policy shall set the agenda and provide general direction to guide the government in achieving the national and international health goals within the spirit of social justice and equity.

Vision and Mission

Vision: Build a healthy and happy nation through a dynamic professional health system; attainment of highest standard of health by the people within the broader framework of overall national development in the spirit of social justice, and equity.

Mission: Achievement of national health goals through sustained provision of quality general and public health services.

Aspirations

Bhutan recognizes health as a prerequisite for economic and spiritual development, poverty reduction, and the road to gross national happiness. The National Health Policy aspires to be congruent with the philosophy of gross national happiness and reflects various inputs ranging from social, spiritual, cultural, and environmental aspects.

It recognizes the values of democracy, transparency, and equity, especially addressing the needs of the poor and underprivileged through partnership in health. It also aspires to further pursue decentralization policy in the delivery of health services to its population.

It aims to promote self-reliance and sustainability by increasing efficiency, productivity, accountability, and ownership in health care interventions and service delivery.

This policy is gender-sensitive, respects the rights of the people, seeks informed consent, and maintains confidentiality in relation to medical decision-making and information sharing.

This policy ultimately aspires to improve the health outcomes by translating these statements into strategic framework through collective national and international efforts.

Medical Care: Traditional Medicines

a. The Royal Government of Bhutan shall continue to preserve and promote the traditional medicine system by effectively integrating it into the overall national health care delivery system.
b. Focused efforts shall be directed towards making Bhutanese "So-wa-rigpa" the centre of excellence in providing quality traditional medical services, including wellness center that is recognizable at an international level.
c. The Institute of Traditional Medicine in collaboration with Tourism Council of Bhutan shall encourage and support the Bhutanese spa and resort industries to institute spa therapies with traditional medicinal practices ("So wa rigpa") and spiritual healing.
d. Identification, demarcation and protection of areas rich with medicinal products for care and management by the relevant Dzongkhag[11] Administration shall be instituted in conformity with Ministry of Agriculture and Forestry.

NOTES

1. Costanza et al. 2007; McKibben 2007.
2. United Nations 2011.
3. The Labour government drew heavily on the inspiration of the economist and historian R. H. Tawney. Passages in Tawney's works *The Acquisitive Society* (1920) and *Equality* (1931) bear a striking resemblance to those of the Bhutanese government regarding GNH philosophy.
4. Ura et al. 2012: 4.
5. DeHart 2013.
6. Khenpo Phuntsok Tashi 2004: 483–84.
7. Quoted in Givel 2015: 23.
8. Wangmo and Valk 2012.
9. The following is excerpted from Planning Commission Secretariat, Royal Government of Bhutan 2000: 16–18. It has been slightly edited to correct some typographical errors and to match the punctuation conventions of this volume.
10. The following is excerpted from Ministry of Health n.d.: 2–3, 17. Punctuation and formatting have been adjusted to match the conventions of this volume.
11. A Dzongkhag is an administrative district of the Bhutanese nation.

18. Using Buddhist Resources in Post-disaster Japan

Taniyama Yōzō's "Vihāra Priests and Interfaith Chaplains" (2014)

LEVI McLAUGHLIN

Taniyama Yōzō (b. 1972) is a Jōdo Shinshū (Shin Buddhist) priest who holds the rank of associate professor at Tohoku University in Sendai, Japan, where he received his Ph.D. in Buddhist studies. Taniyama has emerged as a leading Japanese figure in the application of Buddhism to interfaith initiatives. He was instrumental in founding Tohoku University's Department of Practical Religious Studies and now serves as a principal coordinator of the Society for Interfaith Chaplaincy in Japan (Nihon Rinshō Shūkyōshikai), which he helped establish in 2016.[1] These institutions came out of efforts by Buddhists and other religious activists who cooperated with psychologists, grief care specialists, hospice care workers, and others to provide services for the dead and the bereaved after the March 11, 2011, Great East Japan Earthquake Disasters. Also referred to as "3/11," the combined earthquake, tsunami, and nuclear disasters devastated northeastern Japan. Upwards of 24,600 people were killed, injured, or remain missing, mostly as a result of the tsunami, which destroyed hundreds of communities. The disasters dealt a severe physical and psychic blow to Japan and inspired Japan's largest religious mobilization since the Pacific War.[2]

The 3/11 disasters loom large in Taniyama's account. However, his writing makes clear that Japanese Buddhists had already been at work for decades before 3/11, applying their practices to aid efforts, clinical treatments, and social welfare (see chapter 21 for a pre-3/11 example). Taniyama himself is a "Vihāra priest" (*bihārasō*), a clinician trained to serve the needs of the terminally ill in a palliative-care setting. In the text that follows, he discusses the definition of Vihāra and the potential to extend this care practice beyond end-of-life treatments and its Buddhist origins. The 3/11 disasters provided an impetus for the creation of a new type of licensed caregiver, the role of which builds on Vihāra training and related initiatives. These caregivers are called *rinshō shūkyōshi* (literally "clinical religious instructor"), a term Taniyama prefers to translate into English as "interfaith chaplain." Since 2012, Taniyama has steered an intensive interfaith chaplain training program in which clergy from temple-based Buddhist denominations join Catholic priests, Protestant ministers, Shinto priests, and practitioners from some New Religions (most notably Risshō Kōsei-kai and Tenrikyō) to acquire certification that enables them to work in hospitals or elder care homes. Other medical and social service providers may also undertake interfaith chaplaincy training.

The translation below includes material that Taniyama presents in his interfaith chaplain training program modules. It is excerpted from a chapter by him that focuses on a distinction between "spiritual care" and "religious care." Spiritual care may operate beyond the realm of doctrine and ritual, whereas religious care makes use of explicitly religious resources—although not necessarily only those of the chaplain's own faith. Both care types are enfolded within a broader rubric known in Japan as "care for the *kokoro*": care for the heart, mind, spirit, or core.

Buddhist terms are woven into the explanations Taniyama provides, yet he is clearly eager to move beyond a Buddhism-specific identity as he investigates ways of making Buddhism's full repertoire available to caregivers, no matter their faith or denominational affiliations. To do this, he appeals to a shared Japanese identity called *minkan shinkō*, which can be translated as "common faith" or "folk belief." This is an ambiguous idea Taniyama proposes instead of secularism as a description for the disposition of the Japanese people, who are mostly uncomfortable with "religion" yet remain sympathetic toward spirituality and ritual traditions. According to Taniyama, it is through an appeal to "common faith" that practitioners may hope to carry out spiritual care and religious care in Japan's public sphere.[3]

The extreme caution that Taniyama urges in administering religious care may appear excessive to some readers. After all, why would one object to providing Buddhist or other religious rituals or insights to a suffering person who welcomes them? This anxiety must be placed in a contemporary Japanese context, within a country where memories of religious extremism in the form of sarin gas attacks by the apocalyptic sect Aum Shinrikyō persist, and where the category "religion" took shape only in the late nineteenth century as a component of Japan's transformation into a modern nation-state.[4] We can regard Taniyama's reformulation of Buddhist resources as a deft navigation through Japan's fraught religious landscape. Interfaith chaplaincy, a profession that now enjoys nationally recognized certification, carves out promising new territory for Japan's religious professionals. It clears the way for temple-affiliated Japanese

Buddhists to move beyond their stereotypical funerary roles, and for Japanese religionists of all sorts to potentially escape decades of stigma by building new associations with reassuringly scientific clinical treatment programs. Interfaith chaplaincy also invites questions about what happens to Buddhism when it is disaggregated from sectarian traditions and applied to a biomedical framework. It calls on us to consider the practical limits of Buddhism's adaptability.[5]

Taniyama is a Buddhist priest, but he is also an academic; his Ph.D. in Buddhist studies is not a sectarian designation but an academic degree he earned from Tohoku University, a secular public institution, for research on Buddhism in Bangladesh. His work included here carefully cites Buddhist scholars, Christian academics, and medical researchers, and otherwise uses conventions that demonstrate his academic bona fides. (The circled footnotes in the chapter below represent Taniyama's footnotes, which have been edited for inclusion in this volume, while the endnotes were added by the translator for clarification). At the same time, his work represents a discourse by a practitioner instrumental in shaping a twenty-first-century Japanese Buddhist identity. As such, it challenges a putative divide between primary and secondary sources.

FURTHER READING

Harding, Christopher, Iwata Fumiaki, and Yoshinaga Shin'ichi, eds. 2014. *Religion and Psychotherapy in Modern Japan*. London: Routledge.

Kasai, Kenta. 2016. "Introducing Chaplaincy to Japanese Society: A Religious Practice in Public Space." *Journal of Religion in Japan* 5 (2–3): 246–62.

McLaughlin, Levi. 2013. "What Have Religions Done After 3.11? Part 2: From Religious Mobilization to 'Spiritual Care.'" *Religion Compass* 7 (8): 309–25.

Samuels, Jeffrey, Justin Thomas McDaniel, and Mark Michael Rowe, eds. 2016. *Figures of Buddhist Modernity in Asia*. Honolulu: University of Hawai'i Press.

Watts, Jonathan S., and Yoshiharu Tomatsu, eds. 2012. *Buddhist Care for the Dying and Bereaved*. Somerville, Mass.: Wisdom.

EXCERPTS FROM "RELIGIOUS PRACTITIONERS AS SPIRITUAL CARE PROVIDERS: VIHĀRA PRIESTS AND INTERFAITH CHAPLAINS"[6]

Vihāra Priests

Vihāra is a Sanskrit word meaning "temple" or "resting place." In 1985, Tamiya Masashi proposed this as the Sanskrit term for "Buddhist hospice,"① as a means

---

① Tamiya 2007: 3.

of identifying "terminal care based in Buddhism or a place [for this practice]."[2] Tamiya outlines the following three Vihāra principles:[3]

> Principle 1: For people who have a limited time to live, for people who have been informed of this limit on their mortality, a Vihāra is a place for quiet self-reflection where they may care for themselves.
> Principle 2: The wishes of the recipient serve as the axis for the Vihāra's terminal care and medical treatment. For this purpose, the facility must apply appropriate medical treatment and clinical procedures, where possible.
> Principle 3: The Vihāra is a gathering place for people who care for the dignity of life, a small collective based in Buddhism (though the recipient and the recipient's family, in all circumstances, remain free of the responsibility [to uphold Buddhist precepts], especially in cases where they maintain other beliefs).

From 1984, influenced by a Kyoto Buddhist Youth League trans-sectarian hospital sermon initiative called Bhagavad Kyoto, Tamiya, who is from a Shin Buddhist Ōtani Sect temple family, promoted the trans-sectarian "Vihāra movement." Influenced by this, from 1986 the Shin Buddhist Hongwanji Sect offered a sect-specific "Vihāra activity." In 1988, Tashiro Shunkō initiated a "Vihāra movement" based at the Higashi Hongwanji Nagoya Branch Temple (Ōtani Sect), and in 1994 the Nichiren Sect began its own Vihāra activity. In addition, in various locations across the country, newly founded volunteer organizations undertook independent sectarian and trans-sectarian Vihāra initiatives. There was little difference between efforts that were either labeled a Vihāra "movement" or "activity." The starting point was terminal care, yet since then there have been initiatives for elderly social welfare, care for people with physical or mental disabilities, for children, and for assisting mental health care. In light of these developments, I attempted a redefinition of Vihāra through an internet survey, the results of which I have already published and introduce here:[4]

Narrow meaning: Terminal care, or a facility for this care, founded in Buddhism.

 Broad meaning: With old age, illness, and death as its concern, Vihāra comprises the activities of Buddhists and/or their facilities that provide services in the realms of medical treatment and social welfare.[7]

[2] As of April 1, 2014, there were three Buddhism-affiliated palliative care hospital wards in Japan: Nagaoka Nishi Hospital in Niigata Prefecture (established in 1992, accredited in 1993, trans-sectarian), Kōsei Hospital in Tokyo (established and accredited in 2004, Risshō Kōsei-kai), and Asoka Vihāra Hospital in Kyoto (established in 2008, Jōdo Shinshū Hongwanji Sect).

[3] Tamiya 2007: 6–7.

[4] Taniyama 2005: 39–40.

Broadest meaning: Social engagement centered on Buddhism aimed at disaster relief, youth education, cultural activities, and other undertakings that sustain life[8] or provide opportunities for contemplating life.

Many among the respondents who were clergy, or those with Buddhist ties, supported the narrow and broad meanings of Vihāra, yet the survey results also revealed that almost every respondent believed that the broad and broadest meanings applied. Consequently, it can be posited that the broad meaning of Vihāra should be its principal definition now and that common understanding of the category could be extended to its broadest meaning in the future.

Nagaoka Nishi Hospital, which puts Vihāra into practice, exemplifies the meaning of Vihāra in its narrow sense. There is a Buddhist chapel inside the hospital ward, where every morning and evening time is reserved for ritual observance. The patients are not necessarily active Buddhist believers because they also include so-called nonreligious people, along with Shinto, Christian, and New Religion adherents. In addition to one regular Vihāra staffer, ten or so local Buddhist clergy take part in regular ward activities as volunteer Vihāra priests.

Vihāra 21, a nonprofit organization based in Osaka, serves as an example of Vihāra's broad definition. The group began as a voluntary organization in 2003 and incorporated as a nonprofit organization in 2004. The group maintains a nursing facility and provides a care home for people without families. Its residents include the elderly and those with physical or mental disabilities, as well as students without disabilities. At present, three Vihāra priests are on staff, and a number of other volunteer Vihāra priests are responsible for heart-mind (kokoro) care.

As an example of Vihāra's broadest meaning, I suggest the activities of Vihāra Akita. Founded in 1992 in Akita Prefecture, Vihāra Akita engages practically with various problems that relate to life, such as end-of-life medical care, social welfare for the elderly, death with dignity, brain death, organ transplantation, suicide policies, and environmental destruction.[5] This organization also contributed actively to victim aid after the March 2011 Great East Japan Earthquake Disasters. Though they are known for providing active listening-centered heart-mind care, they focus their efforts on sermons, seminars, and cafés[6]—all activities that match the broadest Vihāra definition.

The definition of Vihāra varies depending on the activity and involves not only clergy but also temple families and parishioners, and even extends beyond Buddhist practitioners. Within this definition, it is Vihāra priests who are responsible for heart-mind care, which can be divided roughly into spiritual care, religious care, and grief care. Each of these divisions includes care for those who confront difficult-to-resolve problems relating to birth, old age, illness, and

⑤ http://vihara.main.jp/.

⑥ http://vihara.main.jp/pdf/63/pdf.

death. The focus of Vihāra priests on hospital wards is principally patients and their families (and the bereaved), but care for hospital staff is also important.

Taking the Vihāra priests at the Nagaoka Nishi Hospital Vihāra ward as an example, the priests support patients and their families, and their bereaved, by taking care of matters around them and maintaining the facilities. They perform as religious professionals by engaging in active listening and chanting *sūtras*; operating within support-providing teams as liaisons and helpers; liaising with ward staff, volunteers, and religious service providers in the area; keeping records; and offering study sessions, educational outreach, and instruction within and outside the hospital.[7] Their duties go beyond heart-mind care to include a wide variety of other tasks.

Interfaith Chaplains

Rinshō shūkyōshi is a neologism that was proposed as a Japanese translation of the English word "chaplain." This proposal emerged to suit the needs of hospice care and those afflicted by the Great East Japan Earthquake Disasters.

After the disasters, religious practitioners in the Sendai municipal area, with the support of the Sendai Buddhist Association (Sendai Bukkyōkai), the Sendai Christian Alliance (Sendai Kirisutokyō Rengō), and the Miyagi Prefecture Religious Juridical Persons' Communications Association (Miyagi-ken Shūkyō Hōjin Renraku Kyōgikai), started up volunteer *sūtra* recitation and a reception desk for the Consultation Room for the Spirit (Kokoro no Sōdanshitsu) at a Sendai city funeral home. These activities coordinated with municipal offices and continued into late April 2011. However, memorial services and grief care were clearly still needed. In order to continue this work, the Consultation Room for the Spirit was established in Tohoku University's Religious Studies Department and was headed by Okabe Takeshi, a local physician who provided in-home hospice care.[8] Not only Buddhist, Christian, and Shinto priests, but also people affiliated with New Religions, religion scholars, grief care specialists, and medical personnel, took part. Determining that relief activities should continue in the disaster area for at least ten more years, it was understood that human resources needed to be cultivated, along with a quickly established administrative office. The Consultation Room gathered donations from various religious groups, a Department of Practical Religious Studies affiliated with Tohoku University's Graduate School of Arts and Letters was established, and the training of interfaith chaplains began.

Rinshō shūkyōshi was a title proposed by Okabe Takeshi. In 2010, Dr. Okabe discovered that he had cancer and announced that he had only ten months to live. Around that time, he appeared to gain a keen awareness of the need for

---

[7] See Murase 2012.

[8] See Taniyama 2013.

"a guide toward descending into the darkness." One of his nurses lost her life in the 2011 disasters. Okabe wrote that "our staff members were greatly shaken up and anguished. The thing that initially calmed them was *sūtra* chanting by volunteer Buddhist clergy."[9] In this way, he became aware of the significance of heart-mind care provided by religious practitioners and welcomed their contribution. Dr. Okabe constructed a plan to connect religious providers who contribute to the public good with medical treatment specialists. After he opened the door to this cooperative venture, he passed away.[10]

So what is a *rinshō shūkyōshi*, an "interfaith chaplain"? This is a Japanese version of "chaplain," a term that points to religious practitioners who offer heart-mind care to people other than their fellow believers in the public sphere. They do not seek to proselytize, and religious cooperation is a necessary presupposition.

Humans require more than scientific and rational understandings: Their lives require support for experiences that go beyond rational explanation. Even when providing medical care, social work, or psychological assistance, it is necessary to understand and respect people's nonrational aspects. Interfaith chaplains are care providers to whom these nonrational experiences may be easily expressed, who welcome and accept these perspectives in support of people's lives. For those who await death, interfaith chaplains may speak about the afterlife, and they can join consultations on postmortem memorial rites and graves. Additionally, in order to develop an interreligious network that extends beyond those fostered to date by chaplains and Vihāra priests,[11] they respond to a wide range of religious needs.

In real-life situations in the public, encounters with people of different faiths or with those who self-identify as nonreligious are common. For religious practitioners, these situations can raise challenging issues. I would like to consider the two-sided difficulty of (1) understanding the other, versus (2) the practitioner's mental and spiritual preparation.

First, on understanding the other: The interfaith chaplain, in order to prepare the way for interreligious cooperation, cannot depend on forging connections via doctrine. To appreciate another person's perspective, the chaplain focuses on "common faith" (*minkan shinkō*). This is the basis for Japanese religion, a faith that one could say survives within the secularized present. It is not a topic that has received extensive attention in Japanese spiritual care discourse, but I propose that people who fit this common faith include those who maintain specific religious commitments, those who profess no religion, and even those who are absolutely removed from historical practices such as ancestor veneration or nature worship. The Dai-ichi Life Insurance Company's Research Institute

---

[9] Okabe 2012: 9.

[10] Dr. Okabe died on September 27, 2012. See Okuno 2013.

[11] Through their training, interfaith chaplains build a foundation for interreligious cooperation as they encounter a variety of contrasting religious practitioners.

publicized the following results from its Survey on Religious Activities and Understandings in Everyday Life:

> It is clear that most of us, rather than basing our beliefs on established religions, maintain a religion-*like* perspective and carry out religion-*like* activities. In particular, while rituals for the spirits of the departed are largely connected to established religions, for concepts such as retribution from the spirit world or divine protection, it is necessary for faith to find purchase elsewhere.[12]

Therefore, I suggest that we must grasp Japanese people's religion not from the perspective of originally promulgated religions (established religions) but from what is termed common faith.

Regarding mental and spiritual preparation: In the public sphere, we do not accept proselytizing practitioners but welcome interfaith chaplains who carry out their activities without missionizing. I can explain preparation for this role in the following way:

Taking baseball or soccer as a metaphor, if one conceives of the sphere created by the relationship between believers and clergy as "home field," the public sphere is, for practitioners, an "away game." While at home, the priest is called upon to operate as an authority figure. If the priest seeks to maintain this kind of relationship with people while away, trouble will readily arise. At the "away game," anguished people seek aid from those who relate to them as allies; those who act as authority figures are not necessarily beneficial. It is absolutely necessary to create intimate bonds in order to serve the others' needs.

Let us also consider the interfaith chaplain's area of operation. Chaplains in the United States are primarily regarded as necessary within the military. Based in this tradition, soldiers leave their local churches and head to the battlefield, where chaplains may carry out such tasks as performing Sunday services and funerals for the war dead, along with providing grief care for families and comrades. No matter the circumstances, it can be said that the U.S. chaplain retains a prerogative to participate in religious ritual. This tradition has given rise to chaplains for police and firefighters, in prisons,[13] on site after accidents and disasters, as well as in schools, hospitals, social welfare facilities, and even in corporations[14] and for athletes.[15] Viewed from this perspective, discourse on chaplains in Japan must be regarded as one-sided.

---

[12] Dai-Ichi Life Insurance Institute 2006.

[13] Chaplaincy directed at prisoners fits the description of Japanese chaplains (*kyōkaishi*); however, in the United States, prison administrations require a chaplain.

[14]. For examples, see U.S. National Institute of Business and Industrial Chaplains: www.nibic .com.

[15]. For examples, see Sports Chaplaincy UK: https://sportschaplaincy.org.uk/.

In Japan, the need for chaplains as participants in the hospice movement and as spiritual care providers has come to be emphasized, so there is a strong image of chaplains as active in palliative care. This can be confirmed in the definitions of Vihāra that I outlined earlier. However, it is easy to imagine that *chaplain* extends beyond a foundational Christian concept of pastoral care to encompass a wide range of possibilities. Not only ministers and pastors but also numerous other religious practitioners provide advice in countless every-day situations. These consultations take place in private settings such as temples, churches, and homes and extend to public places such as hospitals and elsewhere. The practitioner's public face adapted to these situations is that of the chaplain, the interfaith chaplain.

Next, I introduce care for the spiritual responsibility borne by the chaplain, Vihāra priest, and interfaith chaplain.

Spiritual Care and Religious Care

I would like to begin with a discussion of which purposes spiritual care and religious care aim to serve. As I outlined above, spiritual care in Japan focuses on palliative care, yet it can be adapted to a range that extends beyond concerns that surround death. To borrow Buddhist terminology, spiritual care does not only relate to the Four Afflictions of birth, old age, illness, and death, but also extends to the Eight Afflictions, which add suffering experienced when separated from those we love, suffering when we experience that which we dislike, suffering when we cannot attain that which we desire, and suffering because existence does not lie beyond the Five Aggregates; that is, care for suffering when things do not go as expected.[9] Both spiritual and religious care seek to accept the suffering person's difficulties on her or his own terms without aiming to solve these problems. Instead, care is required *because* these are problems that cannot be solved.

Spiritual care emerged from pastoral care intended for Christians, and it also developed out of wide-ranging care offered to non-Christians. Because of this, use of the term can be confusing. It is perhaps not inappropriate to use *spiritual care* within a majority-Christian cultural context, but this is not the case in Japan. Having entered the realms of pastoral care, Vihāra care, and religious care, I have come to emphasize spiritual care as a different category. It is worthwhile considering this emphasis through discussion of the interfaith chaplain.

The two types of care are easily confused, as both are deeply concerned with people's religiosity and value systems. If one were to define basic continuities, both forms of care can "reconfirm and rediscover that which supports the self, and support the reclaiming of power for survival, or self-care."[16]

---

[16] Taniyama 2008: 59.

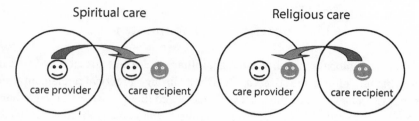

FIGURE 18.1 THE CONTRASTING RELATIONSHIP BETWEEN PROVIDER
AND RECIPIENT IN SPIRITUAL CARE AND RELIGIOUS CARE.
The circles represent the world view or value system of the care provider and care
recipient. In spiritual care, support is discovered within the recipient's world view. In
religious care, support is sought from within the provider's world view.
Source: Taniyama 2009.

The clearest points of difference between the two care types manifest in the nature of the relationship between the person receiving support and the one offering it (figure 18.1).

In the case of religious care, the care recipient has reached a perilous situation owing to an inability to cope based on her or his own religious or value system and, seeking outside support, is open to accepting religious or value-system perspectives. Accordingly, the recipient accepts advice or suggestions presented by the religious caregiver. On the other hand, in the case of spiritual care, the caregiver initiates a relationship without knowing if the recipient is looking to a perspective outside her or his own religious or value system, so the provider must listen carefully to ascertain the recipient's values in order to help. Accordingly, the care provider relies on "active listening"[10] and offers almost no advice. The type of care that is needed will depend on how the relationship between recipient and provider develops, and the understanding between them that forms the basis of their relationship must be reassessed at every juncture.

Self-care is a form of care in which there is no provider and the recipient selects support by her- or himself through discovery—via reading, art, ritual, or other means. For instance, if the recipient enjoys sports, the method will be spiritual care, whereas if it is prayer, the method will be religious care. It is likely that neither care method will be familiar if explained through words but will instead manifest as something the person has carried out throughout her or his life. Self-care is not only for those who face extreme situations such as death but is needed by those who find themselves standing at a crossroads because they have failed an exam, lost love, been fired, suffered illness or injury, been divorced, or are concerned about the future. Every person may potentially become a self-care recipient.

Challenges for Social Implementation

Social implementation is most likely not a familiar phrase, but I use it here to mean "verifying techniques, practices, and systems through practical implementation in society." In lieu of a conclusion, I will identify challenges for social implementation encountered by spiritual care specialists who come from religious backgrounds and operate as chaplains, Vihāra priests, and interfaith chaplains.

For spiritual care, religious care, and implementation of religious resources in the combined area these practices comprise, it is necessary to build up a repertoire of practical methods. However, social implementation is difficult. Every religious practitioner must grow accustomed to specific methods in order to implement them in the public sphere. If I consider my own in-the-field training to date, broad-based interreligious cooperation is required to separate care efforts from suspicions of proselytizing, and the practitioner must become accustomed to public interaction.

The title "chaplain" is most easily recognized as a Christian term, and the title "Vihāra" evokes Buddhist origins. Depending on the region, the local tradition may be the Hongwanji Sect, or perhaps the Nichiren Sect. If an individual practitioner brings to mind a specific sectarian identity, she or he may easily trigger fears about missionizing, even if the individual does not have that intention. Another problem is the fact that definitions of chaplain and Vihāra priest remain unknown within Japanese society. Ultimately, the areas of specialization denoted by these titles are difficult to comprehend. Even if these titles are well known in the religious world, it is difficult to say that they have penetrated into everyday society, and it is doubtful if they are readily understood by care recipients or medical practitioners.

By contrast, the title *rinshō shūkyōshi* [interfaith chaplain] is a new phrase and therefore not well known, but it gives the impression of being similar to *rinshō shinrishi* [clinical psychologist], and it easily brings to mind the image of a religious practitioner who provides care. The meaning of the word *shūkyō* remains ambiguous in practice, ranging from "religion" in general to "cult." Religion retains a bad image among people who are cautious about it, so cooperating with health care providers makes it comparatively easier for religious practitioners to confer services.

Practitioners must avert fears about proselytizing. Traditional modes of perpetuating religious traditions that are practiced in such private spaces as temples and churches are authorized by provisions in the Religious Juridical Persons Law,[11] but it is accurate to say that carrying out these practices in hospitals and other public venues would be regarded as taboo. Unless the practitioner distinguishes an ethical difference between private and public religious conduct, trouble will result. The private realm is the practitioner's "home field," in which she or he may conduct sermons and other practices at her or his discretion. However, the public sphere is an "away game" in which discretionary power is in the hands of others, not the practitioner, such as a chief administrator at a hospital or social welfare facility. Confirming the intent of the care recipient—patient, adherent, or other—remains a necessary precondition, but the practitioner must also, *absolutely*, carefully measure the conditions that surround the caregiving situation.[17]

These matters manifest in practical ways within the public arena, and a pre-condition of practicing in this arena is constructing a mutual relationship based on trust. The cumulative result of this is recognition of the practitioner as a team member by fellow care providers.

It can be thought that religious practitioners' public practice as spiritual care providers in hospitals and related facilities began in Japan within the hospice care movement to suit the social needs of the time. Various initiatives took shape around the advent of hospice care in Japan, and this singular effort developed into a well-regarded institution—for better or worse, a success story that proved to be something of an exception within Japanese society. Thanks to the hard work of our predecessors in the religion and health care worlds, their efforts have blossomed after close to forty years. I do not think I am alone in feeling that the path they forged can finally be clearly seen.

NOTES

1. The Society's website is http://sicj.or.jp/.
2. For studies of the 3/11 disasters in English, see Kingston 2012; Gill, Steger, and Slater 2013. For details on religious responses following 3/11, see McLaughlin 2013a, 2016; Berman 2018. For a vivid journalistic account that includes helpful descriptions of Buddhist care interventions, see Parry 2017.
3. Hori Ichirō, a seminal scholar of religious studies in Japan, theorized on *minkan shinkō* as a means of understanding folk traditions that elude denominational categorization. The term was first standardized in the early twentieth century by Anesaki Masaharu, a professor at Tokyo Imperial University credited with founding religious studies in Japan. See Hori 1968. Taniyama does not cite Hori here, but the legacy of Japanese scholarship on folk religion can be perceived in Taniyama's characterizations of Japanese religious attitudes.
4. Descriptions of the Aum Shinrikyō attacks and their effects on attitudes toward religion in Japan can be found in Reader 2000 and Hardacre 2007. For analyses of the development of the category "religion" in modern Japan, see Josephson 2012; Maxey 2014.
5. Taniyama's organization of Buddhist resources into "spiritual care" and "religious care" can be seen as a Japanese Buddhist contribution to global secularist discourses. For a helpful introduction to debates that swirl around multiple "secularisms," see Casanova 2006

[17] This becomes somewhat complex, as the practitioner must also remain conscious of differences between care practice within a hospital and home care.

and research by scholars at Leipzig University, who in 2016 launched a collaborative project titled "Multiple Secularities: Beyond the West, Beyond Modernities" (www .multiple-secularities.de/media/multiple_secularities_research_programme.pdf).

6. Taniyama 2014.

7. Vihāra's "broad meaning" encompasses the Four Passing Sights: old age, illness, death, and the possibility of escape from rebirth through monastic discipline. Encountering these sights inspired Siddhartha Gautama to renounce the householder's life and seek enlightenment as the Buddha.

8. The term for *life* (Jp. *inochi* or *myō*) in this context extends beyond biological measures to Buddhist meanings pertaining to life-span (Skt. *jīva*) and ethical concerns about livelihood (Skt. *jīvin*).

9. The Buddhist phrase *shiku hakku* ("Four and Eight Afflictions") functions in Japanese as an expression for dire hardship commonly employed outside Buddhist contexts. An exposition on these afflictions can be found in the *Yogācārabhūmi-śāstra* (T. no. 1579.30.289b).

10. *Keichō* ("active listening") is a technique adapted in Japan from predominantly American forms of counseling aimed at treating post-traumatic stress disorder. It has grown in prominence within Japanese Buddhist circles, particularly since the 3/11 disasters, when clergy embarked on "active listening tours" of the disaster area. See Graf 2016.

11. The 1951 Religious Juridical Persons Law (*shūkyō hōjin hō*) guaranteed freedom of religion by designating religious organizations legal persons, thus granting them a material base to conduct free and autonomous activities. The law was revised in 1995 to allow increased government surveillance of religions, a measure taken following the Aum Shinrikyō sarin gas attacks.

19. Medicine Wizards of Myanmar

Four Recent Facebook Posts

THOMAS NATHAN PATTON

This chapter translates four short texts related to the healing powers of Buddhist "medicine wizards" (*hse weikza*) in contemporary Myanmar. The first two are translations from the Burmese of practices involving the recitation of Pāli verses and the drawing and ingestion of sacred diagrams for the purposes of curing a variety of physical maladies. The third is a testimonial of someone who called upon such wizards to help cure his mother's life-threatening illness, while the fourth offers pithy instructions for how to become a medicine wizard oneself. What makes these texts different from others included in this volume is that they are taken from the online social media and networking platform Facebook.[1]

Facebook is so popular and pervasive in Myanmar that it is today considered to be synonymous with the internet for most of the population.[2] Access to the internet, mobile phones, and SIM cards were prohibitively expensive for most of the population under the rule of the military junta. But in 2014, restrictions loosened, and the prices of mobile phones and SIM cards plummeted. Most of the population is now going online for the first time through their mobile devices, and because the Facebook app comes pre-installed on most devices purchased in Myanmar, the app has become the primary portal through which people access the internet. People have begun posting about their diseases or those of their loved ones and asking other Facebook users which Buddhist practices might work to cure them of their ailments.

The circulation of *weikza*-related media on Facebook is changing the patterns of circulation and vernacularization of knowledge, allowing previously esoteric knowledge to become more widespread and accessible. Before Facebook, the most common avenues for obtaining such knowledge were religious magazines and a handful of outdated handbooks and manuals that have been in circulation since the middle of the twentieth century. Governments in power from the 1960s until the early 2000s perceived *weikza* associations to be unorthodox avenues of religiosity that potentially threatened their authority and, as such, went to great lengths to monitor, suppress, and outlaw most of the *weikza* associations, as well as related magazines, printed books, and other forms of media. Individuals interested in learning more about the *weikza*, and perhaps wanting to follow the *weikza* path themselves, were unable to meet freely to discuss and share such knowledge. Even after the persecution of these associations ceased with the installation of a new government several years ago, few people in Myanmar have been keen to form new associations, despite *weikza* beliefs and practices remaining widely popular. Instead, people have become more interested in entering into personal, direct relationships with *weikza* saints and engaging in practices developed through their intimate connections with these saints. Facebook *weikza* groups, like "*Weikza* Branches of Knowledge and Extraordinary Occurrences" and "Worldly Knowledge and the Rosary Bead Path," each with more than one hundred thousand members, help people from all over the country and diasporic communities around the world to come together around a common cause, issue, or activity to organize, express objectives, discuss issues, post photos, and share *weikza*- and healing-related content. Indeed, as illustrated by the examples below, Facebook allows readers opportunities to engage in self-study with online experts so they no longer need to consult experts in their own communities.

I have collected and read through about five hundred Facebook posts, posted between January 2016 and January 2018, associated with various aspects of Burmese Buddhist medicine. I chose the four posts included in this chapter for the current volume for three reasons. First, the posts were shared and copied widely, garnering hundreds of likes and shares, as well as dozens of comments. Second, they include detailed instructions for the procedures and material culture of these practices. Third, these posts are both a suitable length for the purposes of this volume and are broadly representative of the kinds of religio-medical and apotropaic prescriptions found on Burmese-language Facebook pages.

When these posts use the term "medicine wizard," they are referring to a subcategory of *weikza*; that is, a human being—monastic or layperson—who has transformed him- or herself into a semi-divine being through practices of alchemy, *yantra* manipulation, or mastering sacred verses (figure 19.1). Through these practices, it is believed they gain supernatural abilities to cure humans from a host of illnesses ranging from gastrointestinal disorders to cancer, and

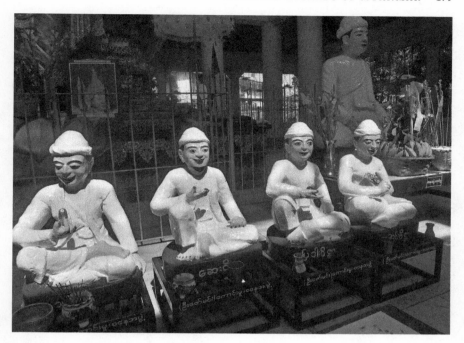

FIGURE 19.1 STATUES OF VARIOUS *WEIKZA* WITH THE MEDICINE WIZARD
SITUATED SECOND FROM LEFT (YANGON, MYANMAR).
Source: Thomas Nathan Patton.

even HIV and AIDS (see chapter 31). At the time of a wizard's death, he or she
leaves this world to reside in an otherworldly abode from which he or she can
continue to help humans in need. Medicine wizards and their devotees understand the world to consist of two kinds of illness: ordinary sickness, caused by
food, climate change, or mental instability, and nonordinary illnesses, caused
by witchcraft, curses, or demons. The Facebook posts translated below deal
with the former to illustrate how healers draw upon, and often combine, a
wide range of therapeutic techniques related to Buddhism and indigenous
medicine to treat illness.

The first post translated below was written by a young man aspiring to
become a master medicine wizard and contains a set of instructions for creating *yantra* (diagrams and drawings using Buddhist syllables, numbers, and
symbols of sacred texts) to be burned, mixed with honey water, and eventually
ingested. The second post is attributed to a Buddhist monk by the name of
Monyin Sayadaw (d. 1964) who is believed by many in Myanmar to have been a
wizard. The post describes a healing practice based upon a popular Pāli verse
(*gāthā*) known as the *Verses of the Perfected Buddhas* (*Sambuddhe gāthā*). One of the

most well-known and widely used incantations for warding off calamities and curing illnesses, it is said to cure even various forms of cancer when recited in the way prescribed in the Facebook post. The third text was posted by a devotee of the medicine wizards who wanted to share his experience of how, in a moment of need, they came to his aid. The fourth post was written by a young woman asking publicly how she can become a medicine wizard so she can cure diseases herself.

The potency of these practices lies, ultimately, in the proper application of Buddhist *yantra* and incantations, for these are the important "ingredients" that imbue the healing techniques with their curative powers. The Facebook posts go to great lengths in describing how one should create *yantra* and accurately recite verses. One can draw *yantra* on various surfaces, the most popular being mulberry paper. The various syllables that make up this type of *yantra* are to be chanted aloud as they are inscribed. For example, the *yantra* prescribed in the second text below has at its core the four syllables CA, DHA, BA, and VA, which represent four separate mantras (figure 19.2).[3]

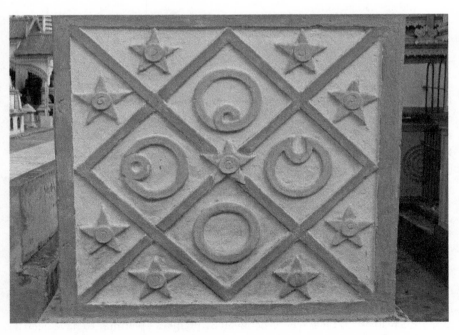

FIGURE 19.2 A STANDARD CA, DHA, BA, AND VA *YANTRA* (MONYWA, MYANMAR).
Source: Thomas Nathan Patton.

FURTHER READING

Brac de La Perrière, Bénédicte, Guillaume Rozenberg, and Alicia Turner, eds. 2014. *Champions of Buddhism: Weikza Cults in Contemporary Burma*. Singapore: NUS.

Foxeus, Niklas. 2016. "'I Am the Buddha, the Buddha Is Me': Concentration Meditation and Esoteric Modern Buddhism in Burma/Myanmar." *NUMEN* 63 (4): 411–45.

Patton, Thomas Nathan. 2018. *The Buddha's Wizards: Magic, Healing and Protection in Burmese Buddhism*. New York: Columbia University Press.

Pranke, Patrick. 2010 [2011]. "On Saints and Wizards—Ideals of Human Perfection and Power in Contemporary Burmese Buddhism." *Journal of the International Association of Buddhist Studies* 33 (1–2): 453–88.

Rozenberg, Guillaume. 2015. *The Immortals: Faces of the Incredible in Buddhist Burma*. Honolulu: University of Hawai'i Press.

1. THE GOLDEN LEAF HONEY WATER *YANTRA*[4]

This method for making a CA-DHA-BA-VA four-syllable *yantra* is intended for all of those good-hearted people who have an interest in such matters. This method is best done in conjunction with using counting beads or sitting meditation. The main purpose of this practice is for health, and it brings great benefit to those who use it. I exhort you to do this practice with confidence and faith.

To begin, offer flowers and fresh water to the Buddha on your home altar, take refuge in the Triple Gem, and take the Five Precepts. You will then need a sheet of paper made from mulberry pulp onto which you will draw the *yantra*. The first *yantra* syllable that you will draw is the CA syllable. That syllable should be drawn on a Tuesday afternoon between the hours of 3 and 4 PM, which is associated with the Wind Element.[5] Facing west, draw the CA syllable on the sheet of paper. That concludes the first day of this practice. After drawing the syllable, place the piece of paper on the Buddha altar.

The DHA syllable should be drawn on a Saturday between 2 and 3 PM, which is associated with the Fire Element, while facing east. Remember to draw it with care. The second day finished, place the piece of paper on the Buddha altar as before. You will draw the BA syllable on the following Thursday between the hours of 1 and 2 PM, which is associated with the Earth Element. Facing south, draw the syllable with care and place it on the altar. The fourth and final syllable, VA, should be drawn on a Wednesday between 4 AM and 1 PM, a time associated with the Water Element, while facing north. At this point, you have completed the part of the practice of drawing the syllables.

On the final day, Wednesday, you should also place the *yantra* piece of paper on the palm of your right hand and chant powerful verses. This will make the *yantra* potent so that you are completely invulnerable to disease, as well as gaining other kinds of supernatural powers.[6] Anyone can draw the syllables on a piece of paper. But this does not make the *yantra* powerful. Only by reciting the following verse aloud, while writing each syllable, will the *yantra* be effective.

First, recite each of the following like so:

BUDDHAM, DHAMMAM, SANGHAM PUJEMI[7] (one hundred times)
BUDDHAGUṆO ANANTO
DHAMMAGUṆO ANANTO
SANGHAGUṆO ANANTO
MĀTĀPĪTUGUṆO ANATO
ACARĪYAGUṆO ANANTO[8] (one hundred times)
ARAHAṂ (eighteen times)[9]

You can then go on to recite other verses and mantras that you like, if you so wish.[10]

When you have finished all of the above, burn the *yantra* paper and set the ash aside. Next, mix pieces of gold leaf and honey water in a jar. The honey should be pure, and the gold leaf should contain at least ten leaves. Place the jar in the sun until the mixture of honey, gold leaf, and water sets. Next, pour the ashes of the incinerated *yantra* into the jar of honey and gold leaf water and shake gently to mix it all together, and place the jar on your Buddha altar for seven days. If the seventh day happens to fall on the day of the week on which you were born, that is particularly auspicious. Regardless of the day it falls on, take a vow to eat only vegetarian food, recite verses and mantras using your counting beads, and send loving-kindness (Pāli *metta*) to all living beings. To really make the *yantra* extra potent with all kinds of powers, spend as much time as you can for the rest of the day reciting your favorite verse, and make offerings to the Buddha and to the pantheon of great wizards.

After reciting verses and mantras with belief and enthusiasm, recite the following nine times: "May all beings be happy and healthy." Then, three times make the tender wish, "May we all be successful in our endeavors."

People who would make use of the golden honey water *yantra* must keep the Five Precepts for each day they use it, as well as refrain from eating meat from large animals and fish. They should have pity and care for all animals. Each day, they must send loving-kindness and make a vow to recite a certain number of verses and mantras on their counting beads each day.

Here is how to use the golden honey water *yantra* mixture:

When waking up in the morning and when going to bed, eat a dose the size of the stem of a betel nut leaf. During the whole week, you will experience all sorts of extraordinary things. For about three to six months, you will be protected from various diseases. Those who are ill will be cured. Use this method according to your own needs, and you will experience various supernatural powers arising related to the use of this *yantra*, and issues related to your worldly life will all be successful.

May all who eat, drink, and use the golden honey water *yantra* become master wizards and saints!

2. A Technique for Reciting the Great Verses of the Perfected Buddhas[11]

You should recite the *Verses of the Perfected Buddhas* at dawn at around 5 AM. Those of you who intend to recite the verses, your body should be clean, as well as your clothes, and your demeanor should be like that of a monk. You should pay homage to all 512,028 buddhas with nine bowls of food, nine cups of water, nine lit candles, and nine lit incense sticks.[12] Then take the Five Precepts. Next, invite the celestial beings in the following way:

> I pay homage to all the 512,028 buddhas and will recite with care the *Verses of the Perfected Buddhas* 108 times.[13] I invite all the spirits of the forests and mountains; guardian spirits of the trees and land; sprits who guard the sky; the spirits who protect the world, cities, towns, villages, neighborhoods, and monasteries; the rain spirits, air spirits, water spirits, [and] moon spirits; all the *devas*; the spirits who guard Buddhism; [the] goddess Sarasvatī and the other groups of seven, nine, and twelve goddesses; Dhatharu, Virulaka, Virupakkha, and Kuvera; and Indra and all the thirty-three royal spirits, noble spirits, and spirit-*devas*. I invite you all to come and listen to a religious discourse. At this time, I will recite the *Verses of the Perfected Buddhas* 108 times. I invite you all to come to this place of refuge to listen to this noble discourse. I entreat you all. Please come to listen to these most revered and holy verses!

After inviting the spirits, *devas*, and so on, sit peacefully in front of an image of the Buddha and clearly enunciate the *Verses of the Perfected Buddhas* 108 times.[14] When finished with the recitation, go on to translate each of the words [from Pāli to Burmese] out loud.[15] Next, offer any merit that you have accumulated from this act to all those beings who have assembled as a result of your invitation. Then try to send as much loving-kindness as you are capable to them all. If you have any wishes or wants, you can request them at this time.

If you do this method in accordance with what I have said, the verses will be instilled with great power. Doing this practice even has many benefits for oneself. If you do it every day, for instance, power will come to you. Everything you do, say, and plan will be successful. You will be free from any and all dangers and misfortunes. You will have power over ghosts, spirits, demons, and ogres. You will be immune to, and be cured of, a multitude of diseases and even various forms of cancer.

People who have done this practice in the past have even been able to make water spontaneously boil by chanting the *Verses of the Perfected Buddhas*, for the water boiled owing to the supernatural power of the incantation. Chanting the *Verses of the Perfected Buddhas* has even caused the sourness of lemon and lime water to disappear and turn sweet.

3. A TESTIMONIAL TO THE MEDICINE WIZARDS' MIRACULOUS CURE[16]

My mother's health was not very good. She could not even walk. She was only able to do *vipassanā* meditation while sitting in a chair and breath meditation while lying down. One day, my sister called me to say that Mom's situation was deteriorating,[17] she was having trouble breathing, and this might be the last time I could see her alive. My sister and I rushed to my mom's house to see her. After paying our respects to Mom, she ordered us out of her room and told us not to cry.

Leaving her home, I said to myself that I would do whatever I could to help her. I immediately placed water and incense on top of a table as offerings. I called upon the chief wizard, Bo Min Gaung, and the medicine wizard, Bo Bo Twe, and entreated them to come and cure my mother.[18] Whether or not they actually came I do not know. I not did see them.

At nighttime, my mother called me on the phone, [saying,] "Son! When you left here earlier today, two wise elders came to me. One was a man with a long mustache and beard. They extracted something from my chest, and I became instantly better!"[19]

The members of my mother's meditation group were amazed when they heard the news. I was so happy and thankful that I immediately made many more offerings to the wizards for the sake of my mom's continued health.

I am relating this event to you all exactly as I experienced it.

4. HOW CAN I BECOME A MEDICINE WIZARD?[20]

[Original post:]
What kinds of religious practice—counting-bead methods and so forth—can I use to cure diseases that afflict me? Please tell me.

[Comment:]
Solemnly vow to do the following for nine days:

Eat vegetarian
Keep the Five Precepts
Meditate for at least ninety minutes each morning
Send loving-kindness to beings
Share your merits with beings

Even if a doctor tells you that you only have three months to live because you have cancer, if you do the above, the cancer will be completely eradicated from your body. Do this all with belief.

NOTES

1. The four posts chosen for this chapter were posted publicly and reposted widely.
2. Potkin 2016; Specia and Mozur 2017.
3. For details on these four syllables, as well as Burmese *yantra* in general, see Patton 2012.
4. www.facebook.com/groups/227601977726343/permalink/277127212773819/, last accessed July 21, 2018.
5. Various forms of Southeast Asian astrology posit that certain times of day are more auspicious than others and pay special attention to the day of the week on which a person was born. The author of this post was born on a Monday, and the time scale he uses in this post is compatible with those individuals born on a Monday. But it is understood that each person must adapt the practice to his or her astrological background. For a detailed analysis of Burmese astrology, see Schober 1980.
6. Such as the ability to fly, walk on water, and pass through solid objects.
7. "I pay homage to the Buddha, Dhamma, and Sangha."
8. "The qualities of the Buddha, Dhamma, Sangha, parents, and teachers are boundless."
9. *Araham* ("Accomplished One") is the first of nine qualities of the Buddha listed in the *Itipiso Gāthā*. The number eighteen is special owing to its numerological properties. Its digits add up to nine, which is an integral element of pagoda building projects and Buddhist sacred diagrams and magical spells, as well as the number most often associated with various rituals of success and prosperity. Its importance presumably comes from numerologically symbolizing the oath of "taking refuge," a standard Pāli chant known throughout the Theravāda world, in which the practitioner takes refuge in the Triple Gem three times (i.e., $3 \times 3 = 9$).
10. Although having different technical meanings, the words *gāthā* and *mantra* are often used interchangeably by Buddhists in Myanmar. Handbooks and manuals of collections of these incantations are popular.
11. www.facebook.com/permalink.php?story_fbid=737091626464138&id=631169490389686, last accessed July 21, 2018.
12. The number 512,028 is numerologically significant, referring to the number of buddhas who arose and died over the course of twenty incalculable eons.
13. Like the number eighteen, the number 108 is a significant number whose digits add up to nine.
14. The *gāthā* is so well known in Myanmar that the author does not even include it. It is as follows: SAMBUDDHE AṬṬHAVĪSAÑCA / DVĀDASAÑCA SAHASSAKE / PAÑCA-SATA-SAHASSĀNI / NAMĀMI SIRASĀ AHAṂ ("I pay homage with my head to the 512,028 buddhas").
15. While an understanding of the meaning of the words being chanted does not usually affect the efficacy of the spell, the author seems to imply that it does or that the translation is done for the benefit of the many beings who have assembled.
16. www.facebook.com/gilbert.htee.9/227601977726343/permalink/330411304112076/, last accessed July 21, 2018.

17. For a discussion of meditation in relation to the path of Buddhist wizards, see Pranke 2010 [2011]; Foxeus 2016.

18. For more on these and other specific wizards, see Rozenberg 2015; Patton 2018.

19. For more cases of wizards extracting illness-causing objects from peoples' bodies, see Patton 2018.

20. www.facebook.com/groups/1573638246261942/permalink/1793686627590435/, last accessed July 21, 2018.

Meditation and Mental Health

20. Naikan and Psychiatric Medicine

Takemoto Takahiro's *Naikan and Medicine* (1979)

CLARK CHILSON

For hundreds of years before the twentieth century, Buddhist monks in Japan cared for the mentally ill. They attempted to allay psychological suffering by performing exorcism, mantra recitations, or ritual prayers or by having the ill sit in hot springs or stand under waterfalls.[1] The one thing they did not do is teach silent meditation to help those who were mentally disturbed.[2]

The first Buddhist-inspired silent meditation widely used for mental health in Japan was Naikan (literally, "introspection"). Its use began in the 1940s. A survey published in 2003 found that twenty-seven medical institutions were using it and that there were thirty-two Naikan training centers.[3]

Naikan involves a person, called a *naikansha* ("person doing introspection"), reflecting on her or his life by asking three questions: What did I receive? What did I give back? What troubles did I cause? These questions are used to examine a relationship with a person with whom the *naikansha* is or has been close (e.g., a parent or spouse) within a specific time frame. So, for example, a *naikansha* may reflect on what he received from his mother between the ages of fourteen and sixteen, what he gave back to her, and what troubles he caused her at that time.[4]

As a daily practice, Naikan commonly involves writing answers to the three questions in a journal. To effect profound change, however, intensive Naikan is often required. This involves doing a week of Naikan at a hospital or training center. During this week, the person does Naikan all day from about 6 AM to 9 PM, sitting behind a screen that forms an enclosed spaced three feet square.

The *naikansha* gets up only to go to the toilet and to bathe. Meals are served and eaten three times a day behind the screen. No reading, writing, talking to other *naikansha*, or any other distraction is permitted.

About every ninety minutes, an interviewer enters into the *naikansha*'s room, opens the screen, bows, and says ritualistically, "What did you examine about yourself during this time?" The *naikansha* then says, for example, "I examined myself in relation to my father between the ages of eight and ten." Then they say what they received from their father, what they gave back to him, and what troubles they caused him during that time. The interviewer then asks what person the *naikansha* will contemplate next. After listening to the answer, the interviewer thanks the *naikansha*, bows, closes the screen, bows again, and leaves.[5]

This practice of Naikan originates in Shin Buddhism (Jōdo Shinshū), a tradition that emphasizes not silent meditation but rather faith in Amitābha Buddha and recitation of his name.[6] Naikan was inspired by a practice called Mishirabe ("self-examination"), which was performed by lay Shin Buddhists in Kansai in the early twentieth century. For the practice, which clergy did not endorse, a so-called sick person (*byōnin*) refrained from sleep, food, and drink while continuously examining the wrong he or she had done in life. About every two hours, the sick person would report to one of the "enlightened" (*kaigonin*) who had successfully done Mishirabe. This continued until the sick person either quit owing to exhaustion or experienced an awakening into their dependence on Amitābha.[7]

The founder of Naikan, Yoshimoto Ishin (1916–1988), performed Mishirabe several times before having an awakening that induced great joy at the age of twenty-one. He wanted others to experience the joy he felt but thought the practice of Mishirabe was too severe. So he decided to offer a modified form of it, which he called Naikan, starting in 1941. For Naikan, Yoshimoto removed the fasting requirements and allowed people to sleep at night. Also, rather than having an unlimited time frame and a goal of achieving an awakening experience, he defined a set period of one week for all practitioners and a goal of simply completing the practice.[8]

When Yoshimoto started working as a prison chaplain in the 1950s, he began describing Naikan in secular language. Correctional officers, as public employees, could offer Naikan to prisoners without breaking the law that prohibited state endorsement of any religion. He argued that Naikan was a self-reflective practice that did not require belief in a deity or adherence to any religious doctrine. Prison wardens accepted this characterization of Naikan, and, by 1965, more than fifteen prisons throughout Japan offered it.[9] Psychiatrists impressed with Naikan's results in transforming prisoners began experimenting with the practice in clinical settings in the 1960s. In the 1970s, a few psychiatrists started to promote it as treatment for alcoholism.[10] One of those psychiatrists was Takemoto Takahiro (b. 1940), the author of the text translated below.

Takemoto has been a leading advocate for Naikan as a psychiatric intervention. In 1976, he established a facility solely for intensive Naikan practice at the mental hospital he had founded in Southern Kyushu. For this, he required some nurses to take part in intensive Naikan training so they could serve as interviewers. He cofounded the Japanese Naikan Association in 1977 and has been involved with the Japanese Naikan Medical Association, which published a journal from 1999 to 2015.

In 1979, Takemoto self-published the book *Naikan and Medicine* (*Naikan to igaku*). The translation below is of three sections from the revised 1994 edition: one on psychosomatic medicine, one on Naikan in relation to psychosomatic medicine, and one on Naikan and alcoholism. The translated sections provide an early example of the medicalization and secularization of a Buddhist-inspired contemplative practice. They show how the medicalization of Naikan was almost concurrent with that of mindfulness in the United States, although it was independent of the mindfulness movement, which had little influence in Japan before 2010. However, unlike many of the early advocates of mindfulness meditation, Takemoto is not a Buddhist modernist. In his numerous publications, he does not refer to the teachings of the Buddha as ancient wisdom congruent with science. In fact, he shows little interest in Buddhism. The translation thus also shows how the efficacy of a Buddhist-inspired meditation has been understood in Japan using scientific concepts and secular language.

FURTHER READING

Blum, Mark, and Robert F. Rhodes. 2011. *Cultivating Spirituality: A Modern Shin Buddhist Anthology.* Albany, N.Y.: SUNY Press.

Chervenkova, Velizara. 2017. *Japanese Psychotherapies: Silence and Body–Mind Interconnectedness in Morita, Naikan and Dohsa-hou.* Singapore: Springer.

Japanese Naikan Medical Association and Japanese Naikan Association, eds. 2013. *Naikan Therapy: Techniques and Principles for Use in Clinical Practice.* Fukuoka: Daido Gakkan.

Onda Akira. 2002. "The Development of Buddhist Psychology in Modern Japan." In *Awakening and Insight: Zen Buddhism and Psychotherapy,* edited by Polly Young-Eisendrath and Shoji Muramoto, 235–44. New York: Routledge.

Ozawa de-Silva, Chikako. 2015. "Mindfulness of the Kindness of Others: The Contemplative Practice of Naikan in Cultural Context." *Transcultural Psychiatry* 52 (4): 524–42.

EXCERPTS FROM *NAIKAN AND MEDICINE*[11]

Medicine of the Mind and Body

Up to this point, I have discussed the neocortex, the paleocortex, and interbrain (i.e., diencephalon, *kannō*). The laudatory, sophisticated science and culture of humans developed as a result of desires that arose in our neocortex. A case in point is electricity. For humans long ago, it was natural to rest at night after the sun went down in the west. Then, when the sun rose and it became light out, people got up and moved around. That, I think, is the primal way of being for humans. But after the invention of electricity, people continued to be active after dark and do various things at night without sleeping. As people started to do such things as study all night for exams and do subway construction work in the middle of the night, we moved far away from that primal way of being. We even started to make convenient things like instant ramen that could be easily eaten with just hot water when hungry at one or two in the morning.

Although our neocortex works hard for our desires, I suggest that we consider our interbrain. For our interbrain, which protects us humans and which is at the core of our brain, night is a time for rest. At night, it works slowly and quietly, and so it slowly moves the heart, lungs, and intestines. But ever since we have started to use electricity, it has been forced to work at night as well. Our stomach is jolted when instant ramen is put into it at an inordinate hour. What I mean by saying it is jolted is that the interbrain is jolted. The interbrain, although exhausted from working incessantly from morning to night, continues to work. The interbrain, the foundation of life, becomes exhausted to the point of torture working for the neocortex.

This is true not only with the stomach, but also with various shocks and stresses in the neocortex. The problem, for instance, of a mother and daughter-in-law fighting creates stimuli that threaten the interbrain. When the interbrain is under constant pressure, a person will start to gradually lose his appetite and not be able to get adequate sleep. This phenomenon is by no means unusual. Stimuli in the neocortex continually and excessively stimulate the interbrain. The academic discipline that studies this problem is called psychosomatic medicine (i.e., mind–body medicine). This is the problem people long ago referred to when they commonly said, "Sickness comes from *ki*." We might say that sickness, or *byō-ki*, is a condition that arises when *ki* becomes *byō*; that is, when *ki* becomes ill. The phrase "sickness comes from *ki*" is one filled with implications.

Owing to the advancements in psychosomatic medicine, we now have a good understanding of the relationship between the neocortex and interbrain. The psyche has various influences on the body that we experience on a daily basis. For example, thunderclaps startle us. At the moment of being startled, our heart starts pounding and our pulse rate increases. Or when we hear about something unpleasant, our face turns pale. Also, when people fight and have arguments, they become excited, their faces turn white, their lips become parched, and they begin to tremble. These physical manifestations clearly show the connection between the psyche and the body.

As psychosomatic medicine continues to develop, we will be able to understand the extent to which the neocortex continually stimulates the interbrain and pressures it. The interbrain is the basis of life. If it does not work, the person will die. If the neocortex dies but the interbrain remains alive, a person will continue to live in a vegetative state. If the interbrain dies, life is over. How we can continue to live in a more human manner is, I think, a problem no different from how we can continue to support in a healthy and refreshing way our primal state of being.

Naikan and Psychosomatic Medicine

Doing Naikan shows us our selfish desires to the point we feel disgusted by them. It also makes us realize the extent to which our selfish desires are causing our interbrains to suffer.

As a result of doing Naikan, however, many people feel lighter in body and mind. There are also many cases in which physical ailments have gotten better. People being cured of constipation, stiff shoulders, or back pain show how Naikan has a major effect that follows a natural course of events. Before doing Naikan, their neocortex created excessive continual pressure on the interbrain. In other words, their self-centered desires, which were squirming and solidifying in the cerebrum's neocortex, are removed one by one as a result of Naikan. Consequently, little by little, the pressure on the interbrain recedes. When the stress and pressure put on the interbrain are removed, the interbrain starts to be able to function freely. Thus, the gastrointestinal tract is vitalized and constipation is relieved. A healthy appetite then develops, and neurogenic gastritis and other illnesses are naturally cured. The same is true with stiff shoulders and back pain. When the interbrain's function is vitalized, blood circulation is smooth, the vasomotor nerve functioning is invigorated, blood vessels expand, and blood flow improves. As a result, stiff muscles are loosened and pain naturally goes away in a convincing manner.

We can say that the interbrain is central to the body and the neocortex is central to the mind. The interbrain is the specific place where the knot is formed that ties the mind and body together. The job of the interbrain is to protect our lives. Therefore, we cannot help but feel happy when the interbrain, which is intimately related to our primal life, is functioning soundly without constrictions. The muscles in our face relax, and we start to smile. Our faces become serene like those of Buddhist statues.

When those of us in psychiatric medicine employ Naikan, we do not aim to cure constipation or improve gastrointestinal movement or loosen tight muscles. Those are secondary byproducts of Naikan. The point of the therapy is to restore to its natural state the cerebral neocortex, which has become distorted by the agglomeration of selfish desires. This is the ultimate aim of Naikan as a psychiatric therapy. Naikan therapy is not for curing constipation, but it is fine if someone uses it to do so. It will certainly meet that expectation.

Naikan and Alcoholism

For those of us in psychiatric medicine who use Naikan, the goal is to get people to achieve their natural state of being human. It is to restore the human state that is in accordance with divine providence[12] and is authentically free and easy. Or, to put it differently, psychiatric medicine for us is something that clarifies the problems with reconstructing a person and with reforming a person.

On the basis of more than 3,500 cases over the last nineteen years, my colleagues and I have validated the psychotherapeutic efficacy of Naikan. Among those cases, there has been some change among 80 percent of them and an effective therapeutic change in about 60 percent. Among patients with alcoholism who have used Naikan, 30 to 50 percent have stopped drinking. This is because Naikan made them conscious of how they had become a bundle of selfish desires and indifferent to all the trouble they had caused. This awareness resonated in their interbrain, and they were able to start to develop a vow to stop drinking.

How this works can be illustrated by thinking about a bottle of potassium cyanide. Hardly anyone who is handed such a bottle would say it looks delicious or that he wants to drink it. That is because the moment he hears it is potassium cyanide, there is a sharp sensation in the interbrain indicating that his life is in danger. Thus, there is no one who will start to drink the potassium cyanide. It is through a similar learned experience that the interbrain stops a person from drinking alcohol.

Sobriety based on reason in the neocortex seems to deteriorate after three months. For the type of person who says, "I know, but I can't stop," the "I know" is reason, and reason is something at the level of the neocortex. Alcohol abstinence that comes from personal experience is an abstinence understood at an interbrain level. It is the refusal of alcohol based on revulsion to it in the interbrain. In other words, the interbrain recoils in response to alcohol and protects the person. It is this disposition that allows for a struggle-free abstinence from alcohol. It is a kind of abstinence void of coercion and based on a natural personal disposition.

This is because when people recall experiences and memories of the past and deeply study them, they come to know themselves while also stimulating their interbrain. They understand with their interbrain. This is what personal experience–based abstinence is. If abstinence is not based on personal experience, it will definitely not continue, and lifelong abstinence will be impossible. Up to now, many people with alcoholism have successfully stayed sober and built peaceful families. Their sobriety has been based on their experiences in Naikan and has been maintained on the basis of emotional personal experiences. Their sobriety is not a result of suppressing desires or restraint based on reason.

Examining our past raises questions about what type of person we should become and what we should now do with our lives. Naikan therapy, I think, is something everyone should do once, because it is a method that allows us to examine such questions as seriously as if we were at the moment of death. Because Naikan is something that involves examining death, it should be done now, while we still have some time to spare and so we can do what needs to be done while alive. The act of looking at death and seriously examining ourselves is Naikan. Introspection in which a person sits aimlessly just passing time is not Naikan and is not what Naikan involves. I hope that you will actually try for yourself Naikan that looks at death and that induces an experience in the interbrain.

NOTES

1. On the history of traditional Buddhist treatments for mental illness, see Hashimoto 2014.
2. The use of mindfulness meditation as a psychotherapeutic intervention developed out of the wider mindfulness movement that started to become popular in the United States in the 1980s. Before this time, silent, seated meditations derived from Buddhism were rarely used to treat stress, depression, or mental illness.
3. This survey can be found in Kawahara 2003.
4. For a more in-depth overview of Naikan and the different ways Naikan is done, see Chilson 2018.
5. For a description of how Naikan is done at training centers in Japan today, see Ozawa-de Silva 2006.
6. Although Naikan advocates often present it as a secular practice or therapy, it still has a connection with Shin Buddhist ideas. For more on this, see Unno 2006. Unno sees Naikan as emphasizing the "utility-value of religion" rather than the "truth-value of religion."
7. On the history of Naikan, see Shimazono 2004: 216–25. Shimazono argues that Naikan can be understood in the contexts of what he calls "psychotherapeutic religions."
8. Yoshimoto Ishin describes how he developed Naikan in his autobiographical account of Naikan. See Yoshimoto 1965.
9. In the 1960s, the sociologist John Kitsuse argued that employing Naikan to reform prisoners was a type of "penitent self-reflection" (Kitsuse 1965).
10. The earliest studies of Naikan as a psychiatric intervention for alcoholism were published by the psychiatrist Suwaki Hiroshi. He points out how both Naikan and Japan's Alcohol Abstinence Society (Danshukai) are based on family relationships (Suwaki 1979).
11. Takemoto 1994: 17–26.
12. The Japanese term *kami no setsuri* is a Christian theological term. Japanese sometimes use Christian concepts even when they are not Christian. The term here should be read as referring to the natural and proper state of something.

21. A Contemporary Shingon Priest's Meditation Therapies

Selections from the Writings of Ōshita Daien (2006–2016)

NATHAN JISHIN MICHON

Ōshita Daien (b. 1954) is a Shingon priest and abbot of Senkōji Temple in Hida, Gifu Prefecture, Japan. He is also a certified music therapist, with nearly three decades of experience volunteering in hospitals and hospices, and the founder of several caregiving associations in Japan. He has authored eleven books to date, most on spiritual care or applying Buddhist teachings in daily life.[1] The selections here come from a few of Ōshita's numerous publications.

Ōshita was born in Gifu Prefecture but, unlike many modern Japanese Buddhist priests, did not come from a temple family.[2] After experiencing a number of deaths in his family by the age of twelve, he began asking his mother many questions about death and the afterlife. She suggested he talk to someone at the local temple, Senkōji. He eventually ordained there, but, unlike other Shingon priests, he also completed Theravāda Vipassanā training at a temple in Sri Lanka.

In 1987, Ōshita Daien's Shingon preceptor became ill with liver cancer. Ōshita began caring for his teacher and became disappointed in the medical treatment of the time for how it prioritized prolonging life over caring for patients' needs. His master eventually succumbed to the cancer, and Ōshita became the twenty-fourth abbot of Senkōji Temple. However, he then found a new calling to combine with his temple duties. He helped found organizations such as the Hida Vihāra[3] and Hida Medical Welfare Volunteer Association, often meeting with doctors, nurses, pharmacists, and others about how to improve daily conditions for the sick and dying. (For more on these types of institution, see chapter 18.)

Ōshita Daien became one of the first modern Japanese Buddhist priests to visit the sick in hospitals. He says he struggled with this early on, since neither hospital staff nor patients were used to seeing Buddhist priests outside of funerals. A security guard once stopped him, saying "The morgue is in the other direction!"[4] If he walked into a hospital room, patients also became fearful, thinking his presence meant death was near. After consulting with nurses and patients, he began wearing an informal brown and yellow uniform (samue),[5] rather than his formal black clerical robe, while volunteering to sit with and care for patients. Over the years, the importance of his work was recognized, and he came to be included in hospital staff meetings.

Not all of Ōshita Daien's work has been based in Gifu Prefecture. In 2006, Koyasan University, a center for training young Shingon priests, reorganized its course structure, and Ōshita Daien led Japan's first Department of Spiritual Care Studies.[6] He was later hired as a researcher and part-time instructor at Kyoto University's Kokoro Research Center. As in his earlier trip to train in Sri Lanka, Ōshita's ecumenical interests showed through during his research in Kyoto. He began learning contemplative traditions from not only other Buddhist traditions but also other religions and looking at how such practices could be applied to health and healing.

Besides continuing to fulfill his roles as abbot of Senkōji Temple and helping in hospitals, he is now a vice-president of the Society for Interfaith Chaplaincy in Japan and leads clinical pastoral education training sessions in numerous cities around Japan.[7] Ōshita Daien's ritual and therapeutic creativity have helped him become one of the leading figures in Japanese Buddhist spiritual care. He combines that creativity and his expansive Buddhist studies with technical knowledge and years of experience in medical care, leading him to play a major role in developing both therapeutic methods and the Buddhist philosophy behind them.

What follows are several short selections from his writings. The first comes from the book *Clinical Meditation Techniques: Four Methods to Revitalize the Mind and Body*. These excerpts illustrate how Ōshita defines the terms "clinical meditation" and "meditation therapy" and how he conceives Esoteric Buddhist paradigms through the lenses of modern psychology and chaplaincy. The next set of excerpts comes from the book *Meditation Therapy Applied to the Care and Support of Others*. This book introduces a wide range of Buddhist meditations Ōshita uses during treatment, and the selection included below presents a brief summary of that range. Finally, a selection from the article "Esoteric Buddhism and Spiritual Care" presents an analogy that details how Ōshita perceives the relationship between caregiver and patient using the example of a terminally ill patient who Ōshita treated. Together, these excerpts show that although Ōshita Daien has adapted to the needs of contemporary treatment settings, he maintains deep roots within his particular Buddhist heritage. The excerpts below also show how meditation is used in a wide variety of therapeutic settings.

FURTHER READING

Giles, Cheryl A., and Willa B. Miller, eds. 2012. *The Arts of Contemplative Care: Pioneering Voices in Buddhist Chaplaincy and Pastoral Work.* Boston: Wisdom.

McLaughlin, Levi. 2013. "What Have Religions Done After 3.11? Part 1: A Brief Survey of Religious Mobilization After the Great East Japan Earthquake Disasters." *Religion Compass* 7 (8): 309–25.

Unno, Mark. 2006. *Buddhism and Psychotherapy Across Cultures: Essays on Theories and Practices.* Boston: Wisdom.

Watts, Jonathan S., and Yoshiharu Tomatsu, eds. 2012. *Buddhist Care for the Dying and Bereaved.* Boston: Wisdom.

Winfield, Pamela. 2005. "Curing with Kaji: Healing and Esoteric Empowerment in Japan." *Japanese Journal of Religious Studies* 32 (1): 107–30.

1. EXCERPTS FROM *CLINICAL MEDITATION TECHNIQUES: FOUR METHODS TO REVITALIZE THE MIND AND BODY* (2016)[8]

When meditation or its techniques are used specifically to help people in clinical settings, I separate this from normal meditation and identify it as "clinical meditation." Most people associate [the term] "clinical" with hospital beds or bedside care, but I am thinking of the term more generally. This usage includes not only the medical field but also the patient support that occurs in psychology, education, and religion. When applying meditation as a therapy, I call it "meditation therapy." Yet more specifically, I mean a psychological and spiritual approach that applies the various functions of meditation to improving factors like the body–mind condition, personality, and spirituality. [. . .]

Rather than continuously avoiding or escaping from self-centered states of mind like personal worries, you look directly into your defilements and spend your life cultivating your human capacities as much as you can. At first, there might be a self-defense mechanism that makes you want to look away from the negative thoughts and feelings. But that is also part of the process of self-insight meditations. It is not about selling yourself short but about being polite in your relationship with yourself. When you are able to forgive yourself through objective self-observation, a peaceful state of mind will eventually arise. In modern thought, concepts such as "resilience" and "sense of coherence" are described to help conquer issues like trauma and post-traumatic stress disorder. But in Buddhism, people have been led through recovery, thoroughly resolving issues through methods of mental training that seek to clearly see reality through insight and observation. [. . .]

Buddhism has phrases such as "birth and death are nondual" (*shōji ichinyō*) and "defilements are none other than awakening" (*bonnō soku bodai*), which mean that both suffering and happiness instruct people during the process of spiritual growth. Instead of removing "the four sufferings and eight sufferings,"[9] you realize the seed critical to developing your "soul" (*tamashī-sei*) by directly facing the suffering. In other words, even if the body becomes sick, you can always try to protect the fundamental health of the soul. When using clinical meditation techniques for spiritual care, while sympathizing with an individual's suffering, you can support their spiritual health with a care that helps them to realize a state of awakening.

2. EXCERPTS FROM *MEDITATION THERAPY APPLIED TO THE CARE AND SUPPORT OF OTHERS* (2010)[10]

Meditating on brilliant light like [that of] the sun or moon carries profound significance, and it is useful because it creates a positive state of consciousness. This is called Illuminating Meditation.[11] Whether in the East or West, and no matter the religious tradition, the presence of light portrays the sacred. Moreover, it is often applied to saving suffering people. There are meditations in which one looks at the morning sun rising in the east or gazes at the setting evening sun [in the west]. In Buddhism, one can visualize the Buddha of the Pure Land of Utmost Bliss in the setting sun. People hope for rebirth in the Pure Land and pray to be saved from suffering in this world. To do this Illumination Meditation in your room, you can also meditate while gazing at an artificial light printed on a poster. I create such an image of light to gaze at and meditate on when I want to release negative states of mind. Prepare your meditative goals (i.e., which suffering to release) while staring at the image and visualizing that image emitting its light.[12] [. . .]

I can probably say that Buddhism is essentially a religion of training through meditation.[13] The teachings of the Buddha's awakening came from a deep meditative state. Thus, Buddhism is nothing more than a "dialogue with oneself" or an "observation of the inner self." From this, a plethora of terms for awakening arose. Whether we look at Buddhist meditation historically or doctrinally, there are many types of meditation. There is *śamatha* meditation, *vipassanā* meditation, stopping-and-seeing meditation, *kōan* meditation, just-sitting meditation, and specific meditations to the Esoteric Buddhist tradition like mandala meditation, A-syllable meditation,[14] moon-disk meditation,[15] and mantra meditation.

One can do mandala meditation while visualizing mandalas and perform A-breathing meditation,[16] A-syllable meditation, and moon-disk meditation while staring at a Sanskrit letter A. A mandala is a pictographic expression of the state of Buddhist awakening. Depending on the type of teaching, there are various types of mandala. There are also mantra meditations through which one can get a taste of the meditative state while chanting mantras or short *sūtras*.

This is a special method for meditation that raises the level of concentration. On the island of Shikoku, when [the founder of the Shingon school of Esoteric Buddhism] Kōbō Daishi Kūkai was still young, he completed a well-known form of mantra meditation known as *Gumonjihō*,[17] in which one continuously chants the mantra of Ākāśagarbha Bodhisattva.[18] He then perceived the morning star and reached a state of awakening. Even when modern people put effort into learning and applying these types of Buddhist meditation practice, they can then embody that practice at any time.

3. EXCERPT FROM "ESOTERIC BUDDHISM AND SPIRITUAL CARE" (2006)[19]

Kōbō Daishi Kūkai sought the human heart's ultimate point of attainment by awakening through yogic practice. Examining Kūkai's awakening through this lens vividly demonstrates the essence of his awakening. Yogic practice refers to meditation aimed at cultivating a perfectly awakened wisdom. From this, we can see the Esoteric perspective on an actualized theory of spiritual care. The harmonizing energy (*enerugi*) of the Tathāgata's[20] immense compassion is like the light of a moon reflected on a lake. The moon is like the self, and the moon's light in the water is like the light in all sentient beings. In a similar way, it is like me and the patient. We are blessed by that energy and unified through the cosmic soul known as awakening. This work unites you and the patient suffering before you through the standpoint of ultimate equality, aiming together for the awakened state. This is what we can call Esoteric Buddhist spiritual care.

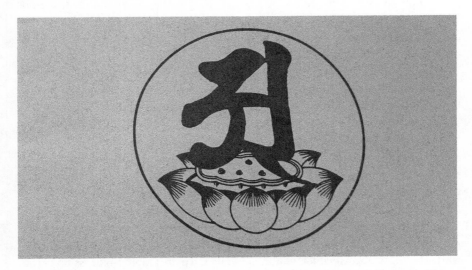

FIGURE 21.1 A TYPICAL *AJIKAN* DRAWING FOUND IN SHINGON MEDITATION HALLS DEPICTING AN A-SYLLABLE ON A LOTUS WITH A MOON DISK.
Source: Miyata 1999.

One concrete example of Esoteric Buddhist spiritual care [comes from] when I worked with Kuriyama Wafu.[21] As a result of ascites, excess liquid bloated his stomach, and he couldn't rest on his side, but he was able to lie parallel to the main altar and practice breathing relaxation. I then used a guided meditation with deep breathing and a visualization of becoming one with the Buddha image on the altar. This was followed by music therapy consisting of guided imagery with a particularly melodic style of chanting called *shōmyō*. At this point, Kuriyama was able to taste a deep state of meditation and experience an expanded state of consciousness. For a little over an hour in this state of mind, he was able to feel free from the throbbing pain of his cancer.

NOTES

1. Spiritual care (*supirichuarukea*) entered the Japanese vocabulary as a *katakana* word (i.e., a word of foreign origin adopted phonetically into Japanese) in 1997. This was a few years after the World Health Organization (WHO) began discussing how to redefine health by including "spiritual health" as a component of overall well-being. Both the WHO and Japanese who deliberated the term afterward were careful to delineate "spiritual" from "religious." For more discussion of the formation of the Japanese term, see Ōshita 2006; Takamatsu 2006.

2. Unlike in the Buddhism of many Asian countries, clerical celibacy is rare in Japan; most Buddhist priests have families. Thus, in contemporary Japanese Buddhism, the leadership of most temples is typically passed down to the first-born son or sometimes the first-born daughter. This wasn't always the case. Japanese Buddhism went through dramatic shifts during the Meiji period (1868–1912), prior to which any act that broke the precepts was considered illegal. A variety of legal, political, and social factors then led to a large shift to married priesthood becoming the norm. For more details, see Covell 2005; Jaffe 2010.

3. Most references to *vihāra* in modern Japan refer to a Buddhist-founded hospice. The primary activity of this *vihāra* early on, however, was a discussion among different caregivers about how to provide the best care to others in different situations.

4. Ōshita 2005: 3.

5. A *samue* is often worn by Japanese priests outside of ceremonies while cleaning or doing other temple chores.

6. This program was revolutionary in Japan but may have been before its time. It ultimately closed owing to a lack of enrollment and was replaced with a single course on spiritual care. However, after 2011, when interest in such programs began to increase, Koyasan University partnered with other programs to allow a concentration in spiritual care by combining studies at its own university with coursework completed in Kyoto and Osaka.

7. Both in the United States and Japan, clinical pastoral education is essentially an internship for chaplains that combines volunteering in a care environment (typically a hospital or hospice) with educational sessions during which a cohort of students can discuss

their encounters with an experienced individual. Especially in Japan, clinical pastoral education sessions often involve role-playing previous experiences of care and then discussing how to improve such interactions.

8. The selections below come from Ōshita 2016b: 28, 55, and 36, respectively. The separation between each excerpt is marked by "[. . .]."

9. *Shiku-hakku*; the term is often used as one word or a set phrase but literally means "four sufferings, eight sufferings." The four sufferings refer to birth, aging, sickness, and death. The first four of the eight sufferings are the same but are then followed by suffering that occurs owing to separation from loved ones, being together with those who are hated, not having what one craves, and attachment to the five aggregates of form, sensation, perception, mental constructions, and consciousness. When the four sufferings and eight sufferings come together as a single term in Japanese, the term can also generally refer to all of the most deep-seated potential sufferings in the mind. (See also chapter 18.)

10. Ōshita 2010: 38–39. Omitted portions are marked with "[. . .]."

11. *Kōmyō meisō*, a visualization of light within the body. In this sense, the word *kōmyō* carries a meaning of not just pure, brilliant light but also a light that awakens and allows for greater wisdom. Although no English word can express this fully, the word *illumination* can at least convey both the sense of light and the arising of awareness. The practice is often combined with the mantra of light in the Shingon tradition. Ōshita Daien simplifies the practice to adapt it for hospital and hospice patients.

12. This meditation is drawn from the Shingon moon-disk meditation. It is common for monks and temples in the Shingon tradition to have hanging scrolls with a painted image of a white disk. Priests practice visualizing the white coming from the scroll and entering their bodies. As they continue the visualization, the disk spreads to illuminate the entire body and then gradually expands to fill the entire universe. The priests then reverse the steps, slowly visualizing the light shrinking back down into the body and then returning to the scroll.

13. Although Ōshita Daien makes this comment, it should be noted that not all Buddhist traditions practice meditation and the degree to which Buddhists of different traditions practice meditation varies.

14. A fundamental meditative practice in the Shingon tradition. The practitioner often sits with a scroll in from of him- or herself, depicting the Sanskrit letter A inside a white disk, which sits atop a lotus (see figure 21.1). The practitioner first visualizes only the letter A inside themselves but then expands the visualization to include the entire picture of the letter, white disk, and lotus. These three parts of the image represent the perfection of voice, mind, and body, respectively. On another level, this can refer to all Shingon meditation practices because the A represents all existence in the cosmos.

15. See note 9.

16. A fundamental meditation learned early in the training of Shingon Buddhist priests in which the practitioner counts his or her breaths in and out. However, on the out-breaths, the practitioner quietly vocalizes a long, guttural "ahh" sound.

17. An intensive meditation practice during which one visualizes oneself as Ākāśagarbha Bodhisattva while chanting his mantra repeatedly for a period of about a month.

18. One of the key bodhisattvas of the Shingon tradition, associated with the Space/Void Element and the subject of visualization during the *Gumonjihō* meditation practice. He is also associated with Venus, the morning star.

19. Ōshita 2006: 121–22.

20. Ōshita Daien uses only the word "Tathāgata" at this point in the text, but he is likely referring to Mahāvairocana Tathāgata, the primary buddha in the Shingon tradition. This buddha is consistently described within the tradition not as a historical or personal buddha figure but as a personification of all light and purity in the cosmos.

21. This is a pseudonym.

22. Mindfulness in Westminster

The All-Party Parliamentary Group, *Mindful UK* (2015)

JOANNA COOK

In the United Kingdom and elsewhere, mindfulness is fast becoming a popular practice. It is now found in British schools, workplaces, prisons, and hospitals. Mindfulness gained popularity as a secular and evidence-based intervention following the development of mindfulness-based stress reduction (MSBR) in the 1970s and mindfulness-based cognitive therapy (MBCT) in the 1990s, and subsequent scientific research into the efficacy of these and other similar interventions. It is now a focus of policy discussion in the United Kingdom.

Beginning in the 1950s in Southeast Asia, reformist monks began to reinvigorate and propagate a form of meditation called *vipassanā*, which is based on the Theravāda Buddhist text the *Mahāsatipaṭṭhāna Sutta*.[1] *Vipassanā* was presented as a "rational" and "authentic" practice, appropriate for monastics and laity alike.[2] Mindfulness (Pāli *sati*) was understood to be an ethically positive perspectival awareness that lay at the core of the practice of *vipassanā*. In the 1970s, Jon Kabat-Zinn developed MBSR, the first modern mindfulness-based medical intervention, at the University of Massachusetts Medical Center. He interpreted mindfulness as a universal human capacity and sought to advance a routinized mindfulness intervention to alleviate some of the suffering experienced by patients facing chronic pain and a range of conditions that were difficult to treat.[3] He famously has defined mindfulness as "paying attention in a particular way: on purpose, in the present moment, and nonjudgmentally."[4]

In the 1990s, Zindel Segal, Mark Williams, and John Teasdale developed MBCT in Cambridge, England, as a psychosocial intervention specifically intended to prevent the relapse of depression.[5] The inspiration for this came in part from the example of MBSR, as well as from a talk given by Phra Ajhan Sumedho, the head of the Thai Forest Tradition in the United Kingdom at the time. Ajhan Sumedho's talk expounded on the Buddha's teaching of the Four Noble Truths (i.e., the truth of suffering, the cause of suffering, the cessation of suffering, and the path leading to the cessation of suffering). In the cognitive framework for preventing the relapse of depression, suffering is understood to be generated, in part, by the ways in which people relate to experience. As such, if patients could learn to relate to experience differently through mindfulness training, they might suffer less.

MBCT and MBSR courses are group-based interventions taught over an eight-week period. Through practice in class and at home, participants develop attentional control, cognitive skills (such as decentering and observational capacity), and behavioral skills (such as embodied or movement-based observation).[6] An MBCT protocol based on this foundation was found to reduce the rate of relapse of depression in three randomized controlled trials[7] and subsequently received a recommendation from the UK National Institute for Health and Care Excellence (NICE) and was mandated by the UK National Health Service (NHS) for people who had experienced three or more depressive episodes but were currently well.

In 2013, mindfulness classes were established in the Palace of Westminster, the seat of the UK Parliament. As of the writing of this chapter, 145 members of Parliament and 250 staff have completed an adapted eight-week MBCT course. In 2014, an all-party parliamentary group (APPG) established an eighteen-month inquiry to investigate the policy potential for mindfulness in four areas of civil society: health, education, criminal justice, and the workplace. APPGs are informal cross-party groups brought together to develop policy recommendations for government on subjects for which there is cross-party interest. Nominally run by members of the House of Commons and House of Lords, administrative oversight is provided by individuals and organizations from outside Parliament. This particular APPG, called the Mindfulness All-Party Parliamentary Group (MAPPG), was supported by the Mindfulness Initiative, an advocacy group composed of professionals drawn together by their professional and personal commitment to mindfulness.

From May to December 2014, eight parliamentary hearings of this APPG were held in Westminster, each focusing on a different area of public life. Following this, a report was produced by the Mindfulness Initiative outlining the character and scale of the challenges identified in each of the four areas and the existing evidence for mindfulness-based interventions. It called for targeted interventions in each area and funding for further research.[8] Significantly, the report mentions Buddhism only a handful of times.

Below, a section of the report (pages 19 to 24 of the original) is reproduced. In this excerpt, the authors present a summary of the health challenges facing the

United Kingdom, the evidence for mindfulness-based interventions, the challenges and costs of implementing mindfulness-based interventions, and recommendations for implementation and further research. The excerpt contains the original footnotes from the report, which have been renumbered, marked with circles, and edited to match the citation style of the current volume. Cited works are listed in this book's references.

FURTHER READING

Cook, Joanna. 2016. "Mindful in Westminster: The Politics of Meditation and the Limits of Neoliberal Critique." *HAU: Journal of Ethnographic Theory* 6 (1): 141–61.

Kabat-Zinn, Jon. 1990. *Full Catastrophe Living: How to Cope with Stress, Pain and Illness Using Mindfulness Meditation*. New York: Delacorte.

McMahan, David, and Erik Braun, eds. 2017. *Meditation, Buddhism, and Science*. Oxford: Oxford University Press.

Mindfulness All-Party Parliamentary Group. 2015. *Mindful Nation UK: Report by the Mindfulness All-Party Parliamentary Group (MAPPG)*. Sheffield, UK: Mindfulness Initiative. www.themind fulnessinitiative.org.uk/images/reports/Mindfulness-APPG-Report_Mindful-Nation -UK_Oct2015.pdf.

MINDFUL NATION UK

Chapter 2: "The Role of Mindfulness in Health"[9]

SUMMARY

Mindfulness-based interventions (MBIs) have a unique role to play in addressing the health challenges facing the country. The NHS is under unprecedented demand, and a new approach to health care is sought by all with a greater focus on prevention of illness, early intervention, and the promotion of health. The strongest evidence for MBIs is in the prevention of recurrent depression. Up to 10 percent of the UK adult population will experience symptoms of depression in any given week,[1] and the rate of recurrence is high—following one episode of depression, 50 percent of people will go on to have a second episode, and 80 percent of these will go on to have three or more episodes.[2] Depression can have tragic consequences for the affected person, with a significantly elevated risk of suicide, and [an] adverse impact on families, friends, and wider society. It also has a steep economic cost in lost productivity, lost earnings, and benefit

---

[1] Singleton. 2002. [Citations corrected and edited to match this volume's usage.]

[2] Cited in Burcusa et al. 2007.

dependence; it has been estimated that in the next decade, the cost of depression will rise to £9.19 billion a year in lost earnings alone, with an additional £2.96 billion in annual service costs.[3]

Depression is two to three times more common in people with a long-term physical health problem than in the general population.[4] There are now more than fifteen million people living with a long-term health condition, which accounts for 70 percent of all our health and care spend.[5] We urgently need effective interventions for the combination of poor mental and physical health.

For people with both physical and mental health problems, recovery from each is delayed, and the effect of poor mental health on physical illnesses is estimated to cost the NHS at least £8 billion a year.[6] Through its mandated Parity of Esteem program, NHS England has recognized that mental health and physical health need to be equally valued, and innovative models of care integrating physical and mental health approaches have been called for as a priority. Mindfulness offers a particular opportunity here, given its integrated mind–body approach and the evidence of its benefits across a range of physical and mental health conditions, as well as supporting well-being and resilience across the population as a prevention strategy to keep people well.

MBIs are inherently participative, inviting an interest in the experience of the body and mind and promoting a different relationship to them. This engaged participation is in keeping with self-management approaches to health that have emerged as important models in health care; mindfulness invites a fundamental transformation of the patient–caregiver relationship into a collaborative inquiring partnership. Mindfulness-based approaches offer great potential for positively transforming cultures of care.

THE EVIDENCE

A meta-analysis of six randomized controlled trials for people who were currently well and who had a history of three or more episodes of depression found that mindfulness-based cognitive therapy (MBCT) reduced the risk of relapse by almost half (43 percent) in comparison to control groups.[7] Since 2004, NICE has recommended MBCT for this group of people. In addition to preventing relapse, MBCT has also been found to reduce the severity of depressive symptoms in people currently experiencing an episode of depression.[8]

---

[3] McCrone et al. 2008.

[4] National Collaborating Centre for Mental Health 2010.

[5] NHS England 2013.

[6] Naylor et al. 2012.

[7] Piet 2011.

[8] Strauss et al. 2014.

There is also emerging evidence from randomized controlled trials support-ing the use of MBCT for health anxiety[9] and for adults on the autistic spectrum,[10] as well as promising evidence for MBIs for psychosis,[11] and that mindfulness-based stress reduction (MBSR) can be helpful in alleviating distress for young people experiencing depression and anxiety.[12] However, there are still signifi-cant gaps in the evidence base for these conditions, and they should be the focus of future research.[13]

One of the most important areas of research has been MBIs and the treatment of long-term physical health conditions.[14] A recent review of 114 studies[15] found consistent improvements in mental health and well-being, notably reduced stress, anxiety, and depression, in the context of poor physical health. In terms of specific physical health conditions, the strongest evidence presented is for the psychologi-cal impact of living with cancer, where 43 studies, including nine randomized con-trolled trials, are described; evidence is also presented from randomized controlled trials for the benefits of MBSR for lower back pain, fibromyalgia, arthritis, HIV, and irritable bowel syndrome. There is also promising evidence that suggests the potential benefits of MBIs in a broader range of other physical health conditions (see list),[16] including conditions that are of pressing concern to policy-makers, such as diabetes and obesity. Whilst most research in this area is with adults, there is also interest in the potential of MBIs for children and young people living with long-term physical health conditions. Finally, there is growing interest in the potential of MBIs in palliative care to support those who are dying and their rela-tives and health care staff, potentially improving the quality of end-of-life care.[17]

[9] McManus et al. 2012.

[10] Spek et al. 2013.

[11] Khoury et al. 2013.

[12] Biegel et al. 2009.

[13] Evidence for the effects of MBIs on mental health was presented at the Parliamentary hear-ing of the MAPPG on 16 Jul. 2014, in the following order, by Tamsin Bishton, Helga Dittmar, Mike Hales, Helen Leigh Phippard, Julia Racster-Szostak, Professor Willem Kuyken, Dr. Clara Strauss, Dr. Kate Cavanagh, Dr. Jerry Fox, Devin Ashwood and Dr. Rebecca Crane.

[14] Evidence for the effects of MBIs on physical health was presented at the Parliamentary hearing of the MAPPG on 5 Nov. 2014, in the following order, by Vidyamala Burch, Dr. Chris-tina Surawy, Dr. Catherine Cameron, Dr. Trish Luck, Dr. Stirling Moorey, Dr. Lana Jackson and Dr. Angela Busuttil.

[15] Carlson 2012.

[16] It includes organ transplant, chronic fatigue syndrome, migraine, asthma, hepatitis, chronic obstructive pulmonary disease, multiple sclerosis, tinnitus, psoriasis, urinary in-continence, insomnia.

[17] Evidence for the effects of MBIs on physical health was presented at the Parliamentary hearing of the MAPPG on 5 Nov. 2014, in the following order, by Vidyamala Burch, Dr. Chris-tina Surawy, Dr. Catherine Cameron, Dr. Trish Luck, Dr. Stirling Moorey, Dr. Lana Jackson and Dr. Angela Busuttil.

While most research has been on MBCT and MBSR face-to-face courses, there is evidence from a recent meta-analysis that self-help mindfulness-based resources such as books and online courses also lead to lower levels of depression and anxiety.[18] This evidence applies in the main to people in nonclinical settings, and so findings cannot be assumed to extend to people experiencing diagnosable mental health difficulties. However, it does suggest potential for a stepped model of care that could extend reach and be cost-effective[19] as an important prevention strategy alleviating subclinical depression and anxiety in the wider population, which in turn has the potential to reduce the need for health service use. The take-up of privately provided mindfulness courses indicates its popularity for this purpose: A YouGov poll for the Mental Health Foundation in 2015 showed 65 percent of people [were] interested in a stress-relieving activity they could undertake daily, and a third of them were interested in learning more about mindfulness. Whilst moderate levels of stress can enhance our performance, excessive or prolonged levels of stress can increase the risk of a range of physical and mental health conditions. A meta-analysis of studies in nonclinical populations indicated that MBSR can significantly reduce stress in comparison to control conditions.[20] Such prevention strategies could be critical to managing demand on health care.

THE CHALLENGES OF IMPLEMENTATION IN THE NHS[21]

There is great interest in mindfulness among health care stakeholders, with 72 percent of GPs [general practitioners] wanting to refer patients to mindfulness courses on the NHS.[22] Yet only one in five GPs report having access to mindfulness courses in their area.[23]

Some pioneering NHS trusts have developed small-scale programs offering MBIs, including Berkshire Talking Therapies, Lancashire Care NHS Foundation Trust, North Wales Cancer Service, Nottinghamshire Healthcare NHS Foundation Trust, Oxleas NHS Foundation Trust, South London and Maudsley NHS Foundation Trust, Sussex Partnership NHS Foundation Trust and Tees, [and] Esk and Wear Valleys NHS Foundation Trust.

[18] Cavanagh 2014.

[19] For example, with pure self-help at step 1, followed by self-help with guidance from a clinician at step 2 and with face-to-face MBCT or MBSR courses at step 3. Such stepped models of care should be a priority for research.

[20] Chiesa 2009.

[21] Barriers and facilitators to the implementation of MBIs in the NHS for mental health conditions were presented at the Parliamentary hearing of the MAPPG on 16th July, 2014, in the following order, by Professor Jo Rycroft-Malone, Val Moore, Dr. Jonty Heaversedge, Paul Bernard.

[22] Halliwell 2010.

[23] Crane and Kuyken 2012.

One such program has been developed by the Sussex Mindfulness Centre, a collaboration between Sussex Partnership NHS Foundation Trust (a mental health trust) and the University of Sussex. The center conducts mindfulness research [and] offers MBCT courses to patients and staff, as well as an MBCT teacher training program. In their adult primary care service in East Sussex (Health in Mind), they offer nine MBCT courses, catering for around one hundred patients each year, with a dedicated MBCT teacher in post to support this provision and ensure its integrity. They are also extending provision into their secondary care adult mental health services and into their children and young people's services.

Another model is Breathworks, a social enterprise founded in 2001 that is based in the Northwest of England and works nationally, [offering] eight-week courses adapted from the MBSR program for people living with chronic pain and other long-term physical health conditions. Their courses are not generally available on the NHS and cost £200 (with some partial bursaries [available] for those who cannot afford to pay). They have also established a program of courses and teacher training.

There are also some excellent examples of courses in NHS physical health services. Three MBCT-for-cancer (MBCT-Ca) courses are run each year in the oncology department at the Alaw Day Unit, Betsi Cadwaladr University Health Board, for people living in North and Northwest Wales. Courses are offered to people with all types and stages of cancer. People with very different prognoses, including those with terminal and advanced disease, are welcome.

However, despite such programs, access to MBCT as recommended by NICE is still extremely limited.[24] One barrier to implementation is that MBCT is recommended as a prevention intervention for recurrent depression rather than as a treatment for current depression. That requires an NHS that prioritizes prevention; the importance of this is well understood in the debate about future health care.

Another barrier to implementation of MBCT is that mental health and physical health are almost always treated by separate NHS trusts, leaving patients and their care teams to negotiate separate systems. Despite the Parity of Esteem principle, availability of psychological interventions within physical health settings is still very limited, and this is true for MBIs, despite the wealth of evidence that they can alleviate symptoms of depression, anxiety, and stress across a broad range of physical health conditions.

The lack of provision within the NHS contrasts with the flourishing and rapidly expanding private provision of mindfulness courses. This restricts access to those who can afford an eight-week course, which typically starts from around £200, or an online subscription, from around £8 per month.[25] The danger is of increasing health inequality, with those who perhaps have the most to gain from MBIs being the least able to access them.

[24] [There is a reference in the original text to note 14 here. This seems to be an error.]

[25] Currently a monthly subscription to the Headspace app is £7.95, and to BeMindfulOnline is £5.

In addition, there is another set of challenges around implementation, which goes to the heart of the effectiveness of those teaching mindfulness. Questions of teacher-training integrity and quality are considered in chapter 6 [not included here].

HOW MUCH WOULD IT COST?

The groundbreaking Improving Access to Psychological Therapies (IAPT) program aims to treat 15 percent of all those with depression and anxiety. Similarly, as a first step, our recommendation would be to get 15 percent of those at risk of depressive relapse and who meet the criteria of the NICE guidelines into MBCT courses by 2020; according to our indicative estimate, this would cost just under £10 million per annum.[26]

Using figures on the cost of depression from the Kings Fund report "Paying the Price: The Cost of Mental Health Care in England to 2026,"[27] this could mean savings of £15 for every £1 spent,[28] with further savings in related health care costs such as [the cost of] antidepressant prescriptions. In line with other mental health treatments, the savings in lost earnings far outweigh the costs.

HEALTH RECOMMENDATIONS

Given the tight financial climate, we have given careful consideration to credible targets as a first stage.

This is an exciting opportunity to develop an innovative treatment to reduce the burden of mental ill health and the added suffering it brings to those facing physical pain and disease. The rate of commissioning within the NHS appears to be slow since the NICE guidelines came out in 2004.

Also disappointing has been the inadequate investment in the high-quality research needed to strengthen the evidence. We urge health care commissioners and the national research-funding bodies to move forward on these recommendations.

[26] MBCT, for a total of 87,000 (the 15 percent target) of the 40 percent who are at risk of relapse from the 1.45 million who meet diagnostic criteria, would cost £9.7 million. £112 per participant (Kuyken et al. 2015). 7,250 courses a year requiring 484 FTE teachers. Burcusa and Iacono 2007 and from McCrone et al. 2008.

[27] McCrone et al. 2008.

[28] Using the target of 87,000 people as per reference 26 above, if they all had MBCT in comparison to not having MBCT, 23,490 of them would be prevented from having a relapse (based on Piet 2011). Based on average estimated lost earnings of £6,338 per person due to depression (McCrone et al. 2008), that is a saving of £149 million to England's economy.

Implementation Recommendations

We recommend that:

1. MBCT (mindfulness-based cognitive therapy) should be commissioned in the NHS in line with NICE guidelines so that it is available to the 580,000 adults[29] each year who will be at risk of recurrent depression. As a first step, MBCT should be available to 15 percent[30] of this group by 2020, a total of 87,000 each year. This should be conditional on standard outcome monitoring of the progress of those receiving help.
2. Funding should be made available through the Improving Access to Psychological Therapies (IAPT) training program to train one hundred MBCT teachers a year for the next five years, to supply a total of 1,200[31] MBCT teachers in the NHS by 2020 in order to fulfill recommendation 1.
3. Those living with both a long-term physical health condition and a history of recurrent depression should be given access to MBCT, especially those people who do not want to take antidepressant medication. This will require assessment of mental health needs within physical health care services and appropriate referral pathways being in place.
4. NICE should review the evidence for MBIs in the treatment of irritable bowel syndrome, cancer, and chronic pain when revising their treatment guidelines.

Research Recommendations

We recommend that:

1. The National Institute of Health Research (NIHR) should invite research bids to evaluate the effectiveness (including maintenance of effects) of MBIs in the following areas:
   - A definitive randomized controlled trial of adapted MBCT as a relapse-prevention intervention for young people with a history of depression to

[29] Of the 1.45 million people meeting diagnostic criteria for depression in any year, 40 percent will go on to have three or more episodes (580,000) based on figures from Burcusa & Iacono 2007 and from McCrone et al. 2008.
[30] This is the target reach used by the NHS's Improving Access to Psychological Therapies training programme (IAPT).
[31] It is regarded as best practice for MBCT teachers to teach on a part-time basis (two days a week), running courses alongside other work commitments. The total requirement of teachers to meet the 15 percent target is 484 FTE teachers, based on them teaching 15 courses of 12 participants per year.

see if the relapse-prevention findings from studies with adults generalize to younger people.

- A definitive randomized controlled trial with full health economic evaluation of MBSR for people living with a range of long-term physical health conditions.[32]
- A program of research exploring the effectiveness of lower-intensity MBIs as a public health preventive intervention for groups and communities at higher risk of mental ill health or indicating preclinical levels of mental health problems. This should include measuring well-being and physical health outcomes, as well as costing health care use.

CASE STUDY: TAMSIN BISHTON, BRIGHTON

In 2008, I was doing a job that I loved in digital communications and working with people I counted as friends. But there was a culture of overworking, pressure, and burn out. I kept going by taking antidepressants, but I stopped them because of the side effects. I hardly slept, and when I closed my front door at night, I was swallowed by panic attacks. One day I realized I just couldn't make myself go back to the office without something changing radically.

My CBT [cognitive behavioural therapy] counsellor suggested a course of mindfulness-based cognitive therapy, and it changed my life. From the first shaky breath, I felt the possibility of reconnecting with my breath, body, thoughts, and feelings. There was something inexpressibly powerful about just stopping, and, having felt trapped and powerless, a pathway opened up. It led me away from my depression, fear, and anxiety by taking me right up close to them. It wasn't an easy path to follow. It's hard to look your demons in the eye and say, "I'm afraid of you, but I am more than you." But instead of feeling overwhelmed, I felt in control for the first time in years—and it all came from stopping, sitting, and breathing.

Finding time to practice every day is still difficult—I'm married with a child— and I never take it for granted. But five years on, I've taken ownership of my well-being and changed how I work. I respond to stress more constructively, and my ambition is to take what I've learned back into the workplace to help others like me.

CASE STUDY: ANU GAUTAM, MANCHESTER

I was a dynamic twenty-six-year-old high achiever when I was diagnosed with advanced-stage Hodgkin lymphoma. I never imagined this would happen to me.

---

[32] This research question would focus on the potential of MBSR as an intervention for multiple physical health conditions within the same MBSR group. Most research in this area is condition-specific (for IBS [irritable bowel syndrome], arthritis etc.), while in practice condition-specific mindfulness-based courses will remain in short supply.

My health deteriorated, and I underwent several years of intensive treatment. It was hard to cope with the physical impact. But I also lost my independence and ability to function, and I felt angry and desperate.

Once the treatment was completed, I tried to get back to what I'd been doing, but health problems kept getting in the way. The Breathworks mindfulness course showed me how mindfulness applied to the difficulties I was facing. The caring environment was important, and so was the inspiration of the teacher, who had really embraced her own health situation.

I learned to get a distance from my thoughts and see that they weren't necessarily true. That had a massive impact. I also saw I didn't have to be pushed around by the ups and downs of illness. I started to experience a kind of peace that was always accessible, whatever was going on.

A couple of years later, I was asked to choose between a bone marrow transplant, which could end my life, or having just a few years without it. It was the hardest decision of my life. After the treatment, I spent six weeks in isolation knowing my life might be ending, but I just stayed with what was going on, including the prospect of dying. It was an amazing time.

My cancer came back last year. That was upsetting, but I knew that it was OK to be upset. I still can't lead a very active life, but my priorities have changed. The most important thing for me is continuing this journey. I feel happier and more whole each day. And it's great.

NOTES

1.   Jordt 2007; Cook 2010; Braun 2013.
2.   Van Esterik 1977.
3.   Kabat-Zinn 1990.
4.   Kabat-Zinn 1994: 4.
5.   Segal, Williams, and Teasdale 2013.
6.   Segal, Williams, and Teasdale 2013: 132.
7.   Teasdale et al. 2000; Ma and Teasdale 2004; Kuyken et al. 2008.
8.   For an extended ethnography of the Mindfulness All-Party Parliamentary Group, see Cook 2016.
9.   This section of the *Mindful Nation UK* report has been reproduced with permission from the Mindfulness Initiative, the policy institute that provides the secretariat of the Mindfulness All-Party Parliamentary Group. The original document can be found at www.themindfulnessinitiative.org.uk/publications/mindful-nation-uk-report and is distributable under a creative commons license. It has been reproduced here with slight editing to match this volume's spelling and punctuation conventions; see Mindfulness All-Party Parliamentary Group 2015.

23. Medicalizing Sŏn Meditation in Korea

An Interview with Venerable Misan Sŭnim

LINA KOLEILAT

The following is an interview conducted in South Korea with the Buddhist monk Misan Sŭnim from the Jogye Order of Korean Buddhism,[1] conducted in the summer of 2017 at his Sangdo Meditation Center (Sangdo Sŏnwŏn). Misan Sŭnim is well traveled and well educated, having completed a Ph.D. at the University of Oxford. Reflecting the wishes of Misan Sŭnim, the interview was conducted in English.

The Sangdo Meditation Center is a four-floor building in a quiet neighborhood of Dongjak-gu Sangdo-dong, near the affluent Kangnam area, in Seoul.[2] Upon entering, one is greeted by a strong smell of coffee, which is made with beans ground at the center and is very popular among young and old lay visitors. Despite its modern design, the interior of the building retains traditional Buddhist elements. A long wooden staircase leads to the huge Dharma hall in the basement, and stone Buddhist statues along the stairs are artfully illuminated with indirect lighting, similar to that used in gallery displays. The center itself represents what Misan Sŭnim is trying to achieve with his recently created meditation program: a modern framework for the Sŏn (Jp. *Zen*) tradition of meditation.[3]

The interview below has been edited for clarity and conciseness. In this conversation, Misan Sŭnim explores ideas of healing, sickness, and suffering and the role of meditation in an effective and holistic therapy he calls "*māha* healing" or "great healing."[4] At the time of this interview, Misan Sŭnim was preparing to market his teachings as a program of prepared courses and practices. He also had plans to design a manual of his teachings, which would accompany a program for teaching instructors in the United States who could implement his program without the need to first become Sŏn masters.[5] Misan Sŭnim has established a complete theological system that he is ready to explain in terms of Buddhist concepts and scripture, bolstered by references to Western science. He portrays his "Heart-smile" program as a perfect melding of mindfulness and science.[6] His description is devoid of mysticism but is peppered with Buddhist terminology, as well as the scientific trappings of medical scans and prestigious research institutions. At the same time, at the end of the interview, Misan Sŭnim describes his modernized teachings as wholly consonant with traditional Sŏn.

In this interview, it is clear that Misan Sŭnim is addressing two global audiences, between which he positions himself as a bridge. On one hand, by seeking international recognition of his meditation program by Harvard Medical School, Misan Sŭnim is addressing a young, modern Korean professional audience who is highly educated and global. This audience is not necessarily interested in the religion of Buddhism per se but rather in a modern practice that is scientifically "proven." Throughout the interview, Misan Sŭnim mentions that he works with a team of qualified doctors, psychologists, and psychiatrists. On the other hand, Misan Sŭnim is also addressing a Western audience. He is seeking international recognition, showing the world the value of Korean Sŏn Buddhism in an academic context. He is also up to date with the popular literature on meditation that is consumed in the West, citing Daniel Goleman and Richard J. Davidson's book *Altered Traits*.[7] By connecting his traditional Korean Buddhist knowledge and practice to Western medical expertise in these ways, Misan Sŭnim offers his followers, both in Korea and the United States, a traditional meditation practice in a global, medicalized package.

As other chapters in this volume amply show, Misan Sŭnim's integration of science and meditation is not new.[8] But the conversation excerpted below deepens our understanding of the medicalization of Buddhist meditation globally, and in the context of South Korea more specifically. It also shows us how leading trends in scientific meditation developing in the West are now impacting the practices taught by monastic Buddhist leaders in Asia and inspiring reforms and reinterpretations of tradition.

FURTHER READING

Buswell, Robert E. 1992. *The Zen Monastic Experience: Buddhist Practice in Contemporary Korea.* Princeton, N.J.: Princeton University Press.

Cho, Eunsu, ed. 2012. *Korean Buddhist Nuns and Laywomen: Hidden Histories, Enduring Vitality.* Albany, N.Y.: SUNY Press.

Goleman, Daniel, and Richard J. Davidson. 2017. *Altered Traits: Science Reveals How Meditation Changes Your Mind, Brain, and Body.* New York: Penguin.

Joo, Ryan Bongseok. 2011. "Countercurrents from the West: 'Blue-Eyed' Zen Masters, Vipassanā Meditation, and Buddhist Psychotherapy in Contemporary Korea." *Journal of the American Academy of Religion* 79 (3): 614–38.

McMahan, David L., and Erik Braun, eds. 2017. *Meditation, Buddhism, and Science.* New York: Oxford University Press.

Park, Jin Y., ed. 2012. *Makers of Modern Korean Buddhism.* Albany, N.Y.: SUNY Press.

Park, Pori. 2014. "Buddhism in Modern Korea." In *The Wiley Blackwell Companion to East and Inner Asian Buddhism*, edited by Mario Poceski, 466–84. Chichester, West Sussex, UK: Wiley.

INTERVIEW TRANSCRIPT[9]

LK: What is *māha* healing?

MS: The Buddha said that there is a fundamental source of pain, and that is what causes suffering. The Buddha is the great doctor and knows exactly what disease is. The Buddha knows the causes of disease. He knows how to remove the causes of the disease and cure it completely, so that it does not return. This is *māha* healing, perfect whole healing. The Buddha himself said you cannot do it half-way and think you are fine. No, you have to have complete healing.

Here in Korea, we developed this Heart-Smile program based on Korean Sŏn Buddhism that says every creature has its own Buddha nature. You and me, we embody the Buddha, so we pass along that teaching in the Heart-Smile training. We train them in a very common and practical way of feeling the smile on your face and bringing that feeling of warmth and tenderness to the center of your heart. As long as you feel that sensation or feeling throughout your body, you can send it out to the people around you, or to creatures around you like birds and trees. You send kindness and warmth and tenderness. Later, you can send your love and kindness to those you really hate, those who really broke your heart. That is the most difficult part, but with this kind of meditation, you should be able to do that.

This is the main program of Heart-Smile. But most people cannot do this, so we develop five supportive practices. First, do some movements with some hand gestures (*mudrā*). The second is meditation for gratitude and acceptance. Many people in the modern world criticize themselves, so in meditation we bring the awareness that you have to love yourself. That's quite a powerful meditation.

In the third, we invite people to relax their body as far as is possible. Our bodies are always full of tension. With tension, you cannot go into deep meditation, so relaxation is essential. We give instruction on how to relax, first lying in meditation with a smile. Just bring your awareness to the whole body and smile, and have that feeling and energy, and scan your body in a particular way. Most programs scan from head to feet, and that is quite common, but our body scan is quite different: We scan the fascia. The fascia is underneath the skin and also is the beginning of the surface of the muscles, which are covered by the fascia like a wrapping. That part is quite important as it contains the emotions of previous lives. If you had trauma on a certain part of the body, the brain recognizes it. The point of scanning the fascia is to relieve that tension and worry. That is one part of relaxation meditation. There is also sitting meditation with the projection of the organs: lung, heart, liver, stomach, and intestines. You sit and imagine that your lungs are in the deep mountain, and they are shining and strong in color. Intestines like yellow, whereas the liver likes blue and kidneys like black. So you imagine that color and some tension on that organ will be released.

The fourth one is sound meditation with OM, and you do a deep Korean bow. You feel the deep vibration and feel the heart center humming. Once you get a calm state of mind, your body is relaxed. Then I tell people to smile and imagine their face is warm like the sun shining. Then, slowly bring that feeling to the heart center and keep it there for twenty or thirty minutes. You will feel all the cells of the body charged with warmth and kindness and compassion. Then clearly imagine your loved ones, then the creatures, and finally that person you really don't like.

Those are the steps. In Korea, we do all this in a program for three days, but in America, we are going to do an eight-week program.

LK: Will you go to the U.S.?

MS: Yes, we are going to do experimental research at the Center for Mindfulness and Compassion at Harvard Medical School. This September, we are going to experiment and teach all these things at Harvard.

LK: Based on the Heart-Smile program?

MS: Yes, we have run this program [for] three years in Korea. We have also published two very important studies in prominent academic journals in Korea.[10] But that is not enough to get international recognition for a meditation program. So, two months ago, I went to America and presented my lecture on this Heart-Smile training to the Harvard Medical School. Next year, I'm going to go back there to teach in English an eight-week course and a six-day intensive course. Based on my teaching, we will create a manual and training program to teach teachers in the U.S. In order to prove that our methodology is valid, it must not be just me who can teach this meditation technique. So we are aiming to train some teachers so they can teach and get good results, so we can show how good our program is. We have been running this program for three years, and it will take us about three more years to produce the manual [and] then train the teachers based on the manual. We will run the teachers' program here in Korea also, but only after we give attention to the English program and reach international standards.

LK: Why did you create this program?

MS: Because the world needs this type of program. People don't know how to love themselves or share with others. In ancient times, they had this well-established method. I realized when I studied in Oxford that Western people had picked up our beautiful things and learned from them, picked up our jewels and put together this necklace, so why don't we learn from them, too? I can teach them, along with the qualified doctors, psychologists, and psychiatrists who work with me to develop this program in Korea.

LK: Is this program good for healing certain diseases?

MS: Yes, it looks at everything. This program will heal you if you are depressed. But that kind of healing is not the end; it is the beginning. For Buddhists, healing is long term.

Buddhist healing is about eradicating the root of suffering and having complete liberation from suffering. If you want shallow teachings, I am not the person for you. I don't want you to take some pieces and spread rumors that this is a hospital. I am not a doctor. I am a recognized *māha* doctor, like the Buddha before me. The government dismisses it, but I don't care. The people have physical fitness, but mental fitness is more important. I am a mental fitness trainer.

LK: How many people have done the program in Korea? And are you collecting data about your participants and their outcomes?

MS: So far, we have done twenty sessions, [and] in each session about thirty people participate, so probably about five hundred people in total. Every session for the last three years, we have been collecting simple data in the area of counseling and psychology. In this field, things are changing very rapidly. But we know that the benefits of meditation are scientifically proven. It took scientists about forty years to prove that. I am currently reading an important book by Daniel Goleman and Richard Davidson called *Altered Traits*. The book is about how meditation changes the body and mind. We are planning to translate that book into Korean this year. The Korean publisher is hesitant because it is a huge volume and it is very scientific, but I think it is worth translating.

LK: What do you think is the influence of Sŏn Buddhism or Korean Buddhism on this new program?

MS: Korean Buddhism has a long-standing authority in Buddhism, and there are still many people who practice it. I am merely the kind of person who can communicate Sŏn Buddhist practice, based on my own study and practice of Zen meditation since my youth. I can bring these traditions to the modern world in the form of a very simple and accessible meditation technique. Meditation should first be understandable. Second, it should be accessible. And third, it should be practical. This is very important.

NOTES

1. For more on Korean Buddhism, see S. Cho 2002; Yoon 2012; Grayson 2013; Gimello, Buswell, and McBride 2014.

2. For a discussion on religious life in Korea among the urban middle class, see K. Kim 1993.

3. For more on Korean Sŏn meditation, see Muller 1999.

4. For more on Korean Buddhist healing, see D. Baker 1994.
5. For more on the experience of a Sŏn master, see Buswell 1992.
6. See, for example, http://heartsmile.org/en/contents/sub01_01_01.php.
7. Davidson and Goleman are *New York Times* best-selling authors.
8. See, among others, Kasamatsu and Hirai 1966; R. Wallace 1970; Hickey 2010; Schmidt 2014. For a useful starting point to the literature, see McMahan and Braun 2017.
9. Interviewed by Lina Koleilat at Sangdo Meditation Center in Seoul, South Korea, August 2, 2017. Condensed and edited for inclusion in this volume.
10. Park, Sung, and Mi San 2016; Sung, Park, and Mi San 2016.

24. Misuses of Mindfulness

Ron Purser and David Loy's "Beyond McMindfulness" (2013)

DAVID L. McMAHAN

Buddhist meditative practices have made a long, circuitous journey from their origins in the ascetic communities of ancient India to the therapists' offices, corporate multipurpose rooms, and neuroscience laboratories of the twenty-first century. The latter phases of this journey were made possible, in part, by new interpretations of these techniques within the framework of modern psychology, medicine, and neuroscience, many of which are discussed in other chapters of this volume. Nineteenth- and early twentieth-century Western interpreters of Buddhism, such as Caroline Rhys Davids and Thomas Rhys Davids, designated its complex treatment of the mind "Buddhist psychology." Mid-twentieth-century enthusiasts explicated Buddhism in psychoanalytic terms, and Gestalt psychologists began to incorporate mindfulness techniques into their therapeutic practices in the 1960s and '70s.[1] It was around the turn of the twenty-first century, however, that certain strains of mindfulness began to peel away nearly completely from their Buddhist roots.[2] This was no accident. Jon Kabat-Zinn, the founder of the enormously popular and influential mindfulness-based stress reduction (MBSR) program, quite deliberately stripped away references to Buddhism in his descriptions of MBSR.[3] This allowed the program access to secular and public institutions like schools, businesses, hospitals, the military, and governments (see chapter 22). Now mindfulness has become ubiquitous, along with a cottage industry of teachers, credentialing programs, books, and commercial venues.

If a single factor has proven pivotal to the acceptance and legitimacy of these programs in secular arenas, it is the recent spate of scientific studies of mindfulness. While advocates of Buddhism have been presenting Buddhism and Buddhist meditation in scientific language for more than a century, only recently have scientists invested a great deal of time and money in the scientific study of Buddhist-derived meditative practices. In the last two decades, the number of studies of mindfulness conducted by neuroscientists, cardiologists, psychologists, and other clinical researchers has increased exponentially, and such studies have suggested that mindfulness can have beneficial effects on immune system functioning, cardiovascular health, and a myriad of psychological problems.[4]

Mindfulness has quickly attained legitimacy in North America and Europe, largely because of the therapeutic and medical benefits suggested by scientific studies conducted at prestigious research institutions. The popular media has seized upon this trend, often presenting mindfulness as a panacea to a host of modern psychological, medical, and personal problems. Such publications have heralded the benefits of mindfulness for stress reduction, increasing the attention span, and a number of health issues, including hypertension and restless leg syndrome. According to the swelling body of popular mindfulness literature, which includes hundreds of books and articles on topics as specific as mindful horseback riding and mindful eating, there is virtually no limit to what mindfulness can help us do better. Mindfulness has also entered the business world. From Silicon Valley tech firms to international banks, corporate mindfulness programs promise to make workers more calm, focused, efficient, and, ultimately, productive.

By the time a special issue of *Time* magazine declared a "mindful revolution" in 2014, however, more skeptical assessments of the benefits and purposes of mindfulness were surfacing. A few meta-analyses of mindfulness studies found the evidence for various benefits less convincing than many had initially suggested.[5] For example, a meta-analysis from the National Institutes of Health found that many trials were beset by problems such as small sample sizes, design flaws, and a lack of clear operational and conceptual definitions of mindfulness.[6] A larger debate had also emerged about what information can truly be derived from functional magnetic resonance imaging (fMRI) scans and other brain-imaging technologies, which have been important aspects of recent mindfulness research. Other critical perspectives coming from the scientific community include research that has recently uncovered many examples of practitioners experiencing disturbing, disorienting, or even psychotic states during meditation retreats, calling into question the assumption that meditation is uniformly good for everyone.[7]

Other critical reflections on recent uses of mindfulness approach the issue from social and political perspectives.[8] These include critiques of the decontextualization of mindfulness from the broader ethical and spiritual environments in which they emerged and flourished for centuries. Few of these critiques condemn mindfulness or meditation outright. To the contrary, they often come from practitioners concerned with how mindfulness has become institutionalized, decontextualized, and commodified. Many are concerned that secular mindfulness programs are unmoored from any ethical orientation and are used in ways antithetical to their earlier purposes.

The publication of the following essay in a 2013 *Huffington Post* blog, by Ron Purser, a professor of management, and David Loy, a Zen teacher, represented a watershed moment of backlash against some of the recent trends of secular mindfulness. The authors claim that "McMindfulness," a "stripped-down, secularized technique" that has been refashioned to be "more palatable to the corporate world" betrays mindfulness's "original liberative and transformative purpose, as well as its foundation in social ethics." They are especially critical of corporate mindfulness programs, which, they insist, have become "a trendy method for subduing employee unrest, promoting a tacit acceptance of the status quo, and . . . an instrumental tool for keeping attention focused on institutional goals." This argument has inspired a lively debate on the use of Buddhist-derived mindfulness practices in corporate, therapeutic, and medical settings. Their essay represents a moment when the discussion of mindfulness began to shift from an exclusive concern with health benefits to the social and systemic issues raised by its new institutional settings.

FURTHER READING

McMahan, David, and Erik Braun. 2017. *Meditation, Buddhism, and Science.* New York: Oxford University Press.

Purser, Ronald. 2019. *McMindfulness: How Mindfulness Became the New Capitalist Spirituality.* London: Repeater.

Purser, Ronald E., David Forbes, and Adam Burke, eds. 2016. *Handbook of Mindfulness: Culture, Context, and Social Engagement.* Switzerland: Springer.

Van Dam, Nicholas T., et al. 2018. "Mind the Hype: A Critical Evaluation and Prescriptive Agenda for Research on Mindfulness and Meditation." *Perspectives on Psychological Science,* 13 (1): 36–61.

Wilson, Jeff. 2014. *Mindful America: The Mutual Transformation of Buddhist Meditation and American Culture.* New York: Oxford University Press.

"BEYOND MCMINDFULNESS"[9]

Suddenly mindfulness meditation has become mainstream, making its way into schools, corporations, prisons, and government agencies, including the U.S. military. Millions of people are receiving tangible benefits from their mindfulness practice: less stress, better concentration, perhaps a little more empathy. Needless to say, this is an important development to be welcomed—but it has a shadow.

The mindfulness revolution appears to offer a universal panacea for resolving almost every area of daily concern. Recent books on the topic include *Mindful Parenting, Mindful Eating, Mindful Teaching, Mindful Politics, Mindful Therapy, Mindful Leadership, A Mindful Nation, Mindful Recovery, The Power of Mindful Learning, The Mindful Brain, The Mindful Way Through Depression,* [and] *The Mindful Path to Self-Compassion.* Almost daily, the media cite scientific studies that report the numerous health benefits of mindfulness meditation and how such a simple practice can effect neurological changes in the brain.

The booming popularity of the mindfulness movement has also turned it into a lucrative cottage industry. Business-savvy consultants pushing mindfulness training promise that it will improve work efficiency, reduce absenteeism, and enhance the "soft skills" that are crucial to career success. Some even assert that mindfulness training can act as a "disruptive technology," reforming even the most dysfunctional companies into kinder, more compassionate, and sustainable organizations. So far, however, no empirical studies have been published that support these claims.

In their branding efforts, proponents of mindfulness training usually preface their programs as being "Buddhist inspired." There is a certain cachet and hipness in telling neophytes that mindfulness is a legacy of Buddhism—a tradition famous for its ancient and time-tested meditation methods. But, sometimes in the same breath, consultants often assure their corporate sponsors that their particular brand of mindfulness has relinquished all ties and affiliations to its Buddhist origins.

Uncoupling mindfulness from its ethical and religious Buddhist context is understandable as an expedient move to make such training a viable product on the open market. But the rush to secularize and commodify mindfulness into a marketable technique may be leading to an unfortunate denaturing of this ancient practice, which was intended for far more than relieving a headache, reducing blood pressure, or helping executives become better focused and more productive.

While a stripped-down, secularized technique—what some critics are now calling "McMindfulness"—may make it more palatable to the corporate world, decontextualizing mindfulness from its original liberative and transformative purpose, as well as its foundation in social ethics, amounts to a Faustian bargain. Rather than applying mindfulness as a means to awaken individuals and organizations from the unwholesome roots of greed, ill will, and delusion, it is usually being refashioned into a banal, therapeutic, self-help technique that can actually reinforce those roots.

Most scientific and popular accounts circulating in the media have portrayed mindfulness in terms of stress reduction and attention enhancement. These human performance benefits are heralded as the sine qua non of mindfulness and its major attraction for modern corporations. But mindfulness, as understood and practiced within the Buddhist tradition, is not merely an ethically neutral technique for reducing stress and improving concentration.

Rather, mindfulness is a *distinct quality of attention* that is dependent upon and influenced by many other factors: the nature of our thoughts, speech, and actions; our way of making a living; and our efforts to avoid unwholesome and unskillful behaviors, while developing those that are conducive to wise action, social harmony, and compassion.

This is why Buddhists differentiate between Right Mindfulness (*samma sati*) and Wrong Mindfulness (*micchā sati*). The distinction is not moralistic: The issue is whether the quality of awareness is characterized by wholesome intentions and positive mental qualities that lead to human flourishing and optimal well-being for others as well as oneself.

According to the Pāli Canon (the earliest recorded teachings of the Buddha), even a person committing a premeditated and heinous crime can be exercising mindfulness, albeit *wrong mindfulness*. Clearly, the mindful attention and single-minded concentration of a terrorist, sniper assassin, or white-collar criminal is not the same quality of mindfulness that the Dalai Lama and other Buddhist adepts have developed. Right Mindfulness is guided by intentions and motivations based on self-restraint, wholesome mental states, and ethical behaviors—goals that include but supersede stress reduction and improvements in concentration.

Another common misconception is that mindfulness meditation is a private, internal affair. Mindfulness is often marketed as a method for personal self-fulfillment, a reprieve from the trials and tribulations of cutthroat corporate life. Such an individualistic and consumer orientation to the practice of mindfulness may be effective for self-preservation and self-advancement but is essentially impotent for mitigating the causes of collective and organizational distress.

When mindfulness practice is compartmentalized in this way, the inter-connectedness of personal motives is lost. There is a dissociation between one's own personal transformation and the kind of social and organizational transformation that takes into account the causes and conditions of suffering in the broader environment. Such a colonization of mindfulness also has an instrumentalizing effect, reorienting the practice to the needs of the market, rather than to a critical reflection on the causes of our collective suffering, or *social dukkha*.

The Buddha emphasized that his teaching was about understanding and ending *dukkha* ("suffering" in the broadest sense). So what about the *dukkha* caused by the ways institutions operate?

Many corporate advocates argue that transformational change starts with oneself: If one's mind can become more focused and peaceful, then social and organizational transformation will naturally follow. The problem with this formulation is that today, the three unwholesome motivations that Buddhism highlights—greed, ill will, and delusion—are no longer confined to individual minds but have become institutionalized into forces beyond personal control.

Up to now, the mindfulness movement has avoided any serious consideration of why stress is so pervasive in modern business institutions. Instead, corporations have jumped on the mindfulness bandwagon because it conveniently shifts the burden onto the individual employee: Stress is framed as a personal problem, and mindfulness is offered as just the right medicine to help employees work more efficiently and calmly within toxic environments. Cloaked in an aura of care and humanity, mindfulness is refashioned into a safety valve, as a way to let off steam—a technique for coping with and adapting to the stresses and strains of corporate life.

The result is an atomized and highly privatized version of mindfulness practice, which is easily co-opted and confined to what Jeremy Carrette and Richard King, in their book *Selling Spirituality: The Silent Takeover of Religion*, describe as an "accommodationist" orientation. Mindfulness training has wide appeal because it has become a trendy method for subduing employee unrest, promoting a tacit acceptance of the status quo, and as an instrumental tool for keeping attention focused on institutional goals.

In many respects, corporate mindfulness training—with its promise that calmer, less stressed employees will be more productive—has a close family resemblance to now-discredited "human relations" and sensitivity-training movements that were popular in the 1950s and 1960s. These training programs were criticized for their manipulative use of counseling techniques, such as "active listening," deployed as a means for pacifying employees by making them feel that their concerns were heard while existing conditions in the workplace remained unchanged. These methods came to be referred to as "cow psychology," because contented and docile cows give more milk.

Bhikkhu Bodhi, an outspoken Western Buddhist monk, has warned, "Absent a sharp social critique, Buddhist practices could easily be used to justify and stabilize the status quo, becoming a reinforcement of consumer capitalism." Unfortunately, a more ethical and socially responsible view of mindfulness is now seen by many practitioners as a tangential concern, or as an unnecessary politicizing of one's personal journey of self-transformation.

One hopes that the mindfulness movement will not follow the usual trajectory of most corporate fads—unbridled enthusiasm, uncritical acceptance of the status quo, and eventual disillusionment. To become a genuine force for positive personal and social transformation, it must reclaim an ethical framework and aspire to more lofty purposes that take into account the well-being of all living beings.

NOTES

1. For a discussion of this history, see Metcalf 2002; McMahan 2008, chapter 7.
2. See J. Wilson 2014.
3. Kabat-Zinn 1990, 2013.
4. Examples of such studies and a few books and articles summarizing some of this research include Davidson et al. 2003; Lazar et al. 2005; Lutz, Dunne, and Davidson 2007;

Wallace 2007; Rubia 2009; Shapiro and Carson 2009; Grant et al. 2010; MacLean et al. 2010; Farb, Anderson, and Segal 2012.

5.   Goyal et al. 2014.

6.   Ospina et al. 2007.

7.   Lindahl et al. 2017.

8.   For a collection of essays in this vein, see Purser, Forbes, and Burke 2016. For examinations of secularized mindfulness in relation to the Buddhist traditions from which mindfulness emerged, as well as social context more generally, see Huntington 2015; Sharf 2015.

9.   The essay is reproduced here in unedited form, except for minor punctuation revisions and the addition of diacritical marks on Pāli-language terms to remain consistent with the rest of this volume. The original can be found at www.huffingtonpost.com/ron-purser/beyond-mcmindfulness_b_3519289.html.

Crossing Boundaries

25. Rediscovering Living Buddhism in Modern Bengal

Maniklal Singha's *The Mantrayāna of Rārh* (1979)

PROJIT BIHARI MUKHARJI

This chapter deals with healing spells used by local healers in the Rārh region of southwestern Bengal. These spells were still being used at the end of the 1970s, and at least some are most likely still in use today. Most of the healers who use them are Hindu, but there are also a smaller number of Muslim and "animist" (śaontāl) practitioners. There are no longer any avowed Buddhists in the region. Surprisingly, however, the spells under discussion can be traced back to Buddhist origins. Their Buddhist character has largely been obliterated, and few, even among those who used the spells, call them Buddhist. It was an amateur Bengali anthropologist and folklorist, Maniklal Singha, who grew up in the region and was fascinated by the spells, who pointed out their Buddhist provenance.

Singha worked mainly from a large corpus of manuscripts collected since the last decades of the nineteenth century in a local repository. But he also toured the region seeking out practitioners who still used the spells. Through close textual study and fieldwork, he carefully correlated the spells, their users, and the specific social geographies where they were found. He succeeded in plotting most of the spells into specific sacred landscapes organized around particular village shrines. Though at the time most of these shrines and their deities had conspicuously Hindu identities, Singha observed discrepancies between the Hindu names of the deities and the statuary or iconography at the shrines. These inconsistencies opened up a deeper history of these sacred landscapes and a deeper social memory inscribed upon them. Pursuing such painstaking methods while working in the region for nearly thirty years before publishing his classic work, Singha gradually identified the names and references in the spells that at first had seemed inexplicable.[1] He was able to identify these seemingly unintelligible names and words with figures from the history of Tantric Buddhism, which had flourished in the region almost a millennium earlier under the Pala monarchs of Bengal.

Singha's efforts also had a longer historical context. General histories of Bengal written in the nineteenth century argued that Buddhism in the region disappeared with the fall of the Pala Empire around the twelfth century. A brief period of Shaivite rule under the Sena kings was followed by the establishment of the first Islamic sultanate of Bengal around 1204. Thereafter there was little trace of Buddhism in western Bengal. In 1894, however, a noted Bengali scholar of Sanskrit, Haraprasad Sastri, claimed to have discovered "living Buddhism" in the region.[2] It was by referring to Sastri's work that Singha was able to establish the historical identity of some of the people and places he had identified in the spells he studied.

By the time Singha worked on the spells, their predominant, though not exclusive, use was for treating snakebites and other stings and venomous attacks.[3] Their Buddhist identity was both deeply embedded and largely unacknowledged or invisible. The specialists who used these spells or mantras were variously called snake charmers (*ojhas*), exorcists (*gunins*), and spell-masters (*mantrajanis*) and frequently belonged to lower-caste groups. These were precisely the kinds of local therapeutic that I have elsewhere described as "subaltern therapeutics."[4] Increasingly, such therapies have either been dismissed as anachronisms or been subsumed within the modernized versions of Āyurveda that are today simultaneously backed by nationalist politics and the postcolonial state.[5] Yet, they continue to be used widely by socially marginalized rural groups, in many ways to retain their distinctiveness.

The very presence of these spells also forces us to rethink the definitions of what exactly is "Buddhist." The figures invoked in the spells are certainly Buddhist. Yet, in the absence of Singha's work and the singular genealogy of that work, no one would have been aware of the Buddhist background to these oral medicines. Most importantly, the users themselves were largely unaware of the spells' Buddhist provenance. Yet, in their usage and invocation, they unwittingly kept alive the memory of a practice of Tantric Buddhism that stretches back almost a millennium.

In what follows, I have translated one of the spells collected by Singha and included his framing text, which established the Buddhist references buried within the text. Through the translation, I hope to illuminate the depth of Buddhist influence in the region's therapeutic culture and Singha's active engagement in making this embedded Buddhist influence visible.

FURTHER READING

Korom, Frank. 1997. " 'Editing' Dharmaraj: Academic Genealogies of a Bengali Folk Deity." *Western Folklore* 56 (1): 51–77.

Ling, Trevor. 1978. "Buddhist Bengal, and After." In *History and Society: Essays in Honor of Professor Niharranjan Ray*, edited by Debiprasad Chattopadhyaya, 317–25. Calcutta: Bagchi.

Shahidullah, Muhammad. 1966. *Buddhist Mystic Songs, Oldest Bengali and Other Eastern Vernaculars.* Dhaka: Bangla Academy.

DHENDHAN PAD'S SPELL[6]

Our discussion of the spells of Rāhr must commence right at the center of the region. Śalda and Moinapur are two ancient villages under the jurisdiction of the Joypur police station in the district of Bankura. Along with a few more ancient villages around them, they constituted one of the most significant hubs of Buddhist Tantrism and its repertoire of spells.

We have collected a number of ancient spells from the Śalda–Moinapur area. These spells throw much light upon the antiquated manuscripts and archaeological remains found in this area. To begin with, let us consider this spell:

Dhānten Lord[7] all four corners DHUNG
Turn around Venom, ANG calls out to you
Place [my] hand on the head
Affliction, leave the body
THADANKA RA RA

[...] The metaled road from Bishnupur to Kotulpur passes very close to Joypur village,[8] and along that road there is a tiny hamlet called Kumbhasthal. A few families of the caste of confectioners and a few from that of milkmen comprise the entirety of the village population. The village gets its name from an eponymous pond in it. This name is highly redolent. In the home of one of the milkmen families of this village, there is a stone image of a meditating Buddha. The image shows the meditating Buddha seated upon a thunder-bed of a fully blossomed lotus flower. Two other meditating figures are upon each side of the Buddha. The long application of regular layers of vermilion upon the head of the image, which bears a topknot, has made it impossible to discern whether there are any other small figures upon its head. The main image most likely represents Akṣobhya, the meditating Buddha of the Epoch of Consciousness. The four images that accompany him are respectively those of Vairocana, Amitābha, Ratnasambhaba, and Amoghasiddhi.

The Lord Tathāgata had been the one to show the way of nirvana not only to the humans wracked by disease, decrepitude, and death, but to the entire family of living creatures. He had directed them all to the nectar of immortality (*amṛta*). The situation of the stone image of the meditating Buddha and the name of the village, Kumbhasthala [literally, "place of the pot"], together insinuate that very "pot of nectar of immortality," viz. *amṛta-kumbha*.

Pot of the Nectar of Immortality [and] venom
Water moves, separates.
Mahādeb[9] orders the venom:
Stay rolled up in a ball.

NOTES

1. Singha 1979.
2. Sastri 1894, 1897.
3. Slouber 2017.
4. Hardiman and Mukharji 2012.
5. Langford 2002; Mukharji 2016a.
6. Singha 1979: 1–2. A section has been omitted in my translation below, marked with "[. . .]."
7. In 1907, when Sastri was the principal of the Sanskrit College in Calcutta, he recognized during a trip to the Royal Library in Nepal forty-seven ancient verses as Buddhist "songs of realization" (Skt. *caryapadas*). These verses, written by twenty-two Buddhist spiritual masters (Skt. *siddhācārya*) in the period between the eighth and twelfth centuries, were believed by Sastri to be the oldest surviving texts in Bengali. His discovery was therefore hailed widely in Bengal, and the verses themselves became a foundational element in Bengali linguistic and literary history. In a portion of the translation that has been omitted below, Singha identifies the "Dhānten Lord" as the author of the thirty-third of these poems.
8. "Metaled roads" refers to roads surfaced with stone chips and tar. These roads are much more conducive to vehicular, especially automobile, traffic than dirt tracks. These roads usually remain open throughout the year, unlike the dirt tracks that become unusable during monsoons. In the 1970s, the Rahr was a rural area with few such metaled roads; thus, the few there became major arteries along which people and things traveled.
9. Literally the "Great Lord"; today, the word is used almost universally to refer to the Hindu god Śiva.

26. Conversations with Two (Possibly) Buddhist Folk Healers in China

THOMAS DAVID DUBOIS

The following text introduces two of the many local religious healers that I encountered during one year of fieldwork in Cang county, a rural and rather poor area of China's Hebei Province.[1] These healers were also farmers or had been in their younger years. Few were literate, and most had lived their entire lives within a day's walk of their home communities.

Rather than using technical knowledge or skills to do their work, these healers channel a power that they identify vaguely with the Buddha. They explain this power in ways that are alternately literal and metaphoric, either closely derived from Buddhist doctrine or more vaguely tied to a complex and eclectic realm of spirits and forces. They also explain the particular relationships of spiritual forces with each other, for example the idea that lesser spirits are servants or avatars of the Buddha.

It is a matter of perception whether to characterize this sort of practitioner as "Buddhist." They all recognize in themselves a unique ability to heal but may be known to clients and admirers variously as doctors or witches (wupo), depending on the circumstances and degree of admiration. One common name for such a practitioner is "head of the incense" (xiangtou; i.e., the person who lights the incense), a vague term that in some places signifies a position of authority in a village ritual setting and in others is the name given to a female spirit-medium.[2] The use of this term for healers alludes to the common role of incense in diagnostic technique but also shows that terminology and titles are very malleable.

Even if the terms sound familiar, something as personal as religious practice will look a little different in every community.

This plasticity also characterizes how people understand Buddhism within their broader religious life. Like most people, Mrs. Wei knew of a deity referred to colloquially as the Medicine King (*Yaowang*; i.e., Bhaiṣajyaguru) but had given little thought to where or whether he would fit into the Buddhist pantheon. She seemed to acknowledge that he is a Buddha of some sort but then advised us to consult a Daoist to find out for sure. Likewise, when asked if his Heaven and Earth Teaching was a Buddhist sect, Teacher Wang responded with a resounding "maybe," characterizing such boundaries as something that would concern only outsiders. Rather than dismiss such responses as demonstrating a lack of specialist sophistication, I suggest we take these explanations seriously as indicative of the contours of lived Buddhism. Even the term "Buddhist" is commonly interchangeable with *religious*. Villagers will casually term any ritual costume "Buddhist dress" (*fayi*) or refer to a sacred text as a "Buddhist scripture" (*fojing*) without any real thought as to whether there is any identifiably Buddhist content.

In these conversations, which I recorded in the late 1990s and have edited lightly for clarity and brevity, the healers explore their eclectic cosmologies of healing, sickness, and suffering and the role of the Buddha in effecting different therapeutic regimens. For them, the Buddha is just one part of an expansive spiritual world that also includes human ghosts and animal spirits.[3] Their points of reference are not scripture but actual events—stories of people who were cured or not, as well as moral and magical sources of divine favor. The individual healers interviewed below offer personalized expressions of this shifting sea of learned and experienced beliefs.

Both healers and their clients accept biomedicine, recognizing distinct categories of physical malady. They reserve Buddhist power to exorcize baleful spirits and for what they believe are essentially spiritual sicknesses—such as physical manifestations of guilt, worry, or stress—and thus beyond the reach of biomedicine.[4] In many cases, people will seek a spiritual solution only after the clinic has failed them.

Sickness is sometimes presented as a result of moral failing, for which the cure consists of repentance and atonement. But the cause is not always seen as divine punishment.[5] Sickness may be a way for a personified Buddha to get a person's attention, possibly to prompt a reform in lifestyle or to send a message, such as a calling to perform a service or even to become a healer. Alternatively, sickness may be viewed as completely depersonalized: The causality between a dissolute or distracted lifestyle and a disordered and diseased body is no more intrinsically moral than the one between overeating and indigestion.

Finally, readers should note that despite their many differences, both interviews are exercises in public relations.[6] To be successful, a healer must build a reputation for being effective and trustworthy. Beyond demonstrating their personal virtues, religious healers are additionally burdened with explicating the theological basis of their abilities in a way that speaks to the expectations of their clientele or, in this case, the ethnographer.

FURTHER READING

DuBois, Thomas David. 2005. *The Sacred Village: Social Change and Religious Life in Rural North China*. Honolulu: University of Hawai'i Press.

——. 2008. "Manchukuo's Filial Sons: States, Sects and the Adaptation of Graveside Piety." *East Asian History* 36: 3–28.

Goossaert, Vincent. 2013. "The Local Politics of Festivals: Hangzhou, 1850–1950." *Daoism Religion, History, and Society* 5: 57–80.

Ownby, David, Vincent Goossaert, and Ji Zhe, eds. 2017. *Making Saints in Modern China*. New York: Oxford University Press.

1. INTERVIEW WITH MRS. WEI

TD: Tell me about yourself.

W: I am Han Chinese, fifty-four years old [lit., fifty-five *sui*]. I was born in Yao Village, in Dulin Township. I moved to Wu Village when I got married. That was when I was seventeen. My son and his wife also live in this same village.

TD: People say that you are a healer.

W: You could say that I am a healer. Mostly people who get sick just go to the village clinic or the hospital in the city.

TD: But sometimes they come to you.

W: Some people do. Mostly people from this village. People who have a problem prefer to reach out to people they know.

TD: I think you are being modest. People say that patients come from far away, even from the city.

W: Sometimes, not often. But I guess I know some tricks. A few days ago, someone brought her little grandson who had a cyst in his throat. Oh, it really hurt him! He couldn't talk, and he wouldn't eat, so I gave him a roll of hot steamed bread with sugar. I told him he could have it, but he had to eat it all in one bite. He swallowed a big mouthful of the hot bread, and it burst the cyst. So now he will start to feel better {laughs}.

TD: That's some trick! Where did you learn that?

W: Oh, it's just common sense. My son was little once.

TD: Do you burn incense to make medicine?

W: That's for a different kind of sickness.

TD: What kind?

W: That's what we call immaterial (*xu*) sickness. Sometimes spirits come and bother people. When someone gets sick, it might be because of spirits, or it might be because of germs. You don't know. If it's an infection or cancer, you send them to the clinic. If it's spirits, then the clinic can't help them.

You can't always tell the difference between immaterial sickness and a material (*shi*) one. Some people know by burning incense. When someone is sick, they go to the spirit tablet and burn three sticks of incense. One stick is for spirits (*shenling*), one is for ghosts (*gui*), and one represents the life of the person. That's how you know where the problem is. I don't burn incense because I don't have the ability to see that light.

TD: In the incense?

W: Yes. If one stick burns brighter, then you know what the problem is. But it's not an ordinary light; only certain people can see it. If the spirit stick is brighter, the [ancestral] spirits are calling the sick person. If it's the ghost stick, then it's evil forces that are coming around to make trouble. If it's the middle [life] stick, then there's nothing to be done. The person's life is going to be over soon. I know of one young woman who went to a see a healer who said that a short life was simply her fate. She died after a few days.

A ghost or animal spirit has to be suppressed. To do that, you write a charm on yellow paper, say a prayer, and burn it. Then the patient takes the ashes home and mixes them in water and drinks it. You can also wear the ashes around your neck. Either way is fine.

TD: Can you write charms?

W: Yes, but I just write a circle and the sick person's name. Usually a charm is enough to make the ghosts go away, but sometimes they just don't want to leave. Then you have to call in a Daoist (*laodao*) in to read a scripture.

TD: Which scripture?

W: Any scripture. You can talk sense (*jiang daoli*) with a ghost. Ghosts don't like it when you read scripture. It makes them feel guilty, and they leave. If the ghost is a really bad one, the scripture scares them away. Animal spirits are the same way; there are good ones and bad ones.

If spirits are calling the person, you have to find out why. Sometimes the person did something to anger them. If you overturn a fox den, you'll probably get sick.

TD: Because of fox spirits?

W: Right. Fox spirits sometimes live with ordinary foxes, and they will definitely seek revenge if someone destroys their home. Then you have to come and apologize, make a sacrifice, and build them a new home.

BYSTANDER: People get sick for doing something bad or insulting the gods. One man from my village took stones from the temple to build a shed. He was killed in a motorcycle crash.

W: Sometimes spirits find a way to tell you what they want. That is how I started healing.

TD: How did that happen?

W: About five years ago, I got really sick. I couldn't get out of bed and soaked through my blankets with sweat. Nothing made me feel better, and everyone thought I was going to die. I actually prepared for my death. Finally, a healer came to burn incense and said that a fox spirit was calling me to work for him. I accepted the fox spirit as my teacher and immediately started to feel better. Now I have an altar to my teacher in my home.

TD: Are the spirits all foxes?

W: It depends. They might be foxes, or they might be the bodhisattva.

TD: Then how do you know which one it is?

W: Honestly, it doesn't really matter. There are good and bad animal spirits. The good ones work for the bodhisattva.

TD: Who is the bodhisattva?

W: The bodhisattva is Guanyin. She works for the Buddha. The Buddha sends her to help people escape from the sea of troubles [i.e., the troubles of this world].

TD: What about the animal spirits? Are they also related to the Buddha?

W: The good ones also work for the Buddha. Spirits also have a life-span, and when they die, they want to be reincarnated in the Pure Land.

TD: What about the Medicine King [i.e., Bhaiṣajyaguru]?

W: That's a different buddha I think, or maybe an avatar of the Buddha. I'm not sure about that. You should ask the Daoists if you want to know about that.

TD: But the Buddha is the one who heals people.

W: All of the good spirits work for the Buddha, so when I heal a sick person using an incantation or giving them incense ashes to drink as medicine, it's the Buddha who heals. That's true even if another spirit helps. They are just using the power of the Buddha. Some people call me a doctor, but I am just channeling the power of the Buddha.

2. INTERVIEW WITH TEACHER WANG

TD: Who was Sister Zheng?

W: She was a teacher of our Heaven and Earth Teaching. She lived in the Xian-feng reign [i.e., 1850–1861].

TD: And she was famous for healing?

W: For healing sickness and for helping women have children.

TD: Is that why people come to her festival now?

W: Yes, that's an important reason. They come and they bring her shoes.

TD: What are the shoes are for?

W: When a woman wants to have a baby, she comes to the temple and asks Sister Zheng for help. After the woman gives birth, she comes back and leaves a pair of baby shoes at the statue to thank Sister Zheng and attest to her power. She also brings a pair of paper shoes. Those are for Sister Zheng, and they're small because she had bound feet. On the last day of the festival, you burn the paper shoes to send them to Sister Zheng.

TD: Can everyone in the Heaven and Earth Teaching heal?

W: No, I am the only one from this area. Some people just have that ability.

TD: But there are lots of other healers. An old lady in this village is a *xiangtou*. Are they fake?

W: {Pause.} Some of the healers are fake, but some people outside the teaching have the ability as well.

TD: What do you do that is different from them?

W: Our teaching heals by confession (*chanhui*). For example [points to a man in the room], Old Wang couldn't get up off the bed. His legs wouldn't work, and his wife came and told me to come and have a look. It turns out that Old Wang had stolen some money from the festival fund, and he felt guilty. His conscience wouldn't let him sleep or eat, so he got weaker every day. I told him to apologize to Teacher Dong [the deified founder of the sect] and return the money, and he got better.

TD: Do you ever burn incense?

W: Another name for our teaching is the Single Stick of Incense (*yizhu xiang*) Teaching. The single stick of incense means that there is only one truth. I also burn incense to heal.

TD: A single stick of incense?

W: Yes, I burn the incense for the patient, and I can tell what the problem is by looking at the light.

TD: Other healers look at three sticks of incense to see if a sickness is material or immaterial . . .

W: Yes, but I need only one. Most of the time, I tell people to go to the clinic.

TD: What if the problem is a ghost or a fox spirit?

W: Then you read a scripture to scare the ghost away.

TD: Where does your power come from?

W: From Teacher Dong.

TD: Is Teacher Dong a reincarnation of the Buddha?

W: No, but he and the Buddha are both children of the Eternal Mother; so is Confucius and your Jesus. They all come from the same source.

TD: Do people think that you are Buddhist monks?

BYSTANDER: We all have hair; you are the Buddhist monk, baldy! {Laughter.}

W: We might be Buddhist-style Daoists or maybe Daoist-style Buddhists {more laughter}. In reality, these names don't matter much. We also worship the Buddha, and he protects all good people.

NOTES

1.   DuBois 2005.

2.   Goossaert 2013, 2019.

3.   Li 1954; Kang 2006.

4.   Fang 2012; Bu 2015.

5.   Christian 1989.

6.   DuBois 2008; Ownby, Goossaert, and Ji 2017.

27. Interview with a Contemporary Chinese American Healer

KIN CHEUNG AND C. PIERCE SALGUERO

The translation below is from an interview conducted with Cheung Seng Kan (Pinyin: Zhang Chenggen), a Chinese American healer in the New York City area. Born in 1955, Cheung emigrated with his wife and son in 1988 from Guang-zhou, China, to Brooklyn.[1] Owing to the large population of Chinese Americans in that city—more than half a million—he and his wife were able to lead their lives without speaking English.[2] Cheung mainly teaches in Cantonese, though sometimes also in Mandarin. He would like to teach to English speakers and laments his inability to do so without an interpreter.

Cheung has practiced Chinese healing arts on himself and his relatives for most of his life. In 2012, he became a community healer when he practiced qigong in a neighborhood park one day and attracted his first student.[3] He now receives regular visits from people seeking treatment for conditions ranging from back-aches and migraines to heart palpitations and even leukemia. Though he usually heals in person, his students also have phoned him to ask for prayers and bless-ings, and he has conducted long-distance healing over the phone for patients as far away as Hong Kong. He does not ask for payment but happily accepts gifts of food and cash offered in red envelopes, according to Chinese custom.[4]

Cheung learned some remedies from two coworkers in the garment factories at which he was once employed.[5] One of his teachers was a medical doctor in China who practiced acupuncture, and another practiced medical arts from the Buddhist Shaolin temple.[6] However, he is primarily an autodidact. Despite having completed only grammar school, he continually incorporates new techniques gleaned from books, radio, television, and, most recently, YouTube videos into his repertoire, which includes many unique combinations and idiosyncratic methods.

In the interview below, translated from Cantonese, Cheung recounts his success in healing balance disorders, short-term memory problems, and facial-bone misalignment for several patients young and old. He uses Buddhist interventions such as *dhāraṇī* incantations, which he also teaches his students to employ for physical healing and for pacifying spirits in cemeteries. He mentions the vows of Bhaiṣajyaguru as a means toward both physical and soteriological goals (on these vows, see *Anthology*, vol. 1, ch. 25), and he incorporates prayers to this and other Buddhist deities in his practice. In keeping with Buddhist teachings, he explains that disease can be caused by internal malfunctions or imbalances, external injuries, or the karmic results of previous actions or lives. The cause of any specific ailment is thus not always clear, and physical and soteriological concerns are not neatly delineated.

Another boundary he blurs is the one between Buddhism and other Chinese religious–philosophical traditions.[7] He talks about his visualization practice of *chan-taiji*, which is a combination of Chan Buddhist meditation and Chinese cosmological principles (*taiji*), learned from internet videos. He speaks of a "sixth sense" acquired through Chan meditation, an unconscious guidance of his hands that he sometimes experiences while giving massage or qigong treatments. The eclectic techniques he uses also run the gamut of Chinese medicine: electro-acupuncture, moxibustion (using local plants gathered from neighborhood parks), therapeutic massage (*tuina*), herbal and dietary prescriptions, an herbal liniment (*diedajiu*) he makes, cupping, scraping (*guasha*), and qigong meditation.[8] Additionally, he employs Daoist visualization meditations, feng shui geomancy, and an arsenal of apotropaic crystals, charms, and amulets.[9] Moreover, to characterize his practices as "Chinese" would be incomplete, as he also employs Reiki, in addition to Japanese and Korean talismans.

Cheung sees himself in multiple roles in his community. He is a healer to those he calls patients, who interact with him primarily when they seek treatment. He is also a teacher (*laoshi*) to his students, who both receive treatment and learn how to heal themselves. Some of his closest students he considers his friends. In this interview, moreover, he plays the dual roles of ethnographic subject and the father of one of this chapter's authors, who served as translator and facilitator of this interview. This familiarity affects the way Cheung answers questions in parts of the interview. For example, he mentions that he is happy not to have to explain in detail much of what he says, since he knows that his son will understand what he means. At times, though, his multiple identities introduce difficulties.[10] Significantly, at one point in the interview below, he mentions that the subject of his self-cultivation, healing practices, and experiences is not entirely appropriate to talk about publicly. While he would normally speak of such things with his son in a personal interaction, in the forum of an ethnographic interview, he demurs, not wishing to publicly appear to be a braggart. Nevertheless, he was willing to answer our questions in some amount of detail, and to publish this material to help researchers. In addition, he adds that there is always good karma in spreading knowledge about healing and Buddhism.

FURTHER READING

Guest, Kenneth. 2003. *God in Chinatown: Religion and Survival in New York's Evolving Immigrant Community*. New York: New York University Press.

Salguero, C. Pierce. 2019. "Varieties of Buddhist Healing in Multiethnic Philadelphia," *Religions* 10 (1), doi:10.3390/rel10010048. Accessed June 16, 2019. https://www.mdpi.com/2077-1444 /10/1/48.

Tsui, Bonnie. 2009. *American Chinatown: A People's History of Five Neighborhoods*. New York: Free Press.

Wu, Emily S. 2013. *Traditional Chinese Medicine in the United States: In Search of Spiritual Meaning and Ultimate Health*. Lanham, Md.: Lexington.

Wu, Hongyu. 2002. "Buddhism, Health, and Healing in a Chinese Community." The Pluralism Project, Harvard University. http://pluralism.org/wp-content/uploads/2015/08/Wu.pdf.

INTERVIEW WITH CHEUNG SENG KAN[11]

CPS & KC: What is your practice?

CSK: My self-cultivation practice has moving and still components. I have practiced Chan meditation, martial arts, and *taiji* in my youth and now *chan-taiji*, which is a combination of Buddhist and Daoist teachings.

CPS & KC: When people who are sick come to you, is this the menu of therapies you use?

CSK: I teach them to practice. I can give them *qi* with Intelligent Qigong (*zhineng qigong*) or Reiki, which are two methods. I can use the buddhas' and bodhisattvas' *dhāraṇī* incantations (*zhou*) to heal. I have, at the very least, these three methods.

CPS & KC: How do you view qigong, Reiki, and *dhāraṇī* incantations? Are these related therapies or three distinct things?

CSK: The three are distinct healing therapies. Reiki practice requires four to five years before [one gains] the ability to heal others. Intelligent Qigong requires only three to four months before one can heal others. It's faster because it's more developed. The founder, Pang Heming, had nineteen teachers, who knew Buddhist teachings, Daoist teachings, and yoga. He combined the essence of those teachings together to create it. That is why this practice has relatively fast results. That is why when I first taught you {addressing KC}, you felt *qi* immediately in your hands.

I practiced *taiji* in my youth. My father started in the 1960s and practiced this until one hundred years of age. My own master taught me *taiji*. *Taiji* can also help heal others. It can regulate mind and body. *Taiji* is known around the world. It starts from the depth and goes to the surface.

The lay Buddhist Huiguang invented *chan-taiji*. It is the combination of the essence of Buddhist and Daoist teachings. He created a thirty-two-style practice. If you practice with sincerity, it is relatively effective for health of mind and body. It is calming and suitable for those who have anxiety, depression, autism, or are in front of the computer all day. This is most suitable. This *chan-taiji* is a new practice.

CPS & KC: Where can one learn *chan-taiji*?

CSK: You can go online to learn.[12] Those with a foundation in self-cultivation can learn this easily. Those without will have great difficulty. It not only has physical movements, like Intelligent Qigong, [but] it also uses conscious intent.

Chan can be practiced while sitting in meditation posture, circumambulating a Buddhist statue, or standing. There is also *chan* while ascending stairs, for example. You can see my movements, but you still need an explanation. First, you need to visualize lifting up the sun, toward the east, right when it rises above the ocean. This is called Moving the Sun Rising in the East. When the sun moves here {gesturing upwards}, it is at its strongest; like the sun at noon, it is very hot. It radiates heat and golden light, penetrating through the entire body, lighting up the body. Light will come out the soles of the feet. So just this movement itself is *chan*.

CPS & KC: Your altar seems to have mostly items related to Buddhism [figure 27.1]; are there non-Buddhist elements here as well?

CSK: It is all Buddhist, except for the picture I received from Japan that looks like the seven [Daoist] immortals. But everything else should be Buddhist.

CPS & KC: What about this red light?

CSK: This crystal light is positioned according to feng shui. Red is used to ward off evil. Yellow is used to invite fortune. Everything else is Buddhist.

CPS & KC: Tell me about your experience with *dhāraṇī* incantations.

CSK: Some can be used to see dead spirits. Since for Buddhism, there are six realms, there must be gods and ghosts.[13] There are so many *dhāraṇī* incantations. Some are used to ask for health; some are to heal disease. For instance, Bhaiṣajyaguru heals disease, right?

CPS & KC: What do you personally chant every morning and night?

CSK: The Bhaiṣajyaguru *dhāraṇī* [see *Anthology*, vol. 1, ch. 25, 28§8], Avalokiteśvara[14] *dhāraṇī* [see *Anthology*, vol. 1, ch. 26], and there's . . . so many, like the one I taught [my student] Mrs. L. when she went to the cemetery, the Cundī Buddha Mother *dhāraṇī*. That one is used to pay respect to the ten directions. Reciting that, wherever the eye gazes, one can see beyond the human realm. That night, when she returned, her practice revealed itself. She is seventy years old. From when she was young until that point, all her past visits to cemeteries came to her as images. She has this type of ability.

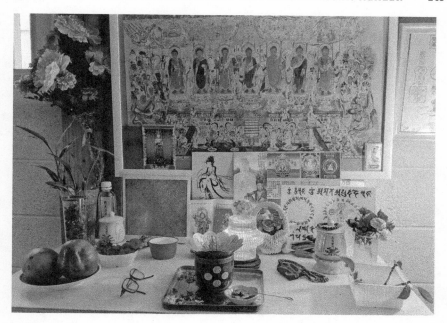

FIGURE 27.1 MASTER CHEUNG'S ALTAR, WITH A VARIETY OF BUDDHIST IMAGES, *DHĀRAṆĪ*, TALISMANS, AND OTHER IMPLEMENTS.
Source: Kin Cheung.

CPS & KC: How do you use *dhāraṇī* to heal? Do you chant for the patient or teach them how to chant?

CSK: Both can be done. *Dhāraṇī* has no distance. *Dhāraṇī* aside, when the Thai guru White Dragon King[15] passed away, and [another of my students] Mrs. F. read that in the newspaper, she had intense headaches. She called me on the phone. She asked for help. I taught her how to visualize looking to the heavens and to use golden water to cleanse her own body. Before even two minutes had passed, her pain had stopped.

CPS & KC: Are you using the buddhas to empower your therapies, or are you teaching people to tap into the buddhas to heal themselves?

CSK: Both. Both are possible because there are different types of disease. When it's cold outside, that causes disease. Going outside, falling can cause injury. Bad eating and drinking habits or lack of rest can cause disease. These maladies are easy to heal. But for some diseases, even though America has good scientific knowledge, there is no cure. These are due to karmic causes, perhaps from a previous life or an action earlier in this life, such as murder or unethical behavior. Those need the buddhas' and bodhisattvas' help to heal, and so one needs to chant *sūtras* and *dhāraṇī*.

CPS & KC: Does that mean the mechanism that the buddhas and bodhisattvas use to heal the patients is by alleviating karma? Is that the only way, or are there additional ways they can help?

CSK: Using *dhāraṇī* is the main way to help. Actually, buddhas and bodhisattvas speak of compassion and saving sentient beings. If you do not know *dhāraṇī*, you can still chant their names. You can just repeat the name Bhaiṣajyaguru or Avalokiteśvara. But the efficacy may not be the same as the *dhāraṇī*. Still, buddhas and bodhisattvas are compassionate and wish to help sentient beings, according to the Buddhist teachings anyway. For instance, Bhaiṣajyaguru has twelve great vows, including to help you have a healthy body, deliver you from the sea of suffering, and alleviate karma. So, once you recite Bhaiṣajyaguru's name, his twelve great vows will arise.

CPS & KC: So are you an intermediary, or a facilitator getting the patient connected to those vows?

CSK: I am helping others, using the *dhāraṇī* of buddhas and bodhisattvas to help others. Others can chant themselves, but if they don't know, then I teach them how to chant. I am teaching them methods. If they have disease, I will teach them how to use Bhaiṣajyaguru. Primarily I teach them how to request help from Bhaiṣajyaguru. I can also chant *sūtras* and send [the merits] to patients. For instance, I ask for my entire family to be safe and healthy. Although my family members are not chanting, they get the protection from my chanting of *sūtras*.

CPS & KC: Do you see yourself in a teacher–student role or healer–patient relationship?

CSK: First, they are learning from me, and that is why they call me Teacher Cheung. Primarily, they are students, and I have a lot to say to them. Not only that, but we can become friends. In America, the teacher–student role includes tuition. If there is no tuition, then it is learning from friends. For instance, if for one lesson I charge ten dollars, at the beginning, they pay. Then, after a while, I tell them there is no need to pay. Then, they find another way. They can give as much as they want. You know that Chinese people use red envelopes. So even though I don't want money, they are sincere in their desire to give to their teacher. So this is a different method, and a different sentiment. Charging tuition and giving red envelopes are different things. There is a different sentiment. Red envelopes mean you can give as much as you want. For example, Mrs. L., I do not charge her tuition. She gives me red envelopes.

CPS & KC: What kinds of conditions do you treat? Are there particular types of disease you are known for?

CSK: Many types of disease. People with diseases look for you. The diseases that hospitals cannot cure lead people to look for you. If hospitals can cure it, they would not look for you because they have medical insurance. For instance, there was a truck driver with back problems who went to the hospital a few times without success, so he came here. Besides back pain, there was Mrs. L.'s large tumor . . . all types . . . I haven't really kept track. As long as they come here, I help them. . . . For instance, there was a young teenage girl who fell on her face. Her jaw was dislocated. She could not use her mouth to chew properly. In the hospital, the doctor said she needed surgery to realign her jaw. Then she needed braces because she could not chew food on one side. She came here and got treatment. I gave her one treatment. I don't know if she has [had] good luck or what, but after one treatment, the doctor said she did not need surgery, just braces.

CPS & KC: What were the therapies you used for the driver and the teenager?

CSK: Some qigong and massage. I have a sixth sense. For a patient, if I just put my hands on them, [they] would move automatically to help them heal.

CPS & KC: Is that guidance coming from buddhas and bodhisattvas? Where is it coming from?

CSK: It has developed from my *chan* practice. During my *chan* sitting, I would automatically start moving. After a while, the movement became an automatic self-healing for me to clear my acupuncture points. Then, when I help heal others with Intelligent Qigong, when I am still, it is like during *chan*. My hands move by themselves to help heal their bodies. But each press of my hand is very accurate because it is not from myself, but from the sixth sense. The number of times I press is not determined. The next movement is not determined. This directs my hands precisely to the spot needed to heal successfully.

CPS & KC: Do you have training in massage that this is built on?

CSK: My massage is not learned. It came out from *chan*. One can learn massage online, consult online about what it is and how to do it. For instance, with Mrs. L., she had headaches for a long time. One time in the nearby park, she asked me to help her. I pressed on a pressure point. It was an automatic pressing. Afterward, she thanked me profusely. [She] just kept saying, "Thank you, thank you." This is because when I pressed her, she felt a long steel needle this long {gestures} going from here {gestures to the top of his head} through to her throat. After this feeling, her head no longer ached, and she felt better. That's why she kept saying, "Thank you, thank you." That's why Mrs. L. keeps coming here. Whenever there is any issue, she will come for help.

CPS & KC: Is *qi* doing this or some other power or force?

CSK: The *qi* moves by itself. The most important is my foundation in qigong. There is also *chan* and the automatic movement. It is *qi* and the sixth sense.

Right before I heal others, this is odd, but I automatically rotate my hips. In my past visit to Chuang Yen Monastery, I did these involuntary movements. In a temple in Taiwan in front of Avalokiteśvara, as well. In Japan, in front of Mahāvairocana on the hill, too. Basically, in front of a major temple, I would automatically move. In front of gods, I would move, and when I was still during *chan*, I would move. Near that temple, just walking along, I didn't even know it was a temple, and I automatically walked into it.

CPS & KC: What is your mental state during this automatic movement?

CSK: There is nothing on my mind. I let go. There is no conscious direction. Like *chan*, what is there? *Chan* is just breathing. I just still myself. You don't have to worry about it. It's like you are just leaving it to the heavens. Or you can say

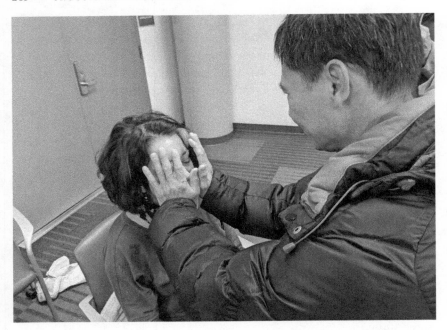

FIGURE 27.2 MASTER CHEUNG GIVING A TREATMENT AT DRAKE UNIVERSITY, IN DES MOINES, IOWA, FOLLOWING A PUBLIC EVENT. *Source*: Kin Cheung.

leaving it to buddhas and bodhisattvas; it's up to you. Like when helping someone heal, at that time I leave it to the buddhas and bodhisattvas and the heavens. If one uses Reiki, one refers to the universal energy to help. If one uses Intelligent Qigong, one refers to Great Nature's *qi* from the ends of the world to return to normal health. If you move, you don't have to worry about it. The reason I just leave it to the heavens is because during *chan*, the movement stretches tendons and opens meridians to heal myself. Of course, I would allow it to move tendons and flesh, *qi*, and acupoints. Whatever it needs, I hand over control to it. That is best; there is no need to think.

Talking about healing reminds me of something. Mrs. F. has a friend who works for a hotel. She ended up in a hospital. The doctor said there is some kind of bacteria in her brain. They are not sure what kind. They treated her like a guinea pig and did experiments. They said there were bacteria because she couldn't remember things. She could remember only small fragments, like, for instance, if an address was 2121, she would remember only 2 and 1. Or, if her room number was 2134, she would only remember 3 and 4. Going up the stairs to the second floor was not possible for her. They said her ear fluids were not balanced. I helped heal her with qigong. During treatment, the sixth sense came out and helped me to press her acupoint. It was not my intention, but from the sixth sense. I knew that pressing this {gesturing behind the ears} would be very painful. I asked if she could stand pain. She said, "I can stand it. I am not afraid of pain." After pressing it, she felt better. Then we left.

After a few days, she asked me to return to help again. She told all of us— Mr. and Mrs. F. and me—that the night after I pressed her acupoint, she felt something in her ear come out. This was just a feeling. But then, there was some small thing that actually fell out of her ear. After it fell out, she could walk up the stairs without getting dizzy. She could remember digits again.

So she got better. In the hospital, with all the X-rays, fMRI, all that equipment, and all those doctors did not know what her disease was. They only said that her brain had some bacteria. After I healed her, she did not dare tell the doctors. She was afraid the doctors would not like the practice of qigong and Reiki inside the hospital. She just knew that she felt better, and that was good enough. No need for surgery or medicine. How wonderful! {He chuckles.}

So, this is a true example [corroborated by] other people. What I say is all true. That is why those red envelopes on the altar are from people I have helped heal. I never asked for money, but they offer it. This is a Chinese custom. When I speak [these words] in front of the gods [on my altar], I speak the truth. I cannot lie about this. All these envelopes are from healing people. This is just a portion; there is more. I am also very grateful for these.

Actually, these things should not be spoken of, broadcast like this. Claiming to be highly skilled: according to Buddhist teachings and as a Chinese person, I should not brag like this. But since you are interviewing me, I will tell you. As an exchange of information, this is OK. But if I were on the streets bragging to strangers, it would not be proper.

CPS & KC: Thank you for sharing.

CSK: No problem. You can ask. Whatever I know, I will tell you. This is for the sake of knowledge and research. This is compassion. This is karmic virtue to help sentient beings. No problem. What you want, I will tell you. If I don't know, I can even find friends and ask for you. We are chatting.

CPS & KC: In what languages are you chanting? Are you pronouncing Chinese characters in specific ways?

CSK: Buddhism teaches separate esoteric and exoteric teachings. Esoteric ones are passed on only by teachers directly from their mouths. Exoteric teachings are not privately taught, so however other people pronounce it, you learn to pronounce it like that. Regarding dhāraṇī, in China they are transmitted mainly through Mandarin, not Cantonese. For Tibet and Nepal, they use the Indian Sanskrit pronunciation. They are mostly esoteric teachings. I try to use the Sanskrit pronunciation. There are many sounds. For instance, for this Cundī Buddha Mother dhāraṇī, the Taiwanese and mainland China pronunciation is slightly different. Northern and Southern dialects are different. That is why Sanskrit is the most accurate. The difference is small, not big.

CPS & KC: Do you have anything more to share or add?

CSK: I encourage people to practice qigong or *chan*. This is my recommendation. People now lead busy lives. Qigong is good; *chan-taiji* is good. Really, *chan-taiji* is beneficial. I believe that, as for China, it is mainly Daoism that is used for longevity and health. And Buddhism is about the heart-mind. I teach both together; I do not separate Daoist and Buddhist teachings. I hope more people can practice to help themselves and others. This project, this interview here, definitely will have karmic merit. Learning about Buddhism will help people be more ethical and less selfish.

NOTES

1. After having lived in Brooklyn for three decades, Cheung moved to New Jersey in 2017, two years after this interview was conducted. His students from New York still visit him regularly in New Jersey.

2. There are Chinese-speaking doctors, accountants, lawyers, and other professionals in the neighborhood to support Chinese Americans. On Chinese Americans in New York City and their religious practice, see Guest 2003.

3. On the modern creation of qigong, see Palmer 2007.

4. On Chinese personal relationships developed through the giving of gifts and favors (*guanxi*), see Yang 1994.

5. Cheung and his wife worked in garment factories for two decades. See Tsui 2009, especially chapter 4 on the changing impact of garment factories on the lives of Chinese Americans in New York City.

6. See Shahar 2008, especially chapters 5 and 6 on the therapeutic goals of martial and medicinal arts practiced at this Buddhist monastery.

7. For more on Chinese American Buddhists, see I. Lin 1996; N. Lin 2001. On Taiwanese American Buddhists, see Chen 2008. On Chinese Buddhists and healing in Boston, see H. Wu 2002. For a broader treatment of Chinese medicine as practiced in the United States, see E. Wu 2013.

8. On the history and contemporary practice of Chinese medical arts in general, see Hinrichs and Barnes 2013.

9. On Daoist visualization and longevity practices, see Kohn 1981, 2000. On feng shui, see Bruun 2003.

10. For instance, when asked questions regarding descriptive characterizations of his past practices, Cheung would answer with prescriptive possibilities for practice. Specifically, when asked if he previously did X or Y, he would answer that both X and Y can be used. Perhaps he is accustomed to talking about healing practices only with his students, in which case his focus would be guidance and teaching. Or perhaps he understands the aim of the interview to be concerned with the prescriptive rather than the descriptive. (Hall and Ames 1987 discusses the differences between the Indo-European descriptive and Classical Chinese prescriptive uses of language.) Another possibility is that Cheung wants to present an image of himself as a healer who can do all the practices in question.

11. Interview conducted by Kin Cheung and C. Pierce Salguero on October 10, 2015, in Cheung Seng Kan's Brooklyn home. The interview was conducted in Cantonese, with questions posed by Salguero and translated by Kin Cheung. It has been edited for clarity, and some portions of the interview that do not relate directly to the theme of this volume have been omitted for space concerns.

12. See, for example, www.youtube.com/watch?v=DUiYqSMi8oo.

13. On the six realms of Buddhism, which are the possible destinations of rebirth depending on the karma or actions of one's life, see Becker 1993. The most common list of destinations includes gods, *asuras* (a type of giant or titan), humans, animals, hungry ghosts, and hell-dwellers.

14. For more on the Chinese context of this deity, one of the most important objects of worship in Buddhism worldwide, see Yü 2001. Avalokiteśvara is mentioned by many other healers throughout both volumes of this anthology. In this volume, see especially the interviews in chapters 28 and 29.

15. A Chinese Thai named Chow Yam-nam, who gained fame as a religious adept through his contact with Hong Kong celebrities. See www.whitedragonking.com/aboutus.htm.

28. "We Need to Balance Out the Boisterous Spirits and Gods"

Buddhism in the Healing Practice of a Contemporary Korean Shaman

MINJUNG NOH AND C. PIERCE SALGUERO[1]

The translation below is an excerpt from an interview with a contemporary Korean shaman named Jung Yonggeum. Jung is active in Seoul, the capital of South Korea, and welcomes her clients in her home shrine at the center of the city. The interview was conducted in Korean on July 21, 2016, at that location. In the interview, Jung offers a first-person narrative of her twenty-year journey as a shaman and healer. She discusses her initiation, her relationship with the ancestor spirits she serves, and her more recent encounter with Buddhist spirituality.

Korean shamanism (*musok*) can be traced back to before the Common Era and represents Korean indigenous religious practice. However, it has long been marginalized, not only under the Confucian rule of the Chosŏn dynasty (1392–1897) but also in the modern republic of Korea (1948–present), where it has been characterized as a "superstitious" or "vulgar" religious belief. Nevertheless, shamanism has played a pivotal role for the socially underprivileged population as an alternative system of healing and communal support. In the latter half of the twentieth century, it started to draw attention from scholars in the English-speaking world, as well as from Korean academics. Laurel Kendall's pioneering work, *Shamans, Housewives, and Other Restless Spirits: Women in Korean Ritual Life* (1985), significantly contributed to the understanding of Korean shamanism by illuminating the place of the female shaman (*mudang*) in the everyday lives of Korean people. Since then, scholarship on Korean shamanism has grown both in and outside of Korea.[2] Today, Korean shamans have their own professional association, the Society of Korean Shamanism (Taehan kyŏngshinyŏnhap'oe, est. 1970), with three hundred thousand members nationwide.[3] Scholars of Korean shamanism have also founded the Association for Korean Shamanistic Studies (est. 1998) and publish the *Journal of Korean Shamanism*. It is important to note that there are active exchanges between the community of Korean shamans and scholars of shamanism, making contemporary Korean shamanism a hybrid field of religious practice and academic discourse.[4]

The interview below testifies to another kind of hybridity or syncretism, namely how Buddhist ideas—especially the figure of Avalokiteśvara (Kr. Kwan'ŭm)—are interpreted and incorporated into contemporary shamanic practice. Four years after her initiation, Jung relates that she accepted the spirit of Avalokiteśvara into her pantheon through a religious experience. However, to incorporate Avalokiteśvara required the reorganization of her spiritual system. Her ancestral spirits, who had been the center of her shamanistic practices of divination, exorcism, and healing, resisted the inclusion of this new deity. Jung describes how she exerted much effort to reconcile the grievances of her ancestral spirits. She also relates how she turned to Buddhist literature to understand this process, in particular the *Thousand Hands Sūtra* (i.e., a name used for a number of versions of a *sūtra* associated with an esoteric form of Avalokiteśvara; see *Anthology*, vol. 1, ch. 26), which was revealed to her when she had a religious experience at a Buddhist temple. In her account of her healing practice, Jung specifically refers to a connection between Avalokiteśvara and an indigenous healing deity named Pulsa Halmŏni.[5] She also describes the unique role of Avalokiteśvara as a source of stability for the restless ancestral spirits in her healing system.[6]

The excerpt below includes Jung's life story, how she understands the different roles of her ancestral deities and Avalokiteśvara in her healing process, and how she perceives the relationship between shamanism and other religions. Her understanding of Buddhism's role in shamanic practice, Korean shamanism's place among "the world's great religions," and the status of both in her own healing practice shows how contemporary Korean Buddhism is always entangled and in conversation with many other discourses taking place alongside the tradition.

FURTHER READING

Kendall, Laurel. 1985. *Shamans, Housewives, and Other Restless Spirits: Women in Korean Ritual Life.* Honolulu: University of Hawai'i Press.

Kendall, Laurel, Yang Jongsung, and Yoon Yul Soo. 2015. *God Pictures in Korean Contexts: The Ownership and Meaning of Shaman Paintings.* Honolulu: University of Hawai'i Press.

Kim, Dong-kyu. 2012. "Reconfiguration of Korean Shamanic Ritual: Negotiating Practices Among Shamans, Clients, and Multiple Ideologies." *Journal of Korean Religions* 3 (2): 11–37.

Kim, Taegon. 1999. "Definition of Korean Shamanism." In *Culture of Korean Shamanism*, edited by Chun Shinyong, 9–44. Seoul: Kimpo College Press.

Sarfati, Liora. 2016. "Shifting Agencies Through New Media: New Social Statuses for Female South Korean Shamans." *Journal of Korean Studies* 21 (1): 179–211.

INTERVIEW WITH JUNG YONGGEUM[7]

JY: I felt a strong energy (Kr. *enŏji*, from the English "energy") in my morning meditation. So I assumed that someone with strong energy would come and visit me. In order to share and communicate my experience with you, I thought I needed to be prepared. So I was very focused this morning. Then, as soon as you came in, I felt the strong energy. You are academics, so I guess you are meant to have those strong energies. {Asking CPS:} Is this the first time meeting a Korean shaman for you?

CPS: Yes, it is.

JY: Such an honor.

CPS: I am very happy to be here, as well.

JY: Before I became a shaman, I taught kids for a while. Then, I had to become a shaman. It wasn't my choice. I was possessed by the spirit that made me a shaman. It was a mysterious process for me. Nobody ever told me about this, and I was twenty-three years old then.

MN: So you had no background of shamanism in your family?

JY: No, I didn't. It is an odd case. Generally, people who study shamanism categorize shamans into two kinds: hereditary and possessed. Hereditary shamans inherit their spirits from other family members, but I am a possessed one. No one in my family was a shaman or had an occupation related to spiritual practice. I was a little peculiar as a child, though. I got sick very often. Also I had a lot of dreams. Some dreams were prophetic, people say. I reflected on the reason why I became a shaman and tried to figure out why this happened to me. When I was born, my father was already fifty years old, and he passed away when I was eleven years old. When my parents had me, since they were at such an advanced age, they were worried about my mother's health and mine. Then, my father had a dream about my birth. In the dream, some beautiful women descended from Heaven, just like those Daoist fairies, and handed a baby girl to my parents. I was born right after that. I was ill from the moment I was born. I could not digest a regular meal until I was six years old. I lived on water, milk, and porridge. Even after I started eating food, I could not eat fish or meat and can't even now. I really can't make myself eat them.

CPS: When you became a shaman, what kind of god or spirit did you have contact with?

JY: It's complicated. When I opened up the "gate of spirits" (*shinmun*) in myself, I had an initiation that is called a possession ritual or descent ritual (Kr. *naerimgut*). People usually think that the spirit a shaman encounters for the first time becomes his or her main spirit.[8] However, just as a person goes through different stages of development as they grow up from a child to an adult, the main spirit or god a shaman serves changes over time. The first spirit a shaman encounters does not have to be her main spirit forever. Of course, usually shamans start with their ancestor spirits. Any shaman would first meet her ancestral spirits, according to my experience and [those of] other shamans I know. But, as I said, there are levels of maturity you progress through as a shaman.

At first, ancestral spirits come into you in the form of the mountain god. My maternal grandfather's spirit plays the role of the mountain god, which people usually imagine as a god who rides on the back of a mystical tiger and appears to people. [. . .] My grandfather's spirit delivers the energy of the mountain god.

My father's spirit mediates my communication with military gods [figure 28.1], such as Admiral Yi Sunsin [1545–1598] or Douglas MacArthur [1880–1964], who helped us Koreans in the Korean War.[9] They were historical figures who later became gods because of their great achievements. Thus, my father's spirit is a military spirit that helps me to channel these gods.

I think there is a very clear division of labor among my ancestor spirits. My [maternal] grandfather's spirit mediates my contact with the mountain god, my father's spirit connects me to the military gods, and my paternal grandfather's spirit gives me knowledge about the academic or literary part of my practice. My paternal grandfather was a schoolmaster when he was alive, so he was a well-learned person. His spirit helps me to write talismans in Classical Chinese characters and connect with Confucius's spirit.

There are female ancestor spirits, as well. First, my paternal grandmother's spirit helps me to do divination and healings for people. Over there on my shrine [figure 28.2], she is wearing her white paper conical hat and has a fan. She connects me to Pulsa Halmŏni, a goddess who looks after my ability to perform divinations for my clients. I was told that my grandmother was a very masculine and vocal woman in her lifetime. Because of that, after I received her spirit inside of me, my personality changed. I became bolder and more boyish than before!

Secondly, my aunt who died when she was only four years old comes to me as a child spirit. When I talk to my clients who have sick children or [who have] lost their children, I am sometimes possessed by my aunt's spirit and talk in a child's voice. She is really accurate. When she talks through me, she points out exactly what was wrong with my clients' kids or how the little ones died.

Therefore, the spirits of my ancestors—[my] maternal grandfather, father, paternal grandfather, grandmother, and aunt—have their distinctive roles in my practice, and I communicate with other spiritual beings and gods through them. This ability to see other modes of existence, or gods, is my shamanic ability. It is a little different from learning from books. We can always meet

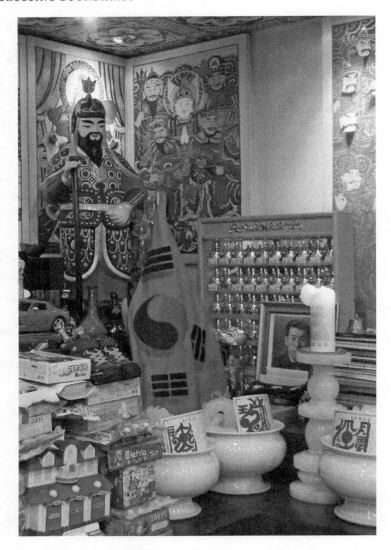

FIGURE 28.1 A STATUE REPRESENTING MILITARY SPIRITS ALONGSIDE OFFERINGS AND IMAGES OF OTHER DEITIES ON THE SHAMAN'S ALTAR. *Source*: C. Pierce Salguero.

Buddha or Jesus through reading books that contain their teachings. Unlike this common learning process, my learning and channeling is about my *qi* [Kr. *gi*]. If I focus and contact the mystic existence of Buddha or Confucius, I can understand their teachings perfectly. I never learned to read Buddhist *sūtras*, for example, but I can recite some lines from *sūtras* and do Buddhist chanting. This directness can be further developed through "spiritual energy" (Kr. *chŏngshinjŏk enŏji*). I have only one body, but I can be a vessel that allows numerous other existences and energies to frequent my body.

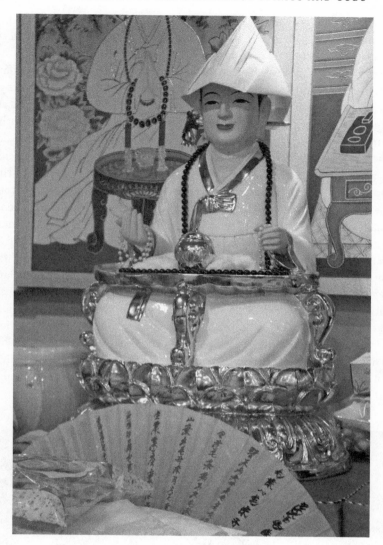

FIGURE 28.2 A STATUE OF THE GODDESS PULSA HALMŎNI ON THE
SHAMAN'S ALTAR.
Source: C. Pierce Salguero.

MN: I am curious about the Avalokiteśvara on your shrine. You have a huge
Avalokiteśvara statue and a Buddhist painting on your shrine [figure 28.3].
How do you understand Avalokiteśvara's power?

JY: Every time I encounter a different ancestor spirit and communicate with
them, I learn something more. For example, when I channeled the admiral
god *Yi Sunsin* through my father's spirit, I learned a lot about the history of
his lifetime during the Chosŏn dynasty. Moreover, I learned about a famous
Chinese military god, Guan Yu [160–220 CE]. I think I was led to learn more

about military gods in general at that time. Just like when I received my grandmother's spirit, my personality became more masculine, and I danced on blades[10] in a different way, more boldly.

In the same way, I think I learned something new and was strongly influenced by Buddhist teachings since I first encountered them. I was twenty-eight years old and had been a shaman for about six years. One night, I had an urge to go on a pilgrimage to Buddhist sites. I went to Namhae, on the southern coast of the Korean Peninsula and then Yŏngju, Gyeongsangbuk-do. There is a famous Buddhist temple in Yŏngju, which is called Pusŏksa Temple. As soon as I arrived at the temple, I started to prostrate myself in the direction of the Buddha statue and crawled all the way into the temple from the entrance. I burst into tears, feeling at home at the temple. Then, when I finally got to the Buddha statue at the main shrine, I called him "Grandfather!" Then I started to recite sentences from the *Thousand Hands Sūtra* and to chant, which I have never learned before. I felt a strong presence of Bodhidharma [a monk from fifth- or sixth-century China] at the Namhae Boliam Temple in the same way. After coming back from the pilgrimage, I stopped eating *ohun* (Ch. *wuhun*; i.e., five acrid and strong-smelling vegetables) just like Buddhist monks do. Moreover, I stopped performing my divination services. My clients were very disappointed and frustrated at that time. This is how my existential crisis started. I wasn't sure anymore whether my divination practice was helpful for people. I kept asking, "What am I doing?

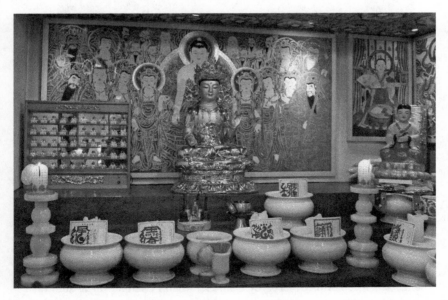

FIGURE 28.3 A STATUE OF AVALOKITEŚVARA ON THE SHAMAN'S ALTAR ALONGSIDE FIGURES AND IMAGES OF SHAMANIC DEITIES.
Source: C. Pierce Salguero.

What are the spirits in relation to my existence? Will my divination be helpful or harmful to others?" By encountering Buddha's teaching, I finally started to see my shamanic practice in perspective.

MN: Then, what does Buddhism do for you now?

JY: I have read about totemism and animism before, and I think my practice is mainly related to these forms of spirituality because I serve my ancestor spirits. In addition, my shamanistic practice, or Korean folk religion, cannot exist without mountain god worship. It does not matter how much I was moved and changed by Buddhism, I am a shaman, so I have to serve my ancestor spirits and the mountain god. I cannot serve Siddhartha as my main god. He has his place in Buddhist temples. Of course, I wanted to serve him as my main god. However, I cannot ignore where I come from. Moreover, my powers, such as healing, divination, and exorcism, were given to me by my ancestor spirits when I began my spiritual journey. Therefore, I made a compromise between my longing for Buddhist teaching and my origins. I am now serving Avalokiteśvara at the corner of my shrine along with my ancestor spirits and Korean folk gods. Buddha and Avalokiteśvara give me wisdom and broader perspective. They calm down my turbulent and selfish mind. Of course, my ancestor spirits also teach me how to live. However, they were commoners after all, when they were alive. Siddhartha, on the other hand, pursued deeper understanding. He definitely has something more to teach me and balance me.

Let me explain a little more. There are great world religions and their countless gods, such as Buddha and Jesus. Ancestor spirits are different from them. They favor their descendants over other people. They are more biased compared with Buddha or Jesus. This is the reason I need to accept greater teachings in my spirituality. I cannot cut off my ties with my ancestor spirits, but for my deeper understanding of human beings and spiritual progress, I need greater energies from Buddhism. I also sympathize with the teachings of Jesus, but somehow, I find Buddha's teaching more relevant for me.

MN: I have another question. You said you serve multiple spirits and gods in your shrine and body. How do they get along? What are their relationships?

JY: I don't think my ancestor spirits are solemn and dignified entities. If we use the word "god" in order to refer to the absolute and transcendent supernatural beings from beyond, my ancestors are definitely not like those beings. Of course, they fight. They were not saintly beings when they were alive. My father, grandfathers, grandmother, and aunt—they were only humans. They have untamed and flawed personalities, even as spirits. They are destined to argue with one another when they coexist in my shrine, since they have different ways of teaching me about spirituality.

Let me tell you a story. I had a problem when I accepted Avalokiteśvara's statue in my shrine. I told you that I stopped divination right after I accepted the Buddha's spirit. I really did not want to do that. With the Buddha's teaching, I started to explain to people about the essence of the universe and the bigger picture. My divination practice seemed petty to me at that time. Once a client came for me and asked me to help her with her sick child. She wanted me to heal the child, but I berated her for being attached to trivial stuff. There is something greater than your sick child, I said. Before then, I used to be a very efficient healer and found a simple reason for people's spiritual illnesses. However, I started to speak too much about abstract principles. When it happened, my grandmother spirit, whom I also mentioned earlier, got mad at me. I told you she had a masculine personality. When she gets mad, she uses strong language. She told me things like this: "Who do you think you are? You are only a shaman! What the hell are you doing, not doing what you should do! You are crazy and useless! Stop this Buddhist crap!" Because of this kind of resistance and backlash from my ancestors, the situation was difficult for me when I decided to include Avalokiteśvara's spirit in my shrine and accepted Buddhist teachings.

So, I had to negotiate and cajole my ancestor spirits. I told them nicely, "I know you, Grandma and Daddy, always care for me. All the ancestors care for me and cherish me. I appreciate it. However, you are no saints! You are not as great as Buddha or Jesus. I need greater teachings along with your powers. You need me as much as I need you. I would like to learn from Buddha, and you will have to learn from Buddha, as well. We will grow together spiritually." And it worked. For me, spirits or gods are not the main subjects. I, the shaman, am the main character. We need to balance out the boisterous spirits and gods. I live with spirits and gods together in harmony. There are other spiritual existences in the universe, but they are not absolute, and they never dominate me. Neither do I [dominate them]. We are in reciprocal relationships. I feel them because they feel me. They need me to exist. We are partners who develop spiritually and progress hand in hand. We can't stop learning. That's the reason I came to serve Avalokiteśvara in my shrine.

CPS: How, specifically, do you heal people?

JY: You have to diagnose first. It is all about energy and *qi*. There are different causes of illness. I can heal people who are sick owing to the acts of spirit and soul and soul (Kr. *chŏngshin, hon*; Ch. *jingshen, hun*). However, if someone is ill because of genetic diseases or merely physical reasons, I cannot heal that person. I have to really tell which case is which. In other words, I can heal people who are possessed or "mounted" by the wrong spirits but not people who are sick from other natural causes. That is my first step when I heal people: discerning if the person is ill because of spirits or not.

I am a shaman, and my body is unusual. I can accommodate more than ten different spirits in my body, and they can frequent my body without any resistance thanks to my spiritual talent. However, normal people cannot do this. They are not equipped with the kind of spiritual energy that can take the existence of the spirits in the body. Even a single extra spirit in a normal person's body can cause great illness. The person might behave differently or experience mental illnesses. If the misplaced spirit in a patient's body stays for too long, it cannot be healed. Timing is important. You have to come quickly after you are possessed. There are many different and complicated cases. I usually recommend to treat a patient along with Western medicine. People should go to the hospital for their illnesses derived from natural causes, but I can help people for other kinds of diseases. For example, one of my recent clients was a terminal cancer patient. She was being treated in a hospital, but she came to me because she could not eat anymore, and the doctor could not help her. I saw her having multiple problems. Her body needed treatment using Western medicines, but she needed additional help from me to keep eating, because that issue had spiritual causes.

I control spiritual energies and *qi*, and this is how I heal people. I specialize in incantation prayers (*kyŏngmun*). I often use my shamanic musical instruments, such as a gong [figure 28.4]. When I hit this gong, I communicate with the possessed person and the spirit inside. I don't necessarily need the sound, but it facilitates my spiritual concentration. I have walked on blades and done other kinds of practice, but a gong works the best for me to extract extra spirits from a patient's body. Spirits circulate in our bodies through the nervous system; that's where I track them and treat patients. I recite incantation prayers and play a gong to invite the spirits out.

CPS: Do you sometimes have to force them out of a patient's body?

JY: Of course. There are many cases in which a spirit may not come out. Ancestor spirits of a patients are the easiest because they care about the patient. Also, some weaker spirits are not too difficult to treat. I can easily seduce them with food and offerings. If they like the offerings, they immediately leave the patient's body. That being said, there are some cases that involve strong and angry spirits. In these cases, the situation can be messy. I cannot force them out in one go. I usually have to do an incantation prayer ritual several times. It also depends on how much spiritual energy the patient's body can handle. If the patient's body is waning, I really have to be careful. It can be dangerous for the patient. They often pass out during the ritual. I sometimes invite other shamans to pray together in difficult instances if I think my spiritual energy cannot take the spirit's strong energy.

CPS: Whose authority do you use to drive out the spirits? Does Avalokiteśvara provide you power, or extra protection, or any other kind of practical thing when you heal people?

JY: There is nothing I can do by myself. There are certain roles I play and the gods and spirits play. The spirit of my father and the admiral gods exert the most power in subduing a spirit in a patient's body. After overpowering the spirit, Pulsa Halmŏni intervenes. She hears out the wretched spirit in a patient's body and persuades them to come out, eventually healing the patient. She is over there on my shrine, wearing a white conical hat. She is connected to Buddhism.

The energy of Avalokiteśvara and the energy of Pulsa Halmŏni are the same for me. Therefore, shamans always say that if you serve Pulsa Halmŏni, it is very difficult and tiring, because we have to keep some Buddhist rules, such as dietary restrictions and abstinence, when we serve Pulsa Halmŏni.

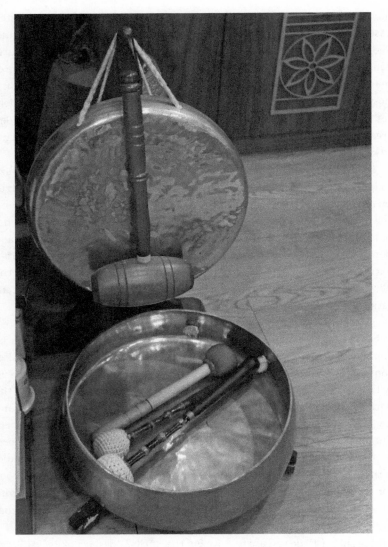

FIGURE 28.4 THE SHAMAN'S GONG, USED TO HELP HER CONCENTRATE WHEN COMMUNICATING WITH A POSSESSED PATIENT'S SPIRIT.
Source: C. Pierce Salguero.

NOTES

1. This study was funded by the National Research Foundation of Korea (grant number NRF-20141342).
2. The debate regarding the applicability of the Siberian term *shaman* to Korean shamanism is a compelling example of the intellectual maturation of scholarship on this subject. See T. Kim 1999.
3. See www.mudang.org.

4. For instance, as an American anthropologist working on Korean shamanism since the 1970s, Laurel Kendall witnessed changing perceptions about shamanism throughout the latter half of the twentieth century. She recounts how Korean nationalism and the search for "Koreanness" propelled vigorous research and led Korean academics to re-create a new discourse on Shamanism as an essential part of Korean national culture. Consequently, shamans themselves have employed this academic language and have claimed a position as the adherents of a legitimate religion and the bearers of "authentic" Korean traditional culture. See Kendall 1998, 2009a.

5. In popular Korean shamanism, Pulsa Halmŏni has often been identified with Śakra or Indra, a guardian deity in Buddhism. However, the iconography of this deity is decidedly female. Below, the shaman equates her to Avalokiteśvara, and her statue bears some visual resemblance to the female representation of that deity common in East Asia.

6. In this respect, the shaman's acceptance of a Buddhist deity and modern discourse of religious studies can be seen as a negotiation of "practices between shamans, clients, and modern competing ideologies," as Dong-kyu Kim argues regarding the matrix of meanings in Korean shamanism (D. Kim 2012: 32).

7. Interview with Yonggeum Jung (b. 1969), conducted in Korean at her home near Kunkook University in Seoul, South Korea, by Minjung Noh and C. Pierce Salguero, July 21, 2016. Translation by Minjung Noh.

8. Here, the shaman uses the Korean word *shin* (Ch. *shen*) to refer to her ancestral spirits. In contemporary Korean language, *shin* broadly indicates spirits, gods, and various kinds of supernatural entity in popular parlance. Here, we translate *shin* as "spirits" when she refers to ancestors. In other cases, when she mentions more general religious entities from Buddhist or Daoist traditions, we translate *shin* as "deity" or "god."

9. It is common among contemporary Korean shamans to serve the spirit of General MacArthur, nationally recognized as a hero of the Korean War. A number of scholars have witnessed this intertwined relationship between twentieth-century Korean history and shamanism. See, for example, Knecht 2003: 1; Kendall 2009b: 305–26; Choi 2010.

10. In Korean shamanism, shamans often ride or dance on sharp blades to demonstrate their spiritual power. Once a shaman successfully dances barefoot on sharp metal blades without any injuries, the shaman is recognized as having special protection from the spirit he or she serves.

29. Among Archangels, Aliens, and Ascended Masters

Avalokiteśvara Joins the New Age Pantheon

C. PIERCE SALGUERO

It is well known that European and North American encounters with Asian religious symbols, ideas, and practices significantly influenced the development of Western occultism in the nineteenth and twentieth centuries.[1] Beginning with the development of Theosophy in the 1870s, many popular Western spiritual movements and esoteric religions have appropriated meditative, tantric, and yogic practices particularly associated with Hinduism and Buddhism. One of the most significant contemporary descendants of these nineteenth-century trends is the New Age movement (today often referred to as "Western Esotericism"). Originating in the 1970s in Britain and North America, this tradition weaves together several strands of nineteenth-century occultism along with twentieth-century popular cultural phenomena, including UFOs, neopaganism, neoshamanism, popularized notions of quantum physics, and some aspects of the counterculture of the 1960s and '70s. Simultaneously eclectic and universalizing, New Age adherents have always welcomed healing traditions with putative origins in Asia (e.g., meditation, qigong, Reiki, *taiji*, yoga) as integral parts of their syncretic mix. These connections have often included close ties and significant crossovers with Buddhism.[2]

This chapter presents an ethnographic interview conducted in the summer of 2015 in the Bay Area of northern California with Melissa Halsey, a Caucasian woman whose practice might be described as New Age, while also intimately involving Buddhist practices, ideas, and symbols. Referring to herself as a "spiritual channel," Halsey describes communicating with a range of spiritual beings to bring their blessings, teachings, and healing advice to her clients and students. In the excerpt below, she describes how the bodhisattva Avalokiteśvara, whom she calls "Quan Yin," first appeared to her during a channeling session. She has continually channeled the bodhisattva for about twenty years now, particularly focusing on health-related issues. In the interview, Halsey discusses her methods for accessing Quan Yin, the benefits her clients have received, and her own subjective experience while she is doing these "readings."

One of the questions Halsey addresses in the interview is that of her religious identity. As is typical among adherents of the New Age tradition, she is clear in disassociating herself from organized religious groups or labels, rejecting any categorization and even eschewing the label "New Age" itself. Despite admitting that her practice is "very Buddhist"—she has studied extensively with the Dalai Lama, and her chief spirit guide is a bodhisattva—she also rejects the label "Buddhist." Instead, she calls her practice simply "universal." Taking this stance outside of official religious orthodoxy allows her a high degree of flexibility in her use of Buddhist concepts, which she incorporates into a syncretic framework of doctrine and practice that also includes certain aspects of gnostic and Catholic Christianity, neopaganism, and American space-alien pop culture. (In this regard, this American channel offers an interesting point of comparison with the Korean shaman presented in chapter 28, who likewise tells of how she retrofitted a developing personal relationship with the same bodhisattva into a preexisting non-Buddhist healing practice.)

Over the past two decades, the New Age tradition has attracted much attention from scholars of religious studies, and it is now taken seriously as an influential New Religious Movement with a large number of adherents around the world.[3] However, syncretic Western forms of Buddhist religiosity such as are presented in this chapter rarely have warranted close study by scholars of Buddhist studies, who on the whole have exhibited a marked preference for more classical forms of Buddhism. When they have been noticed at all within Buddhist Studies, adherents of Western Esotericism, New Age, and other similar traditions have too often met with an air of dismissiveness or disdain.[4] In contrast, this chapter takes Halsey's practice to be an example of a legitimate religious or spiritual practice that is deeply meaningful to a large segment of contemporary North Americans. It also takes the channel's practice seriously as a contemporary "translation" of Buddhism into a new culture, and as an indication of the mobility, influence, and explanatory power of certain elements of Buddhism within the contemporary Western religious landscape. Halsey mentions not only the figure of Quan Yin but also the Dalai Lama, meditation, mindfulness, impermanence, the Middle Way, mantras, and other aspects of Buddhism as key concepts in her understanding of health, well-being, and how best to thrive as a human being in the twenty-first century.

FURTHER READING

Cush, Denise. 1996. "British Buddhism and the New Age." *Journal of Contemporary Religion* 11 (2): 195–208.

Gutierrez, Cathy. 2015. *Handbook of Spiritualism and Channeling.* Leiden: Brill.

Hanegraaff, Wouter. 1998. *New Age Religion and Western Culture: Esotericism in the Mirror of Secular Thought.* Albany, N.Y.: SUNY Press.

Urban, Hugh B. 2015. *New Age, Neopagan, and New Religious Movements: Alternative Spirituality in Contemporary America.* Oakland: University of California Press.

Wilson, Jeff. 2008. " 'Deeply Female and Universally Human': The Rise of Kuan-yin Worship in America." *Journal of Contemporary Religion* 23 (3): 285–306

INTERVIEW WITH MELISSA HALSEY[5]

CPS: Do you consider yourself Buddhist? Or, maybe it would be better for me to ask it this way: What role does Buddhism have in your practice?

MH: What I call myself is a spiritual channel. I didn't want to use the word "psychic," although I am clairvoyant. I call myself a spiritual channel or a spiritual teacher.

I "woke up" in 1987—that's what I call it. I think the process was happening since the early 1980s, but it was during something called the Harmonic Convergence that I actually felt it. I thought it was kind of bunk then, but I could feel something coming in my life. It was huge, like the universe opened and I saw the world and the planet, and I knew that I wasn't doing what I was supposed to be doing. So I had this tremendous kind of opening that changed my life in a big way.

The first being that I ever channeled was Sananda, which is the Christ Consciousness. Quickly after that, St. Germaine came in and different archangels. So, mostly angelic forces and ascended masters . . . and space beings {laughs}.

I eventually had to put it all together. How do you put it together? You need something . . . a practice. And so for me, even though I am not officially Buddhist, because my guidance indicates that I should not be, my practice is very Buddhist. Impermanence, the Middle Way, and mindfulness all make a lot of sense to me, and are things that people seem to be able to embrace. I think those are huge parts of being balanced in this world right now. And they come, of course, from Buddhism.

I teach mindfulness meditation and loving-kindness meditation a lot. And I do use a mantra sometimes. There is a Shambhala center nearby here, and I've gone once or twice for meditation. And there's also an ashram here that I've gone to once or twice to get very spiritual energy. But I tend to feel my practice is my own and do not really get into groups.

I don't like categories. I guess I would say my framework is "universal." It's kind of like His Holiness [the Fourteenth Dalai Lama] always says, "Don't become a Buddhist." He must say it every single time he's talking: "Stay with your own tradition." I think he's focusing on the idea of being a better human being. Be the best balanced being you can possibly be, and use all the material that you have that brings wisdom. And Buddhism, to me, brings a lot of wisdom of how to be in the world as the better human being, so that's why I use it.

CPS: So, tell me a little about how you started to work with Avalokiteśvara.

MH: I don't have formal Buddhist training, so it started from intuition. Quan Yin simply became present when I moved to Charlottesville [Virginia].[6] There was a new energy when I was doing a healing session one day, just in the corner of the room. The first time I saw her, she was a column of light, just shimmering, and her name came into my head, "Quan Yin." But I didn't know what that meant.

I guess it was 1995 or something, so Quan Yin wasn't as prevalent as she is now. I mean, these days, you can search on the internet and Quan Yin is everywhere, it seems like. But before that, most people didn't know who Quan Yin was, including myself. So, I was sort of starting to try to find out who she was, and then randomly somebody sent me a statue. They said it was the Buddha, but it wasn't. I opened up the box, and it was a carved female deity. I turned it over; it said, "Quan Yin, Buddhist Goddess of Compassion."

So, like that, she just started appearing in my life. As she came more and more often in my channeling, I would see her in different ways. Lots of times she comes in the Chinese white-robed form. Or, she has come on a white elephant or with other auspicious animals. She has come with many arms a few times. Sometimes, she comes in a space-alien form, wearing something almost like Japanese samurai armor, with coal-black almond-shaped eyes—all black, no whites. She comes in different forms, which are different aspects of her, but her presence is always the same. It's a presence that's filling, like the ocean is. You wouldn't describe the ocean as one thing. She's more like that.

When she appeared to me, my guidance indicated that there was an outside teacher waiting for me, a female teacher in India. So, I started visiting female gurus and connecting with them. I was enjoying their energy and their light, but kept sensing "no, no, no." Then, I was in New York at a workshop, and the elevators were loaded because a lot of people were coming in, so I had to go up the stairs. On the stairs, there was a shelf with everybody's flyers for workshops they were doing at this center, and I picked up a bunch of them and stuffed them in my bag. The day after, I felt a strong presence that said, "Your teacher is in your briefcase." So I started looking through the papers, and among the fliers there was a picture of the Dalai Lama. I felt like, "Oh, this is my teacher!" But my mind was like, "Wait a minute, he's not female, he's not Indian, I don't get it." But I read a book about him, and it said he's an embodiment of Quan Yin, and living in India, and so that started my journey.

I started taking a lot of teachings with His Holiness. I probably have done about forty at this point. I usually see him somewhere twice a year, and that brought me in more contact with Buddhist teachings. I was at a Kalachakra ceremony with him in Toronto when my mind really opened up to the Diamond Light teachings. I've used that a lot with my students to give them a practice to help them move through all the openings that I feel are going on with the planet.

CPS: So let's say you're going to work with her in a healing session. Do you call on her to come, or is she just there? How do the mechanics of that work? Do you do something to invoke her?

MH: Do I sit down and formally access her before I do a reading with somebody? Nine times out of ten, no. I have a little prayer that I got from an elderly healer that I open all my sessions with to ask for help from the Divine Mother, Divine Father, Ascended Master, archangels, guides, guardians, Quan Yin, or Mary Magdalene, or someone who has something to do with the patient. And then we go through about six minutes of breathing to balance the electromagnetic body, nerve impulses, and nervous system. I picked this up from another healer. So that's kind of how I start, and then a reading happens.

I feel Quan Yin's presence most of the time. I have images of her around, and I talk to her a lot. Her presence is there, and I feel the light of her in my being. She's not there when I'm out of balance—or rather, she's always there, but at times I forget. What do the Buddhists say . . . the Diamond Mind is always there, although it can be obscured by the clouds of your thinking? And the Compassionate Heart is always there, as well, but it's buried, or we push it away? So, the healing is kind of getting to that light and helping people find it. She's been brilliant, I think, in doing that.

Quan Yin gave us the gift of a garden, which is a place where you can go for refuge and compassion. It is a fifth-dimensional energy that's above the dual world, the physical world, and you get there through the heart. She says that the garden is real, and when she gave it to me, she said that the garden could be transferred into any space just by opening your heart and calling on her.

She also gave me a prayer, which I've probably said nine million times:

Dearest Lady Quan Yin,
I call on you to help me love and accept myself fully.
I ask that you grant me a full measure of compassion for myself and for others.
I pray that those suffering in the world can see and feel your loving presence.
I pray that the hardened hearts will melt
in the presence of your compassionate understanding.
I pray that the waters of grace and compassion that you pour on the earth
will nourish the seeds of love and compassion in all hearts,
creating gardens of beauty within all living beings.
It is my intention to nourish the garden within myself through prayer,
meditation and right thinking.

In my heart my garden flourishes,
spilling over and filling my world with the fragrance of the garden.
Thank you Dear Lady Quan Yin for your presence in my life and in my world.

Invocations or prayers like that will come to me literally in two seconds. And I'm the kind of person who sits there trying to write a letter for an hour, so I know that they're coming from her. I've had that prayer for maybe ten years now, and I share it as much as possible. I feel like the prayer is a giant teaching that helps access the garden, and that's the vehicle that I use a lot with people.

So, that is how I work with Quan Yin. I believe she's always there, and I believe she's here for everybody. Because we need compassion.

CPS: I'm wondering what your own experience is like when you channel her. What happens to you?

MH: My personality is still there, but this bigger part is there that's just in the moment with that connection. Channeling is kind of like that. I do not trance-channel. Trance-channeling is when you completely leave the body and you don't know what happened. I'm what's called a conscious channel. So I'm bringing the energy in, and it's huge.

Internally, it's interesting. If I'm doing a group channeling, rapid awareness and pictures come through. I just open my eyes and mouth, and it's like, "Blah, blah, blah." I can't stop, and I can't keep up with it. I'm "see-feeling" it, and I'm "see-understanding" it, and I'm having to put it into words, and it's really sometimes hard to. My mouth just opens, and it goes, and I will see many, many things. I'll be in a different place seeing it, but I'm still there.

CPS: I'm sorry if that question didn't make sense. I've heard from some people I've interviewed that when I start asking these kinds of questions, I force them to put into words things that they just feel or that just happens. Maybe I'll ask something that's more tangible, like if channeling exhausts or energizes you?

MH: I will feel completely different after a group channeling than I do before. It's very energizing. If I had a headache before, or if I was stressed before, it's all gone and I feel great, and sometimes kind of high for a while. These days, the more balanced I become, the more the experience is centered—Middle Way rather than high and low. In the beginning, it was really high and low, but the practice has brought me to realizing I want to meet it all with that sort of calm presence of awareness.

I prefer to do the teachings in a group. But I never organize myself enough, so my main income comes from individual channeling sessions. That can be draining. You have to be involved with the psychic body of the other person to do the reading, and that's tiring. If I'm with someone who's just had chemotherapy, for example, they'll leave feeling really good, but I will throw up afterward. And that will last for a while. It's especially draining when you're working with people who are resistant, who are not really wanting to be open. So I pretty much ask for people who want to be open, who are on a path, and I pretty much get that. I don't work with people who are not wanting to be clear, or who are not wanting someone else to help.

CPS: When you do sessions with people who are sick, are you trying to cure them? Are you trying to use some kind of energies to help them? Or are you trying to teach them to help themselves? And, is the healing about the physical body, or is it more about something else?

MH: That's an interesting question. So, this one local doctor actually sends patients for my input on what I see. Sometimes a patient will come and say, "The doctor doesn't know what to do with me anymore. He doesn't know what protocol to use. Should we work first with the herbs, or should we work first with the blood transfusions?"—or whatever it is. Other times, it's about helping them to understand and not fight the body or fight the illness.

Sometimes people will come for a reading and it'll be very clear: "Upper-right-hand side of your mouth; you need to go to the dentist." And they'll go, and they need a crown. Sometimes people have called me up afterward and said, "You told me I had precancerous cells in my uterus. I looked, and I did, and now I'm cured because of it." Sometimes you find out the reason for the shoulder pain has to do with some trauma, like a rape or childhood molestation or something. And only then can the physical healing start.

Aside from when I help a person to make a specific choice, for the most part my work is helping them to start healing the origin of the physical illness—which sometimes does seem to change the physical symptoms and sometimes not. So, it's not about *curing* cancer, but a lot of times it's about what choices they can make once they have it, and about openness. Surrendering, not resisting. And I think a lot of times, the energy helps people do that.

Sometimes, you'll get information that's actually specific: "Go do this. Go do that. Look this up." But I don't feel confident enough to be the only source of somebody's medical healing. I will scan the body, and I will tell you in a reading if I see something. For example, one patient came because he had a hurt ankle. He kept telling me about hurting his ankle, and I kept saying, "This is your kidney. You have a kidney problem." And he said, "No, it's my ankle." And a couple of days later, he called me up and said, "Well, sure enough, I have a kidney infection." It's not always that exact, but guidance is guidance, and I think it's given to people to help bring them to what they need. Does that make sense? They are like little treasures along the way—keys, so to speak.

CPS: And what is Quan Yin's role in that? Is she the source of the energy? Is she giving you the answers when there's a question about what should be done?

MH: Quan Yin's main role is compassion. We all need balance and compassion, and she is teaching us about the waters of compassion that she pours on the earth. She does bring physical healing, but more than physical, we need spiritual and emotional healing. The planet right now is in a healing crisis.

So, all these messages are being given to us about healing. All this stuff is coming up—you know, medical problems, universities and institutions breaking down, and how many African American young men are in prison—all these wounds that are not healed that have been shoved under the rug are resurfacing. And all our fears are resurfacing. I think this is great, because it's the only way we can heal. You can't get light without seeing more darkness. So, I think that we're getting clearer and lighter.

Quan Yin and the masters in the past five or six years have given a lot of gifts and are constantly reminding us that we have the ability to bless and to heal. They are talking about praying, talking about blessings, reminding us to use the Violet Flame, the Violet Cloak, the Garden, whatever their gifts are. There's been a lot about using your own power and not focusing on the illusions that we've bought in to. So there's Buddhism again, teaching you to calm the mind, to step out of your perception of things, to move beyond these obscurations, and to see the light. That's why I keep doing what I'm doing. To help individuals be empowered to make personal choices that bring them peace and happiness is, I think, ultimately what's going to bring it to the planet. I don't think there's any other way.

NOTES

Thanks to Ben Joffe for his feedback on drafts of this chapter and for his contributions to the chapter's references.

1. Prothero 1996; De Michelis 2004; Urban 2007; Cheah 2011: 19–35; Hackett 2013; Djurdjevic 2014.
2. Cush 1996, for example, discusses parallels and entanglements between British Buddhism and New Age movements.
3. See, for example, Lewis and Melton 1992; Kyle 1995; Heelas 1996; Brown 1997; Sutcliffe 2003; Pike 2004; Urban 2015. This author has personally witnessed the importance of New Age thought and practice—and the influence of Buddhism on both—in places as diverse as Argentina, Bulgaria, France, India, Thailand, and Uruguay.
4. Quli 2009.
5. This interview was conducted by the author on August 6, 2015. It has been edited for conciseness and clarity, and has been read and approved in this final format by the interviewee.
6. Charlottesville boasts a sizable community of relocated Tibetans, meditation centers, and Western Buddhists.

Buddhist Healing in Practice

30. Buddhism and Resistance in Northern Thai Traditional Medicine

An Interview with an Unlicensed Thai Folk Healer

ASSUNTA HUNTER

T he translation below comes from an interview conducted in 2009. These are the words of an unlicensed folk healer, Mo ("Doctor") Somboon (a pseudonym), a teacher and practitioner specializing in the treatment of HIV. He is an unlicensed traditional medicine practitioner in his late fifties, and although he is both well respected and widely known in his local community and in Chiang Mai Province, his practice is technically illegal. Unlicensed practitioners are generally not prosecuted in Thailand; however, they cannot advertise or promote their practices, and they are not legally allowed to charge fees for their services.

Mo Somboon describes practicing traditional medicine without a license as a form of resistance to the control of Central Thai officialdom.[1] In the interview, Mo Somboon compares himself to Khruba Siwichai (1878–1939), a revered monk and teacher in northern Thailand. This comparison is striking. It is a marker of his perception of himself as a good Buddhist, one whose controversial actions are making merit and helping others to earn merit. Khruba Siwichai developed a substantial following, was widely believed to have supernatural powers, and had strong local support. He practiced a local form of Buddhism known as Yuan Buddhism, a regional tradition that emerged in the Lanna kingdom of northern Thailand. Khruba Siwichai was known in the North for his extensive program of building and repairing religious monuments, both a community-strengthening activity and a form of Buddhist merit-making. His popularity at the time was looked on with great suspicion by Central Thai officials who were attempting to unite the diverse local cultural traditions of Thailand under Central Thai authority. It was feared that Khruba Siwichai might lead a local revolutionary movement to maintain the independence of the Northern Thai regions.

Concern about independent northern Thai voices peaked in the early years of the twentieth century when the Lanna kingdom came under Central Thai control as part of the cultural consolidation that created the modern Thai state. The assimilation of the Yuan sect into Central Thai Buddhism during the reign of King Chulalongkorn (1868–1910) placed all Theravāda Buddhists under one centralized administrative structure located in Bangkok. The reforms established the principles of a national religion through the Sangha Administration Act of 1902. This act drew regional monks into a national structure and consolidated the central powers of the Thai state. Khruba Siwichai resisted the increasing central state regulation of the monastic order, the promotion of standardized and revised religious teachings, and a centralized and bureaucratized ecclesiastical organization that drew Yuan Buddhism under the control of the Central Thai Buddhist *sangha*.

The introduction of Central Thai as a national language and the suppression of local languages such as Lanna Thai had an immediate impact on traditional medicine practice, because medical manuscripts were written in these local languages using the Yuan script.[2] In addition, oral transmission, a key aspect of the transmission of medical knowledge until the mid-twentieth century, used northern Thai language to refer to plants, practices, and rituals. Thus, the transmission of traditional medicine knowledge in both text-based and oral forms was significantly disrupted in the twentieth century by the decreasing literacy in regional languages.[3] The Thai government actively suppressed the use of regional languages, texts, and manuscripts (including medical texts) to such an extent that medical manuscripts were often hidden or destroyed in the period leading up to the late twentieth century when a revival of Lanna culture and language occurred.

Mo Somboon laments the marginalization of local traditions of medicine. But he also speaks of the parallels between Khruba Siwichai's religious dissent and his own defiant practice of traditional medicine, which he sees as a form of resistance to current laws regulating traditional medicine. Mo Somboon's use of Khruba Siwichai as a model for his own behavior highlights the Central Thai suppression of many local practices of traditional medicine, and illustrates the continuing entwinement of Buddhism with traditional medicine practice.

Mo Somboon's altar includes plastic flowers, Buddha statues, and silver offering bowls, and on one side is a photograph of Khruba Siwichai smoking a typical northern Thai cigar. Photos on the walls show the opening ceremony for the HIV clinic established by Mo Somboon. The clinic is housed in a temple and provides a hospice for people with HIV. He started this project by himself in 1992 but gradually involved the assistance of many people from his local community.

In the process, he has managed to decrease the prevailing stigma against HIV in his local area.

When Mo Somboon first announced that he was going to build a temple to support HIV-positive people in his community, many thought this was a "crazy" idea. He retreated to the village temple wearing white (indicating his retreat into Buddhist prayer), meditated, and talked with the old people of the village about his plan. He eventually gained their support for building a temple for the HIV-positive population, enlisted the help of the community to build a hospice, and used the last of the money donated by the community for a Buddhist ceremony to consecrate the temple. Mo Somboon's integration of Buddhism into his medical practice is evident throughout the interview.

FURTHER READING

Bamber, Scott. 1998. "Medicine, Food and Poison in Traditional Thai Healing." *Osiris* 13: 339–53.

Brun, Viggo. 1990. "Traditional Manuals and the Transmission of Knowledge in Thailand." In *The Master Said: To Study and . . .*, edited by Birthe Arendrup, Simon B. Heilesen, and Jens Ostergård Petersen, 43–65. Copenhagen: East Asian Institute, University of Copenhagen.

Cohen, Paul T. 2001. "Buddhism Unshackled: The Yuan 'Holy Man' Tradition and the Nation-State in the Tai World." *Journal of South East Asian Studies* 32 (2): 227–47.

Chokevivat, Vichai, and Anchalee Chuthaputhi. 2005. "The Role of Thai Traditional Medicine in Health Promotion." In *Proceedings of the Sixth Global Conference on Health Promotion*. Bangkok: Department for the Development of Thai Traditional and Alternative Medicine, Ministry of Public Health, Thailand.

Weisberg, Daniel. 1984. "The Practice of 'Dr' Paep: Continuity and Change in Indigenous Healing in Northern Thailand." *Social Science and Medicine* 18 (2): 117–28.

INTERVIEW WITH MO SOMBOON[4]

AH: Mo Somboon, tell me about working as a traditional medicine practitioner in a rural community.

MS: I was thinking about Khruba Siwichai, the famous Northern monk. He was the ideal monk. He had strong ideals about his practice. And when they wanted to combine Northern Thailand together [with Central Thailand], he was the one who went against the rules of the new monastic practice. He disagreed. He broke the rules, and they did not give him papers. He was jailed, but he just continued to do what he had done. He didn't care about that; he was Khruba Siwichai. He did that, and people respected him until he died. He is famous still. Meanwhile, other monks who have followed the orders of Bangkok, no one remembers them.

So I have no license [to practice traditional medicine]. I believe that if I have good karma, they will come, [and] they will learn. Now I have a mouth but cannot speak; I have eyes but cannot look for many people. I cannot promote what is good about herbal medicine, about my ideas, my concepts about herbal medicine. What I try to do now is keep quiet. Sometimes the Lord Buddha says it is better not to say anything. So people who come learn about this. And when I die, I will finish my karma and live only with the goodness of what I have done.

AH: How did you learn to use traditional medicine?

MS: I started to learn about herbs at eight or nine years old by walking from here to Lamphun with my father to take herbs to get powdered. He used a grinding machine there in a factory, and then he brought the herbs back here. My grandfather and father were herb doctors (mo yaa); my great-grandfather was a healer, and his father was a healer. My father would ask me to get herbs from special places. He would say, "The herb looks like that; it is at this house," but he did not teach me directly.

In the beginning, I learned herbal plants. Later I learned to make herbal medicines, and my father brought me with him to help him. After a while, when I knew the places to pick herbs, my father told me to make things on my own, and I started doing that for myself. So I started to work by myself.

AH: How did you start treating HIV-positive patients?

MS: In 1992, HIV started. I saw many patients. At that time, the doctors said to patients, "You can only wait until you die." I felt that this was something very sad. So I asked my father about treatments. In the past, there were serious diseases like cholera. He said that at the time of cholera, there was only one hospital in the North, and many people got this disease. My father said that if you got this disease and died, people did not come to your funeral, and people would not even go past your rice fields for fear of infection. So I asked how he treated this. My father taught me the treatments. I followed his treatments, and I followed the survivors. I found survivors, and I asked them how they felt and why they survived when other people died. They told me that the people who died did not listen to the healer. Survivors told me that fear made them do exactly what they were supposed to do, because they were scared of dying.

When I started treating HIV patients, they were there on site in this clinic, and I was treating them and watching them. I am proud of that and what I learned, and I felt lots of support from my father.

My father said, "When you are a healer, all diseases will come to you. You have to pray, you have to meditate, [and] you cannot be scared to treat. You have to support the patient. If patients commit to the treatment, you have to continue to treat them; you cannot stop, [you] cannot leave them alone. If you stop, the gods will punish you, and it will be very bad. If you ask for money for treating, that is bad."

You must do ceremonies and meditation and have good karma to support the patients getting better. No matter how rich or poor the patient is, it is the same price for the medicine. Herbs are 10 baht per packet. For patients who do not have money, I ask them to bring herbal medicines in exchange for treatment [i.e., they bring raw herbs for Mo Somboon to process into medicines].

My father had texts in the Northern dialect, and he taught me that. I studied Thai traditional medicine and medical practice, but I have not passed the exams. It is difficult for me to pass the exams because I know the names of all the plants in the Northern dialect, but when they do exams, they use Central Thai.

AH: How is your traditional medicine work connected to Buddhism?

MS: The learning of healers is never ending. They always have to learn more. I have to understand about practice and Dharma, and if I understand, it will help me to treat people better. I must treat people according to their minds and their hearts. Their minds and their feelings as well as the physical. We call it *dharma yaa jai* . . . treating with Dharma, herbs, and the feelings, as well.

I am not a monk, but I [entered the monkhood] for three months. I understand the Dharma of the Lord Buddha. I practiced meditation a lot, even when people said that I was crazy. Dharma is good. I practiced, practiced and then could obtain an empty, clear mind. Sometimes when I sleep, I wake up at midnight with a very clear mind and am very energetic, very comfortable, and then something comes to me.

I am not rich, not poor. The last words the monk said to me before I left the temple [were,] "Rich or not rich, you will have difficulties. Famous or not famous, you will also have difficulties."

AH: How do you see the future of traditional medicine?

MS: I worry how the future will be. Herbal medicines are becoming hard to find. The number of folk healers is getting smaller and smaller. Many older healers are dying, and many people do not really care about them. People in the family do not continue the study of folk medicine. Folk healers do not get support from the government to study; they are not recognized. So they do not keep on with the study. The people in government do not recognize folk healers' importance, and so the family does not recognize their importance [either].

In the future, it will become like a mountain where all the trees are cut down. So they will have a mountain but no trees. The mountain needs the trees of the forest. This is the same for the folk healers. Many of them are dying. It used to be each village had one or two or three healers, [but there are] much fewer now.

NOTES

1. See Cohen 2001, which discusses the concept of a man of merit (*ton bun*) in relation to Khruba Siwichai (1878–1939). *Ton bun* is a term used to describe a person who uses their great store of accumulated merit (*bun*) to work for humanity, thus providing opportunities for others to acquire merit. Cohen argues that Buddhist revivalism established a local history of dissent in Sipsongpanna (the cross-border area bounded by Southern China, Northern Thailand, Myanmar, and Laos) through the stories of Khruba Bunchum and Khruba Siwichai. Their temple-building and merit-making activities led to what he describes as the establishment of a Yuan Buddhist kingdom, a sacred kingdom that extends beyond the boundaries of the Thai nation-state and into Sipsongpanna.

2. The Northern Thai or Lanna language (*Kham muang*) belongs to the Tai language family but is considered a distinct language.

3. See Weisberg 1984 and Bamber 1998, which both discuss the changing pattern of folk medicine and the use of local languages to describe plants and medicines.

4. This interview with Mo Somboon (a pseudonym) was conducted by Assunta Hunter with the assistance of a Northern Thai interpreter, Amporn Boontang. It took place July 11, 2009, in a rural area on the outskirts of Chiang Mai city, in Chiang Mai Province, Thailand. It was conducted as part of doctoral research on traditional medicine practitioners in Northern Thailand. I have slightly edited the language as necessary for readability, but this editing has not affected the meaning of Mo Somboon's responses.

31. Burmese Alchemy in Practice

Master U Shein's Healing Practice

CÉLINE CODEREY

This chapter consists of a translation of an interview conducted with Master[1] U Shein, the most well-known Burmese alchemist, who died in 2014,[2] and one of his main disciples. The interview took place in 2009 in U Shein's house in Yangon, a majestic building filled with images of the Buddha, Hindu–Buddhist devas, powerful beings released from the cycle of rebirth, and territorial spirits. This predominance of Buddhist elements is very common among healers and largely reflects the central role Buddhism plays in society as a provider of a cosmological system and a value system.

During the interview, the master relates how he received his knowledge and healing power from a deity and how he uses this power to cure people affected by all sorts of disorder, including life-threatening diseases such as HIV and AIDS. The disciple also present during the interview describes the long process through which U Shein's medicines are produced and highlights the importance of "gold ash" (*shway pya*), the dust deposit produced by a "ball of energy" (*datlon*)[3] created by combining and burning mercury, lead, bismuth, and silver.[4] To provide us with objective proof of the legitimacy of U Shein's practice and of the efficacy of his treatments, we are shown several documents: international medical diplomas and awards, reports from scientific labs attesting the nontoxicity of his remedies, and some patients' HIV and AIDS test results that turned from positive to negative. The need to prove one's legitimacy by resorting to scientific or biomedical tools is very common among this kind of healer and is clearly related to the hegemonic position biomedicine has come to occupy in contemporary Myanmar. U Shein also testifies that he has long been ingesting his own medicines and that this has contributed to keeping him young and strong.

Although U Shein's fame is exceptional, his practice is not. Alchemy, "the art of fire" (aggiyat pyinnya), and in particular the use of "gold medicine" (shway hsay),[5] has been widespread since the eleventh century.[6] According to tradition, alchemy is one of the four weikza practices (from the Pāli vijjā, meaning "knowledge"), the other three being esoteric yantra diagrams, mantra, and remedies.[7]

Paired with the practice of concentration meditation,[8] weikza practices are supposed to contribute to the accomplishment of both worldly and otherworldly aims (see also chapter 19). On one hand, they are used to prevent and cure of different kinds of disorder and disease, especially those believed to be caused by spirits, witches, or sorcerers. On the other hand, they are used by the practitioner him- or herself to gain supernatural powers,[9] such as seeing the future and communicating with deities. Weikza practices especially can be used to extend one's life and to release oneself from the cycle of rebirth.[10]

Traditionally, weikza techniques can be learned in two ways: through revelation from a deity or weikza (as in the case of U Shein) or, more commonly, through an initiation into one of the congregations of weikza practitioners that are widespread across the country.[11] These groups have been feared by state authorities (first colonial and more recently military) as potential threats to their power. This is all the more so given that in periods of political crises, some of these groups have taken a messianic and millenarian turn.[12]

Since 1952 (a few years after Burma was granted independence in 1948), the government has sought to marginalize alchemy and other practices through the formalization and institutionalization of traditional medicine.[13] Given the dominant status of biomedicine in the latter half of the twentieth century, the reform of traditional medicine has been accomplished largely through adapting to biomedical standards and exterminating aspects that seem not to fit those standards. The institutionalization of traditional medicine in this period aided the government's aims of nation building, homogenizing the population, and taking control of peripheral areas.[14] The standardization of medicine also helped to neutralize or integrate potential threatening forces, such as those related to the spiritual and esoteric forces associated with the weikza.

The version of traditional medicine formalized by the government focuses on herbal medicine and astrology, with weikza practices being greatly marginalized. In 1996, the government also decided to regulate the circulation of traditional medicines through the introduction of a production license that banned toxic substances such as heavy metals. These regulations completely excluded alchemical products from the authorized market. Other limitations have also been imposed on practitioners of traditional medicine, including interdictions on injections and operations, as well as on involvement in treatments for cancer and HIV. If alchemy has retained any role at all, it has been reduced to a form of chemistry, purified of any esoteric or supernatural aspect, and its purpose reduced merely to curing diseases.

Although the practices of most traditional alchemists and other healers who could not meet the government standards were rendered illegal, many healers have remained convinced of the power of their techniques and continue to practice. Many alchemists defiantly try to cure diseases that biomedicine is unable to, particularly HIV.[15] U Shein was the most high-profile of these practitioners in recent times. According to a couple of his close friends whom I have interviewed, the government was especially threatened by his charismatic personality and had on many occasions tried to stop him. However, owing to the fact that "his treatments have really proven to be effective," the government eventually came to accept him into the official traditional medicine association. Of course, the integration of U Shein into this group could be interpreted as a strategy for the government to better control him. However, it is the former narrative that circulates, thus spreading the idea that the power of alchemy is so strong that even the government and medical authorities can do nothing to stop it.

FURTHER READING

Brac de la Perrière, Bénédicte, Guillaume Rozenberg, and Alicia Turner, eds. 2014. *Champions of Buddhism: Weikza Cults in Contemporary Burma*. Singapore: NUS Press.

Patton, Thomas. 2016. "Buddhist Salvation Armies as Vanguards of the *Sāsana*: Sorcerer Societies in Twentieth-Century Burma." *Journal of Asian Studies* 75 (4): 1083–1104.

Pranke, Patrick. 1995. "On Becoming a Buddhist Wizard." In *Buddhism in Practice*, edited by Donald S. Lopez, 343–58. Princeton, N.J.: Princeton University Press.

Tosa, Keiko. 1996. "A Consideration of *Weikza* Belief in Burma: The Meaning of *Làwki* and *Làwkoktăra* for the *Gaìng*." *Mizokugaku Kenkyu* 61 (2): 215–42.

INTERVIEW WITH MASTER U SHEIN[16]

CC: Master, may I know, how did you acquire your healing powers?

US: I was born on October 7, 1926, in Pylulwin, not far from Mandalay. My horoscope at birth already revealed that I was fated to be gifted with special powers. And indeed, from very young, at the age of ten, I was able to make predictions about other people's lives, and they always turned [out] to be right. At sixteen, I entered the army and stayed for twenty years. I received many signs pushing me to withdraw, but I never understood them, not until later, when they became very explicit. I seriously injured my hand and knee as the result of an incident involving a grenade and gunshots. One night, I was visited in my dreams by a deity, who had been my sister in a previous life. She suggested that I visit a hermit who was staying in a cave near my hometown. I went and found him. He said he was my father from the realm of the deities and that he wanted to transmit his knowledge and healing powers to me. He then put the palms of his hands on mine and told me, "You have to respect and follow the Buddha's commandments. [. . .] If you do so, in one year from now, signs will appear on your palms, and from that moment onward, you should work as a healer."

Look {showing me his right palm and indicating a triangle formed by the lines of the hand}. This is the Shwedagon Pagoda [i.e., the most famous and venerated pagoda in Myanmar], [. . .] and this {showing me a little protuberance on the palm of his left hand} is the Kyaiktiyo [i.e., the famous golden rock in the Mon state]. The Shwedagon represents my supernatural power, the power through which I cure supernatural disorders; the Kyaiktiyo represents my natural power, the power to cure natural disorders.

Then the hermit gave me a fruit to eat and some water to drink. [. . .] A glass of water suddenly appeared in my hand. [. . .] After I drank it, the hermit proclaimed, "Now you have the powers." Then I fainted, and when I woke up, the hermit was gone. [. . .]

CC: So the hermit was [. . .] a *weikza* [here meaning a person who has acquired extraordinary powers, including the ability to extend one's life and release oneself from the cycle of rebirth]?

US: Indeed, he was a *weikza*.

CC: But you did not study in a congregation?[17]

US: No, I don't belong to any congregation. [. . .] Since the encounter with the hermit, I have been visited in dreams by devas who gifted me a ball of energy and instructed me on how to use it to produce "gold ash," which became the essence of my medicines. Even after that, they often contacted me to provide me with instructions about how to improve the medicine. I first cured myself from the several injures I had received in the army, and then I started to cure people affected by both natural and supernatural disorders. [. . .] This medicine is very powerful; it has regeneration properties. Since taking it, I no longer need glasses, my eyesight has improved, my hair turned black again, my muscles are strong, [and] I feel full of vitality. {To convince me of this, the master's assistants show me some photos in which the master is arm wrestling some muscular Western men.} By ingesting this powder, my body has become hard and cold, like gold. {While saying this, he stretches his arm toward me and invites me to touch it to testify to the truth of his words.}

CC: Can you tell me more about this gold powder and how it is produced?

ASSISTANT: The production process is very long; it takes up to twenty years. It involves heating, melting, mixing, drying, [and] burying several ingredients, including metals, fruits, and honey. The first step is carried out by monks in the forests of Shan State. It consists of heating and melting five metals: gold, silver, copper, zinc, and mercury. This process is conducted 108 times for each metal and aims to make the metals absolutely pure. Handling the mercury is particularly difficult because when heated, it tends to evaporate [. . .], yet this process allows it to transform into a solid state.

The metals are then mixed together in a clay pot with pieces of apples, pineapples, oranges, grapes, and honey. The honey is of a very high quality and has many healing properties because it is made with the nectar of innumerable flowers collected from remote mountainous regions. The pot will be alternately kept underground and outside in year-long cycles for twenty years. Every time the pot is taken out, it is filled with some new fruits and honey. This is the food for the metals [and is] responsible for their transformation and purification. The final product is then washed, dried, melted again, and then processed into very thin foils. These foils are chopped up and heated up together with the energy ball until a white powder appears. The powder is then blended with the fruits and honey and buried for another year. The substance resulting from this process is then dried in a special oven for two to five months. The result is gold ash. This is then combined with some binding agent and rolled into pills.

Western doctors [i.e., doctors practicing biomedicine] say that the metals we use in this alchemical process are toxic and dangerous to human health. We know they are toxic. [. . .] It is true, but the toxicity is entirely neutralized by the alchemical process. {While saying this, another assistant hands me reports of lab tests proving the nontoxicity of the medicine.} I give clear directions to my patients on how to take this medicine. It is very important that they follow my directions.

CC: What kinds of disorders do you cure with this medicine?

US: I have been curing people for more than forty years now [. . .], people affected by natural and supernatural disorders. My medicine has cured people affected by the most serious diseases, including those incurable by Western medicine, such as HIV. My medicine is much more effective and much cheaper than Western medicine treatment.[18] I have cured a Burmese, a German, and a Swiss affected by this disease. And also another Swiss, a woman, who was suffering from drug addiction. [. . .] She was a relative of mine in a previous life. {One of U Shein's assistants passes me some documents of testimonies from the patients to whom the master is referring.}

ASSISTANT: The master is very famous. He receives visitors from all over Myanmar and also from other Asian countries—Thailand, China, Singapore, Japan—and even from Europe. On several occasions, the master has been invited to Germany and Austria to attend international conferences on traditional healing methods. In 2006, he was awarded a doctorate in natural medicine by the University of Colombo in Sri Lanka.

CC: Do you cure here, in the house?

US: Most of the time, yes, but I also cure in my clinics. [. . .] I have five clinics around the country [run by disciples]. I have three thousand disciples in total, who are curing following my methods and oftentimes using my medicine.

CC: You mentioned "natural" and "supernatural" disorders. Can you tell me more about them? How do you differentiate? What are the causes of these disorders?

US: There are two kinds of disorder: *yawga* and *payawga*. According to Buddhism, *yawga* is a normal, ordinary disorder caused by one or more causes: karma, the mind, food, or the seasonal or climate changes. Karma is the most important. There are three kinds of karma: mental action [i.e., thought], physical action, and verbal action [i.e., speech]. All of them have consequences in both this life and the future life, in accordance with the law of cause and effect. Some consequences of karma can be avoided, but others—those of actions of very serious gravity, such as killing—cannot be. At best, they can be attenuated. Karma is really important. You have to keep the Three Gems [i.e., the Buddha, the Dharma, and the Sangha] constantly in your mind in whatever you are doing, [whether] eating, urinating, [or] having sex. There are ninety-six kinds of [natural] disorder in all.

    The second kind of disorder is *payawga*: disorder caused by aggression from witches, sorcerers, or spirits. It is a disease that comes from outside, *pa* meaning "outside," and *yawga* meaning "disease." Despite being caused by invisible forces, these disorders are often translated into visible symptoms. {The master's assistants now show me X-rays of patients affected with *payawga* clearly displaying some anomalies, such as white spots.}

CC: How do you know if a patient is affected by a natural or supernatural disorder? How do you make your diagnosis?

US: To detect if the disorder affecting the person is a natural or supernatural one, I give her this. {He shows me a small laminated piece of paper inscribed with esoteric symbols.}[19] If the person starts trembling or feels strange, unusual sensations, it is because she is affected by *payawga*, whereas if nothing happens, it is a sign that the disorder is a normal, natural one.[20] Sometimes, to complete the diagnosis, I call a "deva-girl" [i.e., a young woman who can be possessed by a deity] and have her possessed by a deva I then have a dialogue with [. . .] in order to obtain the information I need. Daughter [i.e., an expression used to refer to women of a younger generation], come please! {A young woman comes and sits close to us.} One, two, three! {He says this in multiple languages. The girl then replies by emitting some sounds, the language of the deities, I am told. The master extends his hand toward the girl, who suddenly faints. The master shakes her, but she does not move. But she revives as soon as the master makes another gesture with his hands.}[21]

CC: So, do you cure all kinds of disorder only with this medicine? {I ask this because, around me, I see the master's assistants taking care of patients and making use of other objects and remedies. I also notice that a bottle of honey is given to many visitors.}

US: I use gold ash for all kinds of disorder. Yet there are other remedies that are used. Each factor involved in the disorder is addressed. You can fix, increase the karma, by making an offering to the Three Jewels. The mind can be controlled, improved, [and] calmed by keeping in mind and reciting the formula of the Three Gems. You can counter the effects of the weather by moving to a cooler [or] hotter place; [you can] neutralize the effect of a food through other food. I also use my own power, inscribed in my hands, to release people from *payawga*.

CC: I have heard from other informants that during the full moon of November, you host a major medicine-making ceremony. Can you tell me about this? What kind of medicine is this?

US: Many healers from all over Myanmar and even from abroad gather here for that event; together, we produce the most powerful remedy to cure *payawga*. This medicine, however, is efficacious only for women, as its power is conditioned by the nonconsumption of alcohol and cow meat—something that men can't avoid. All participants then leave this place carrying with them some of this medicine they will then use to cure *payawga*.

CC: And what are those dolls? {I refer to little dolls hanging from a stand placed in the center of the room.}

ASSISTANT: These are amulets [. . .] for people to have with them for protection. People can purchase them. The master was advised to sell these amulets by his sister [meaning the sister from his previous life, the deity].

CC: I have heard from some visitors that you help people to create a connection, [to] get in touch with relatives from the previous life. [. . .] How do you do that, and why? Is this related to the healing practice?

ASSISTANT: Yes, it is so. The cure may also involve making offering to relatives from a previous life. Indeed, it can happen that a debt or an unsolved problem from a previous life might affect this present life and hinder the process of recovery from a disease. It is thus important to solve this problem through an offering that appeases the relatives' minds. But some people want to make offerings simply because they want to get help from relatives from a previous life.

NOTES

1. The term *hsaya gyi* is a title of respect used to address and refer to a senior (and supposedly very powerful) healer.

2. Since the death of U Shein, it is his granddaughter, previously one of his main disciples, who continues his work.

3. This is the product of the alchemical transformation of metals; in Western literature, it is often referred to as the philosopher's stone.

4. Rozenberg 2010: 93–94.

5. "Gold remedy" refers to the remedy produced through the alchemic transformation of metals and their combination with fruits and honey. This is the main remedy the master uses to cure natural and supernatural diseases.

6. Rozenberg 2010: 87.

7. The term *weikza* refers to both the practices used to reach the status of *weikza* and the people who have reached that status. *Weikza* practices comprise esoteric diagrams (*in*), alchemy (*aggiyat*), mantra (*mandan*), and remedies (*hsay*). One becomes a *weikza* when one

has acquired supernatural powers allowing one to be released from the cycle of rebirths and to extend one's life until the arrival of the next Buddha. By paying respect to the next Buddha, one will then gain direct access to Nirvana. The most studied among the *weikza* techniques is the technique of esoteric diagrams. (See Spiro 1967: 36; Tosa 2005: 160; Coderey 2011, 2014, 2017; Patton 2012.) The same technique is attested to elsewhere in Southeast Asia.

8. Burmese *thamahta*, Pāli *samatha*. For studies on meditation practices, see King 1980; Houtman 1990; Rozenberg 2001.

9. Burmese *teikdi*, Pāli *siddhi*. See Spiro 1971: 166; Pranke 1995: 350; Tosa 2009: 298.

10. The expression used is *htwetyat pauk*, which means "a place through which one leaves the cycle of rebirth in order to attain enlightenment." See Schober 1988: 14.

11. Schober 1988; Rozenberg 2010; Coderey 2011.

12. Mendelson 1963; Ferguson and Mendelson 1981; Schober 1988; Foxeus 2011.

13. The vernacular term for traditional medicine is *taing-yin hsay pyinnya* ("knowledge of the remedies of the country" or "indigenous medicine"); this is in opposition to *ingaleik hsay pyinnya* ("knowledge of the remedies of the British" or "Western medicine").

14. Aung-Twin 2010; Coderey 2011, 2018.

15. Coderey 2018.

16. This interview was conducted in Burmese and has been slightly edited for inclusion in this volume.

17. I ask this question because the vast majority of healers of this kind acquire their knowledge by being initiated into a *weikza* congregation.

18. I didn't dare ask the cost of the medicine, but I have been informed by other visitors and healers who know U Shein that the full treatment for a serious disease costs approximately $1,000 USD.

19. Inscriptions of letters or numbers referring to Buddhist, astrological, and cosmological concepts are empowered by the recitation of mantras and by summoning the power of the Buddha, the *weikza*, and the deities. See Patton 2012; Coderey 2017.

20. During the several hours spent in the house, I saw a couple of patients who were undergoing this test, which, in their cases, gave a negative result.

21. I am invited to do the same, with the master holding my hand, and the same effect is reproduced. This is possible, they tell me, because the physical proximity of the master grants me a temporary supernatural power.

32. Mental Illness in the Sowa Rigpa Clinic

A Conversation with Dr. Teinlay P. Trogawa

SUSANNAH DEANE

T he following interview was conducted with a Sowa Rigpa practitioner, Dr. Teinlay P. Trogawa, at the Chagpori Tibetan Medical Institute (CTMI) clinic in Darjeeling in May 2012.[1] A second-generation exile whose family moved to India from Southeast Tibet, Dr. Trogawa studied Sowa Rigpa in India with his uncle, the renowned practitioner Dr. Samphel Norbu Trogawa Rinpoche (1932–2005). He also acted as his uncle's translator on his visits to Europe, eventually gaining his own medical certification in 2004. Founded by Trogawa Rinpoche in 1992, the CTMI has its own Sowa Rigpa training college and runs five clinics in the Darjeeling Hills and South Sikkim. Recognized as the incarnation of a renowned lama physician[2] at an early age, Trogawa Rinpoche followed the tradition of the original Chagpori Institute in Lhasa, emphasizing religious practice in his teaching and giving Buddhist transmissions to his students, as well as producing "jewel pills" (see *Anthology*, vol. 1, ch. 60). This focus on Buddhist practice remains, with CTMI students instructed in both rituals related to Bhaiṣajyaguru and other healing-related Buddhist teachings.[3] Today, Dr. Trogawa is the director of the CTMI and president of its governing board. While there are several Sowa Rigpa practitioners working at the Darjeeling clinic, at the time I interviewed him, Dr. Trogawa continued to see patients there, particularly those with a long-standing connection to either him or his late uncle.

As outlined in the *Four Tantras*, Tibetan medical theory describes various aspects and functions of the mind and body using the concept of the *tridoṣa* (Tib. *nyépa*).[4] Defects are said to ultimately arise from the three mental factors (Tib. *nyön mong*) of the Buddhist tradition: ignorance, attachment, and aversion.[5] One of the *tridoṣa*, Wind (Tib. *lung*), is said to be responsible for the inhalation and exhalation of the breath, as well as for the physical movement of the body. The fundamental role of these "mental factors" in the formation of Wind is described in the *Four Tantras*.[6] Wind is also understood to be intimately related to the consciousness—the mind is said to "ride" the wind as a person rides a horse—and the manipulation of Wind is therefore a fundamental aspect of many Tibetan Buddhist tantric practices, undertaken in pursuit of enlightenment.[7] Owing to this relationship between Wind and consciousness, any disturbance in Wind is believed to have the potential to affect the mind and the senses, and vice versa. (Wind illnesses and therapies are discussed in *Anthology*, vol. 1, ch. 41–43.) If conducted incorrectly, tantric practices aimed at manipulating Wind may therefore lead to psychological disturbance. Indeed, in Darjeeling, I heard several narratives of Wind illness caused by incorrect tantric practice or other practices related to the manipulation of energies in the body, such as yoga or qigong.

Certainly, it is the Wind that is the focus of much discussion of mental health and illness. While disturbance in any of the *tridoṣa* can lead to mental illness, as Dr. Trogawa explains, it is the Wind that is most often implicated. Wind disturbances are sometimes described as manageable through both medicine and Tibetan Buddhist meditation.[8] In addition, other factors, such as the interference of spirits, may also be involved in a case of mental ill health, as discussed in the interview below. In such cases, while the *Four Tantras* describes numerous medical treatments, Sowa Rigpa practitioners may in fact recommend the consultation of a Tibetan Buddhist lama, whose spiritual power is understood to be necessary to subdue such spirits.[9]

The apparent lack of division between physical and psychological ailments in basic Sowa Rigpa theory is one of the most often mentioned differences between the Tibetan and biomedical systems. Many conditions listed in the *Four Tantras* encompass both physical and psychological symptoms, and the text does not separate mental and physical ailments into different sections. In the following interview, Dr. Trogawa discusses several Sowa Rigpa categories of mental illness, including Wind disturbances and insanity, describing the different causes of these illnesses according to the *Four Tantras*. He explains some Sowa Rigpa perspectives on the interplay between body and mind in relation to mental illness, describing the ways in which the body can affect the mind, and vice versa, and highlighting the importance of behavior (e.g., diet or sleep patterns) alongside Sowa Rigpa medication. As Dr. Trogawa makes clear, taking care of the mind is also a question of taking care of the body, owing to the fact that their functioning is so closely intertwined.

Dr. Trogawa's many years of experience treating both Tibetan and non-Tibetan patients and his travels to Europe have allowed for a significant engagement with Western notions of mental health and ill health, evident in his explanations below, in which he uses biomedical terms such as "schizophrenia," "depression," and "bipolar" to describe the illness known in Tibetan as *semné*. Indeed, Dr. Trogawa draws equivalences between several biomedical and Sowa Rigpa diagnostic categories.[10] However, highlighting the problematic nature of such cross-cultural endeavors, he also notes the difficulties of trying to draw such analogies, when, for example, the symptomatology of one Sowa Rigpa category overlaps with several biomedical ones.

Alongside his descriptions of long-standing Sowa Rigpa concepts of causation and treatment, Dr. Trogawa also flags some contemporary issues facing both practitioners and patients in Darjeeling and beyond. He describes, for example, treating patients who are already taking biomedical medications for mental illness. He also discusses changes in Tibetan culture, including increased access to biomedical and Sowa Rigpa practitioners but a decline in the number of spirit mediums in the Tibetan community. He also discusses some potential problems of cross-cultural interactions, describing, for example, Wind conditions Westerners may face as a result of engaging in unfamiliar practices without sufficient guidance. Indeed, these were topics raised by a number of interviewees in Darjeeling, where discussions often encompassed issues of cultural and medical pluralism, as Tibetan and biomedical concepts of mind, body, health, and illness collide in the contemporary sphere.

FURTHER READING

Adams, Vincanne, and Fei-Fei Li. 2008. "Integration or Erasure? Modernizing Medicine at Lhasa's Mentsikhang." In *Tibetan Medicine in the Contemporary World: Global Politics of Medical Knowledge and Practice*, edited by Laurent Pordié, 105–31. London: Routledge.

Clark, Barry. 1995. *The Quintessence Tantras of Tibetan Medicine*. Ithaca, N.Y.: Snow Lion.

Epstein, Mark, and Sonam Topgay. 1982. "Mind and Mental Disorders in Tibetan Medicine." *ReVision: A Journal of Consciousness and Change* 9 (1): 67–79.

Millard, Colin. 2007. "Tibetan Medicine and the Classification and Treatment of Mental Illness." In *Soundings in Tibetan Medicine: Historical and Anthropological Perspectives. Proceedings of the Tenth Seminar of the International Association of Tibetan Studies (PIATS), Oxford, 2003*, edited by Mona Schrempf, 247–82. Leiden: Brill.

Schrempf, Mona. 2011. "Between Mantra and Syringe: Healing and Health-Seeking Behaviour in Contemporary Amdo." In *Medicine Between Science and Religion: Explorations on Tibetan Grounds*, edited by Vincanne Adams, Mona Schrempf, and Sienna R. Craig, 157–84. New York: Berghahn.

INTERVIEW WITH DR. TEINLAY P. TROGAWA[11]

SD: Can you tell me about the different kinds of illness related to the mind?

TPT: For mental illness, we say semné. It's a general name for all, a real umbrella term. Also, sometimes people may say that the doṣa or the Wind Element is high, so some people may refer to that, too. Normally, we say that when the mind is in an undisturbed state, that's best. But when the mind is disturbed or worried—as a result of family worry or work stress or whatever it is—that would disturb the energy of the Wind, and then illness would manifest. Also, if one has had physical illness for a long time, then that could also bring a burden on the mind.

In terms of the different kinds of semné, as per the text [i.e., the Four Tantras], we have different types: those that are predominantly caused by the energy of Wind, Bile, Phlegm, or some combination [of these]; illness resulting from mental worry; illness caused by external factors—[for example,] some kind of toxin, poison, or chemical effects; or illness caused by evil spirits.

SD: Can you tell me about the illness known as "Life-Holding Wind" [Tib. sok (zin) lung]?

TPT: Life-Holding Wind is a kind of Wind disorder. One could roughly say it's like patients who come with schizophrenia or some patients with a case of depression. Patients will sometimes have this high and low [mood]; some people get a blocked feeling in the chest region, or, sometimes in a closed room, they think that they are getting suffocated. Sometimes they'll have disturbed sleep, [and] if you press their Wind points,[12] they will be very sensitive and tender. In patients who have a little mental tension for a short time, maybe this would be some kind of Blood Wind[13] or normal Wind; we'd say it's some imbalance of the Wind energy. But for Life-Holding Wind, there needs [to be] a major cause, maybe a very big shock or mental worry or too much stress or burden on the mind over a long period of time.

[In addition,] sometimes, when some people do different exercises that are related to breathing and the energy level, if it's not done under proper guidance, that could also cause Life-Holding Wind. For example, there may be a normal [healthy] university student doing some kind of qigong and all these kinds of exercises [related to manipulating the energies within the body], but when they are not under proper guidance, that also causes Life-Holding Wind. Of course, [qigong] is also a good form of exercise, at the physical level and also at the mental or the energy level. But in the past, when I was traveling in Europe with my teacher, Trogawa Rinpoche, I saw that many European patients used to come who had Life-Holding Wind after such exercises. Also, there are patients who have had substance abuse [problems] and are trying to recover. There are different causes [of Life-Holding Wind] that you can see in Europe: substance abuse, experimenting with different kinds of exercise, mental-level [meditation] exercises, and so forth.

SD: Can you treat Wind problems and Life-Holding Wind with Sowa Rigpa?

TPT: One can treat it properly, but it should be treated well, not only with medicine but also the patient should take care of their health, in food and drink and in one's daily habits. [For example,] sometimes some people change their body clock—working late in the night or working night shifts—and then they sleep during the day. That also causes Wind disorder. At the time, when one is working, and one is young, one doesn't feel pressure. But later on, when one gets a bit older, maybe in their thirties [or] mid-forties, then one comes to realize that something is not in balance.

SD: Can you tell me about nyö né?

TPT: Nyö né is insanity. It is more severe [than the conditions already discussed]. There are seven causes: an imbalance of any one of the three tridoṣa; the combined effect [of more than one of them]; worry or mental pressure; external substances; and the influence of evil spirits. Some spirits are just like the nāgas; they will just have a negative effect on the patient that will cause illness. But sometimes, in severe cases, the patient gets possessed by the spirit, [and] somebody else's spirit enters the patient's body. [In addition,] when people don't do proper Dharma practice, according to their level [of study or attainment], then this can also be a cause of nyö né.

Usually, we diagnose this through the checkup. Of course, it depends how severe the illness is. If the illness is at the onset, then of course one can easily make the diagnosis—especially with these illnesses caused by evil spirits, the symptoms and the heartbeat, everything, will change very often. And of course, in severe cases, the patient would not be like themselves at all, so then that's very clear. In such cases, the treatment from the spiritual side has to be done by the lamas. Then, from the medical aspect, we doctors can help the patient, but from the spiritual aspect, it is necessary for the lamas to treat [the condition]; otherwise, it's difficult. Medicines alone will not work on the patient.

SD: Would Tibetan patients in Darjeeling also consult a Tibetan spirit medium in the event of a spirit-caused illness, or even a local Nepali spirit medium?

TPT: Whichever faith one follows, it's best to treat [the condition] according to the patient's own personal inclination. Usually in the Tibetan system, there are of course spirit mediums and all these things. Before, when there was not much good communication, transport, and so on, there were all these sorts of religious healers, so people in the particular locality would go to that kind of healer first. One reason was that [in the past,] they had no other option, because for the other options, they had to travel very far. But nowadays, communication is easy, [and] one can travel by train or car easily compared with before. So in serious cases, we would recommend, if the patient is Tibetan, or Buddhist, to go to a good lama—one whom the patient has faith in—and then take further advice or further treatment. Even if it's diseases caused by evil spirits, or whatever it is, then it's best to follow the lama's advice. In the past, in the Himalayan regions, there was this custom of having spirit mediums, but the realm of the god [i.e., the spirit that possesses the spirit medium and from whom the power for healing is drawn] is also within the cycle of Saṃsāra, so this god can only assist to a certain level; beyond this, it's not possible for them to help.[14] And nowadays, in Tibetan communities, we don't see many spirit mediums like before; they used to say that each and every village used to have many such spirit mediums. But nowadays, it is decreasing with the new generation. These kinds of ritual [conducted by the spirit mediums] were a part of the tradition that was passed on through the centuries in the Tibetan community. In remote places, especially in the places of outer Tibet, like Ladakh, throughout the Himalayan region, many such healers were quite prevalent I believe—even in the 1960s, '70s, and '80s. Now still there are some in Ladakh, I believe, but that also is slowly declining. [In addition,] with the introduction of Buddhism [into Tibetan cultural areas], people came to know that Buddhism is the correct way, that spirit mediums' practices are helpful [for treating some conditions], but only to a certain extent; no more than that. So in the Tibetan community nowadays, you will not see many spirit mediums.

SD: Can you describe the symptoms of nyö né?

TPT: When nyö né is on the mild side, according to the text, if it is caused by a disturbance in the Wind, then the person will become thin, and they will foam at the mouth and be very talkative, or maybe they will cry for no reason. The whites of the eyes will sometimes become very red, and their symptoms will get aggravated the moment they have digested a meal. If it's caused by Bile, then the person will become angrier, more ferocious in their way. The first [Wind type] nyö né has more of a passive nature; this [Bile type] has more of a wrathful nature, you could say. One will prefer to stay in a cooler place, and the tears will be more yellowish. Or one will see just fire, flames, or stars, or something like that in front of their eyes. If the nyö né is caused by Phlegm, then the person will not speak a lot, wanting to be all by themselves. They will have no appetite, will feel very sleepy, and will have lots of saliva and excretions from the nose. And if [the nyö né is caused by] a combination of the three [doṣa], the patient will have the symptoms of all these three.

If nyö né is caused by mental sorrow, then, when the person remembers the cause, they will become very depressed; they will have the symptoms, or they will feel very uneasy or very unhappy. If it's caused by some chemical effect or poisoning, then at that time, we would say that the aura of that person will diminish, and one will become physically weak and have a disturbed mind.

If [the madness] is caused by an evil spirit's influence, then the patient will act in the habit of that particular spirit. So if the patient is a man, but he is possessed by the spirit of a deceased woman, then that man will speak more like a woman, and vice versa for a female patient; it can happen like this. Normally, when such patients come, they are physically very strong—sometimes jumping around—but normally, the family first will take such patients to a monastery to [see] a lama for a blessing. Sometimes, for some patients, they will only get well with blessings, but if they have got other physical illnesses, too, they can also take [Sowa Rigpa] medicines.

SD: How do you treat cases of nyö né and semné in the Sowa Rigpa system?

TPT: When the [nyö né] illness is not very severe, one can easily completely cure the patient, but again, the patient must be careful of their food and drinks and their daily habits. If it's a very severe case—those patients have these on-and-off periods—you give them medicines, and they feel better for some time, but when they stop taking it, then after some time again, it recurs. For some patients, it's like that, so it depends on how severe the case is; because for some schizophrenic patients, it's not easy: on, off, on, off—it comes and goes. For semné, you could just say it's a mental illness, so it can have this high [manic] period, too—not only the low period. This low period may be like depression, because in the low period, you have mental sorrow.

The thing is, with these mental illnesses, one should take proper care, because even if one has a lot of mental work[15]—not real illness, but maybe just a lot of mental work—if one can't take proper care of oneself, then in the future, [this] could cause some Wind disorder that in the long run could have some effect not only on the mind but also on the whole body. So one has to be careful.

There are also "jewel pills" for mental illness, but nowadays, we don't make these much. Before, our late [Trogawa] Rinpoche used to make jewel pills, so he used to give them [to patients]. These jewel pills would dispel the suffering of the mind. You would prescribe it to be taken once a week; usually with the jewel pill, you take it at a particular [time] on an auspicious day, the full moon or new moon, [for example,] and that was also helpful.

SD: From your experience of treating Western patients, do you think there are similarities between sok lung or nyö né and categories such as schizophrenia, psychosis, or bipolar disorder?

TPT: I'm not totally sure, because with nyö né, it's difficult to find the correct Western term for the medical term we have in Tibetan medicine. So I think it is best, when you try to translate it, not to find the exact Western medical term for it. In our text, many symptoms and indications are mentioned, so if you mention those, then the reader can sort of think, maybe it's more like this [condition] than that [condition].

Here, we don't get [conditions like bipolar disorder] much, but in the West, sometimes such patients do come; they say that sometimes they're very high and [other times are very] low. We would consider this to be a kind of Wind illness for sure. But the treatment for that illness depends very much on the constitution of that person; we will make the diagnosis considering the base constitution of that patient. When we prescribe herbal pills, we also give diet advice, and so on. Normally, these kinds of illnesses are caused by Wind, but, as I said, sometimes it will be in combination with some other [causative] factor, because of the base constitution of the patient. So for illness more related to the mind, if you give not only medicines but also advice to help calm the mind, that will also help the patient a lot.

SD: When you traveled with your uncle in Europe, did you see many Western patients with these kinds of conditions?

TPT: Usually when the patients come to us, they have [already] tried different kinds of [non–Sowa Rigpa] treatment, and then when nothing helps, they hear of us and they come. And then there are more serious patients; normally these are patients with [mainly physical] illnesses, but some also have mental illnesses. So some people complain of having these highs and lows; some are people with schizophrenia, or they are recovering from substance abuse. [. . .] Different kinds of patients come.

For these mental illnesses, how to treat the illness depends, because some patients have been taking [biomedical] antidepressants and [similar] medications for a long time. For them, they have to continue with those drugs; otherwise, if they just stop the next day, then again, all their symptoms will get aggravated. Everything flares up, like a fire. The patient who has the symptoms but who has not been on other chemical drugs, for them, our medicines can help easily. But for these other long-term patients, of course our medicines will help, but at the same time, they have to take their other pills. Sometimes when they have been taking these [biomedical] antidepressants for a long time, the same dosage does not work on them [anymore], [and] they have to go on increasing this. But our herbal pills can help them to stop at that dosage; they won't have to go on increasing them forever. So, we can help like that.

SD: Do you see many patients with these kinds of mental illness here in Darjeeling?

TPT: It depends, I think, on which area you are in. Here, of course there will be Tibetan and local Indian patients who have some kind of mental illness who come [to the clinic]. This is quite common. But if you go to the West, and places where people are working under a lot of stress, I think then it will be more common to have such *semné*—mental illness. It's not only Westerners; nowadays, so many Tibetans are going to the West and to America. I've not been to America to see patients, but I'm very much sure that there will also be such patients there, in equally high numbers. It depends on the surroundings; I think maybe when people worry, or whatever, it's quite common for people to have [these kinds of illness]. That's common; for Tibetan, Western, and local Indian patients, it's common.

NOTES

1. This interview was conducted as part of my doctoral research project exploring perspectives on mental health, illness, and healing within a Tibetan exile community in Darjeeling, Northeast India. This project was conducted at Cardiff University between

2010 and 2015, with funding provided by the Cardiff University School of History, Archaeology and Religion, the Body, Health and Religion Research Group, and the Wellcome Trust. This research is more fully described in Deane 2018. The interview was conducted in English and was lightly edited for clarity.

2. The practitioner Drag Lhong Gomchen Paljor Gyaltsen, part of a Tibetan Buddhist Kadampa lineage said to date from the eleventh century.

3. See the CTMI website: www.chagpori.org/college.htm.

4. Although the Tibetan term *nyépa* is often translated as "humor" by both Tibetan and non-Tibetan practitioners and scholars, it is better translated as "fault," "weakness," or "energy" (Samuel 2001: 255; Yoeli-Tlalim 2010: 319; Ozawa-de Silva and Ozawa-de Silva 2011: 104). Some contemporary practitioners translate this instead as "defective energies" (Kloos 2010: 17n20).

5. Epstein and Topgay 1982: 71.

6. Ga 2010: 182.

7. It is important to note that the Tibetan notion of Wind involves two different Indian or Sanskrit concepts: *vāta*, one of the *tridoṣa* of the Ayurvedic medical system, and *prāṇa* (often translated as "life-force" or "breath"), part of the "subtle body" system of Indian Tantra (see discussion in *Anthology*, vol. 1, ch. 42). As such, in the Tibetan context, the concept of Wind spans the spheres of medicine and religion, with the manipulation of Wind through Tantric practice therefore important in relation to both health and spiritual liberation.

8. Dorjee 2005: 167.

9. While in the past, many Sowa Rigpa practitioners were also highly skilled Tibetan Buddhist ritual specialists who could conduct rituals for healing, today this is less common, and medical practitioners may instead advise patients to consult Buddhist specialists for such treatments. Nevertheless, contemporary Tibetan Buddhist monastic practitioners may study Sowa Rigpa, and, in 2011, CTMI's most recent group of graduates consisted of a majority of Tibetan Buddhist nuns.

10. Jacobson 2002, 2007; Millard 2007.

11. Interview conducted on May 31, 2012, at the Chagpori Tibetan Medical Institute clinic in Darjeeling, India.

12. These are particular points on the body associated with Wind.

13. *Trak lung*, often likened to high blood pressure.

14. The spiritual power of Tibetan Buddhist lamas is understood to be stronger than that of spirit mediums. The lamas' Tantric Buddhist practice gives them access to the spiritual power of enlightened Buddhist deities, unlike spirit mediums, who may only access the power of unenlightened deities through their possession by them. Lamas are therefore thought to have a greater ability to deal with such problematic spirits and/or deities who may be causing difficulties for humans. This is a foundational understanding of Tibetan Buddhism, which emphasizes the supremacy of Buddhist knowledge and practice above all other forms and which is reflected in such explanations of health, illness, and healing.

15. This phrase often refers, as here, to mental activities such as thinking and worrying.

33. Biographical Interview with the Tantric Meditator Tshampa Tseten from Bhutan

With a Translation of His "Edible Letters"

MONA SCHREMPF

The Buddhist meditator Tshampa Tseten (figure 33.1) belongs to a group of lay tantric practitioners from Bhutan locally known as "great meditators."[1] He is a speaker of the Dzala language from the remote Khoma valley in the far northeast of this small Himalayan country.[2] Tshampa Tseten is a follower of the Nyingma or "Ancient" school of Tibetan-style Buddhism that is well established in the eastern part of the country.[3] *Tshampa* are meditators who practice within hereditary or teacher–student lineages of the Nyingma school, acquiring their knowledge through classical Tibetan Buddhist methods of empowerment, teaching, and oral transmission. *Tshampa* play an important yet often underestimated social role in the everyday life of rural communities, including through their attention to the health and well-being of individual patients.[4] Tshampa Tseten uses both ritual techniques and medicinal herbs to heal his patients and thus is also part of a large and diverse spectrum of ritual healers found throughout Bhutan.[5]

As modernity increasingly reaches into remote rural areas such as the Khoma valley, outmigration is on the rise, while government-supported modern education and public health care services—both of which are free in Bhutan—have become more available to village dwellers. In part owing to these developments, the number of *tshampa* and other tantric practitioners in Bhutan is in decline.[6] Today, Bhutan balances on a tightrope between trying to advance modernization and economic development in a sustainable way (see chapter 17) while also wanting

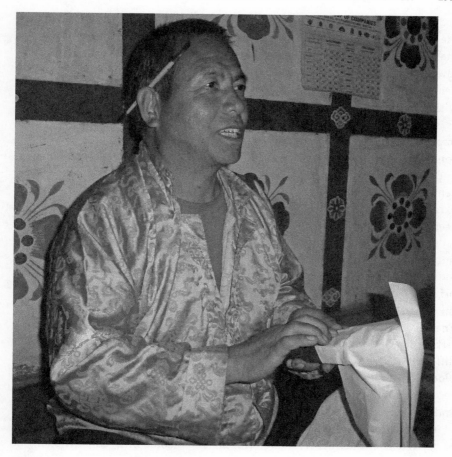

FIGURE 33.1 TSHAMPA TSETEN AT HIS HOME IN BABTONG VILLAGE, BHUTAN.
Source: Mona Schrempf, 2011.

to preserve the diversity of its rich cultural heritage. Local healing practices have only recently become recognized and classified as part of the government's initiative of the *Intangible Cultural Heritage of Bhutan*, under the auspices of the United Nations Educational, Scientific and Cultural Organization (UNESCO), and are now subsumed under the heading of "folk knowledge and technology."[7] Nevertheless, despite falling outside the domain of government-subsidized, institutionalized medicine and public health care, as well as existing outside organized religion, local ritual healers remain popular among patients.[8]

At the time of my field research, Tshampa Tseten was the sole healer serving the rural communities of the Khoma valley where he lives.[9] His specialty is the use of so-called edible letters (*zayig*),[10] a rather secret and exclusive type of healing knowledge that belongs to the Nyingma "treasure" (*terma*) tradition.[11] This tradition holds that the famous eighth-century Indian tantric master

Padmasambhava hid religious treasures throughout the Himalayan region and the Tibetan Plateau in the form of texts and sacred objects.[12] The point was for these to be discovered and made public once again by so-called treasure revealers[13] during future times of general moral, physical, and environmental decline.[14] Both the treasures and the places they were found are connected with promises of salvation and remedying the ailments of the present age, such as natural disasters, social disorders, and diseases that are difficult or impossible to cure. Even though Tshampa Tseten does not mention a direct connection between the Nyingma treasure tradition and his natal place during our interview, in Khoma today, there are traces of the famous fifteenth-century Tibetan treasure revealer Ratna Lingpa, whose collected works include extensive texts with edible letters for healing of the type used by Tshampa Tseten himself.[15]

Tshampa Tseten's knowledge and practice are a classical example of how intertwined Buddhism, healing, and medicine can be.[16] Edible letters consist of individual letters[17] written in the Tibetan script and engraved upon a wooden printing block known as an "engraved seal" or "stamp" (yigkö).[18] These blocks are inked and then used to produce paper copies that patients can directly consume. The inked letters are also used for printing upon a patient's skin. Individual letters can be combined into different mantras,[19] each of which serves to heal different maladies. Tshampa Tseten is equipped with several wooden printing blocks (figure 33.2) to produce his cures, a small manuscript (figure 33.3) recording a narrative of the tradition's origins, and a key to the mantra sequences and the diseases these can treat.

The contemporary use of edible letters in Tibetan healing practice appears to be derived from much earlier Indian traditions connected with "edible charms."[20] The practice also shares affinities with the use of magical spells and charms in medieval Chinese Daoist and Buddhist contexts, as well as with older shamanic techniques for healing and well-being.[21] While some forms of mantra healing are practiced widely among ritual practitioners today, including within Sowa Rigpa,[22] the authentic edible letters practice has become very rare.[23] Nevertheless, the healing technique is still practiced in Bhutan, Tibet, Mongolia, and in some weikza (wizard) cults in Myanmar (on the latter, see chapters 19 and 31).[24]

The first translation below is an interview conducted by the author in which Tshampa Tseten provides biographical details of his life, training, and practice. The second text is a translation of his handwritten manuscript folio. The left half of the folio provides a grid-square copy of his main printing blocks, a key to the corresponding mantras, and his notes on diseases and their symptoms. The right half records a short origin narrative for this healing tradition as a treasure text purportedly brought forth by an eighth- or ninth-century treasure revealer named Nyangban Tingdzin Sangpo.[25] In this short narrative, the temporal framing, prophesied future revelation, and other clues all strongly imply that the wording is meant to be understood as spoken instructions from the great tantric founder of the treasure tradition himself, Padmasambhava.

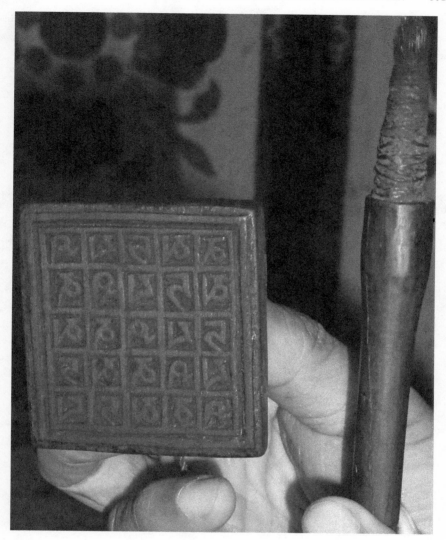

FIGURE 33.2 TSHAMPA TSETEN'S ENGRAVED WOODEN SEAL FOR *ZAYIG* ("EDIBLE LETTERS") WITH INK BRUSH. THIS WOODEN SEAL IS IDENTICAL TO THAT DISCUSSED IN DOUGLAS 1978: PLATE 16.
Source: Mona Schrempf, 2011.

FURTHER READING

Douglas, Nik. 1978. *Tibetan Tantric Charms and Amulets*. New York: Dover.

Drungtso, Tsering Thakchoe. 2008. *Healing Power of Mantra: The Wisdom of Tibetan Healing Science*. Dharamshala, India: Drungtso.

Garrett, Frances. 2009. "Eating Letters in the Tibetan Treasure Tradition." *Journal of the International Association of Buddhist Studies* 32 (1–2): 85–114.

Samuel, Geoffrey. 2014. "Healing in Tibetan Buddhism." In *The Wiley Blackwell Companion to East and Inner Asian Buddhism*, edited by Mario Poceski, 278–96. Chichester, UK: Wiley.

Schrempf, Mona, and Nicola Schneider, eds. 2015. "Women as Visionaries, Healers and Agents of Social Transformation in the Himalayas, Tibet, and Mongolia." *Revue d'Etudes Tibétaines* 34 (special issue): 1–217.

Taee, Jonathan. 2017. *The Patient Multiple: An Ethnography of Healthcare and Decision-Making in Bhutan*. New York: Berghahn.

1. INTERVIEW WITH TSHAMPA TSETEN[26]

MS: How old were you when you began to heal, and what kind of healing do you do?

TT: I began to heal when I was about thirty years old.[27] I received personal instructions and healing knowledge directly from my root lama, Yangma Rinpoche, during the 1960s and early 1970s.[28] He was a very famous healer from Kurtö, and many patients came to see him.[29] He mainly gave edible letters and performed healing rites that were very effective. Yet, most of the time, Yangma Rinpoche meditated in secluded retreat. I was fortunate to receive his training in both edible letters and traditional medicine by way of his empowerment, oral transmission, and personal instruction.[30] I also practiced meditation in retreat for several years. Even though Yangma Rinpoche had many students, he taught medicine and healing only to two of us, and I was one of them. The other one has already passed away. Yet today, nobody is interested in continuing this kind of knowledge anymore.

I practice two different types of diagnosis. I use the pulse-reading technique from traditional medicine, and sometimes—in case my healing was unsuccessful, or if I am in doubt about the cause of a disease—I also use divination.[31] When the wearing of protective amulets and healing rituals for expelling disease-causing spirits[32] do not help the patient either, I use as a last resort the Dorje Gotrab protection mantra[33] together with moxibustion.

There are 404 diseases. Many can be healed by either edible letters or medicine. It depends upon the cause of the disease. If it is a disease caused by poison, I use aconite.[34] But mostly I use edible letters. Healing with edible letters is especially useful for the treatment of paralysis and epilepsy caused by malevolent planetary beings,[35] affliction by water spirits, jaundice, heart-related disorders,[36] as well as back problems, swellings, and nerve disorders.[37] Also, I use edible letters for extending a patient's life-span, to improve tingling or bad blood circulation problems, to stop bleeding in case of menstruation problems, to make the placenta come out, and for use against curses and against gossip. There are also edible letters against demons and an edible letters charm for invoking a deity in a temple to turn an enemy of an enemy against the latter.

MS: How did you learn these techniques? From your teacher? What was your method?

TT: I learned everything from my teacher through direct instruction. I also wrote down his words and copied my teacher's wood block seals with the engraved edible letters and learned how to apply them. One needs a special Indian ink for printing the letters onto the patients' swollen or sore body parts, or for printing on paper. The paper is then eaten by the patient. This is Padmasambhava's healing method.

I made special notes on how to produce edible letters. First, you need to write down the edible letters depending on the disease. Then I perform a ritual, and last, I consecrate the paper with the Dorje Gotrab mantra.[38] However, edible letters are not a simple "trick" or printing technique but require visualization techniques based on years of tantric meditative training and dedication. It is a secret practice that is only rarely passed on, usually within a lineage of treasure revealers, certain tantric practitioners, and to chosen students.

MS: Did you also have a personal experience through practicing healing rituals?

TT: I believe that without meditation and my longevity ritual practice,[39] I would not be alive anymore. My life-span was said to be only forty-nine years. Now I am fifty-five, and I attribute that to the benefit of my meditation practice, which is also necessary for maintaining and improving my healing powers.

MS: Did you also encounter contagious diseases during the past?

TT: Yes, there was a lot of tuberculosis and malaria. Now people get many injections against TB over a period of eight months. But there are diseases that hospitals cannot heal. For example, at the hospital, they cannot heal epilepsy. I can heal that with the right edible letters.

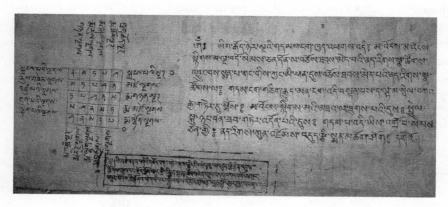

FIGURE 33.3 TSHAMPA TSETEN'S MANUSCRIPT OF THE ORIGIN NARRATIVE OF THE TRADITION (RIGHT) AND THE KEY TO THE TWENTY-FIVE CARVED LETTERS AND HEALING MANTRAS (LEFT).
(The small block print on the lower margin of the manuscript is not relevant to the present subject and is not translated here.)
Source: Mona Schrempf, 2011.

MS: What about patients with mental problems?

TT: Yes, they come to me, too. Then I give them the edible letters of Pekar and
Dremo.[40] Mental problems can also be caused by demons, for which I have
special edible letters. They roam around and are not bound to a particular
place. People believe that invisible demons[41] eat the patient's body, [and the
patient] feels that as pain. The edible letters treasure by Tertön Jigme Lingpa
[from Tibet] helps in this case. But these evil spirits can attack us only when
our personal powers are low.[42] Other types of disease, such as stomach pain,
headache, eye problems, or unconsciousness, all this can also be caused by
them. In those cases, I give special edible letters and expel demons with a
smoke offering, Indian myrrh, and white mustard seeds together with a special mantra for expelling these obstacles. This is the simple version; a more
wrathful and powerful one is done by way of a larger expulsion ritual. And
all my patients are healed.

2. SPIRITUAL INSTRUCTIONS FOR THE
TWENTY-FIVE CARVED LETTERS[43]

Translation of the Right-Hand Side of the Folio

OṂ—This is the excellent spiritual instruction of the twenty-five carved letters.
In the future, the future [age] of Rampant Fivefold Degeneration, all types of incurable illness will emerge to [afflict] sentient beings. Thus, it will be a time when even
physicians are unable to help. With regard to all the types of incurable illness,
since the spiritual instruction [to cure them] is taught here as an oral transmission
lineage, it has not been spread at the present time. Conceal it as a sealed instruction treasure! At the end of the future degenerate [age], at the time of a benevolent
one, when Tulku Nyangban causes the profound treasure to come forth [from con-
cealment], these instructions will subdue every type of illness of transmigrating
sentient beings. May it be a supreme medical elixir! May it be virtuous!

Translation of the Mantra Chart

TRANSLATION OF INSCRIPTIONS AROUND THE MANTRA CHART

	1	2	3	4	5	
20	NA	MA	TA	PA	SHA	6
19	MA	TA	PA	SHA	NA	7
18	TA	PA	SHA	NA	MA	8
17	PA	SHA	NA	MA	TA	9
16	SHA	NA	MA	TA	PA	10
	15	14	13	12	11	

TOP SIDE (READ TOP TO BOTTOM)

NA MA TA PA SHA—mantra for inflammation[44]
MA TA PA SHA NA—mantra for infected sores that have reached the bone[45]
TA PA SHA NA MA—mantra for dried sores[46]
PA SHA NA MA TA—mantra for pustule sores[47]
SHA NA MA TA PA—mantra for blood-covered sores[48]

RIGHT SIDE (READ RIGHT TO LEFT)

SHA PA TA MA NA—mantra for swellings
NA SHA PA TA MA—mantra for leprosy
MA NA SHA PA TA—mantra for inflamed sores
TA MA NA SHA PA—mantra for leprous sores
PA TA MA NA SHA—mantra for ulcerated sores

LOWER SIDE (READ BOTTOM TO TOP)

[illegible]
[illegible][49]
MA NA SHA PA TA—mantra for ulcerated sores
NA SHA PA TA MA—mantra for varieties of sores
SHA PA TA MA NA—mantra for sores on the cheeks and jaws

LEFT SIDE (READ LEFT TO RIGHT)

SHA NA MA TA PA—mantra for large cancerous ulcers
PA SHA NA MA TA—mantra for infections of the tongue
TA PA SHA NA MA—mantra for smallpox
MA TA PA SHA NA—mantra for acute bone pain
NA MA TA PA SHA—mantra for swellings

NOTES

My ethnographic research on ritual healers in the east Bhutanese districts of Trashigang and Trashiyangtse from 2010 to 2012 was funded by the German Research Foundation (SCHR 733/4-1). In Bhutan my research has been facilitated by the Centre for Bhutan Studies with the support of Dasho Karma Ura and my interlocutor, Dorji Gyaltsen. I thank them all wholeheartedly for their support.

1. *Tshampa (mtshams pa)* is a local term used for a Buddhist practitioner who specializes in meditation retreat. *Gomchen (sgom chen)* literally means "great meditator." On how *tshampa* and *gomchen* are defined by the Bhutanese state as part of the country's intangible cultural heritage, see Jagar Dorji 2015: 97.

2. Bhutan is an independent Himalayan country. Its first state was founded by Zhabdrung Ngawang Namgyal (1594–1651), a Tibetan Buddhist lama from the Drukpa Kagyu school. He also introduced the Tibetan dual system of political and religious governance, institutionalizing the monastic Drukpa Kagyu tradition as state religion.

3. On the history of the Nyingmapa in Bhutan, see Aris 1979: 153–64. For their transnational history, see Düdjom Rinpoche 1991, vol. 1.

4. Aside from *tshampa* and *gomchen*, ritual healers in Bhutan include more well-known groups of spirit-mediums, in particular *pawo (dpa' bo*, lit. "hero"), *pamo (dpa' mo*, "heroine"), *neyjom (rnal 'byor ma), jomo (jo mo)*, and *terdak (gter bdag*, literally "treasure owner") who heal through possession by distinct local and Buddhist deities, such as the Tibetan-deified King Gesar (Schrempf 2015a,b). On a female ritual healer in Eastern Bhutan and her at-times problematic encounters with various other ritual healing specialists who belong to or are legitimized by institutionalized religion, see Schrempf 2015a,c.

5. Ritual healers, sometimes also called "village" or "traditional" healers (cf. "alternative healers" in Taee 2017), share the locally adapted Tibetan Buddhist term *rimdro (rim gro*, "ritual") to designate their ritual healing practices. The term does not include physicians' practice of "traditional medicine," who are known as *drungtsho* in Bhutan and are part of Bhutan's integrative public health care system (even though they may also, at times, use ritual healing techniques). On the diverse spectrum of healers in Bhutan, see Schrempf 2015a.

6. On the influence of modern education, see Jones 2014. On declining numbers of *gomchen*, see Rigyal and Prude 2017. On declining ritual specialists known as *bon po* in Bhutan, see Huber forthcoming.

7. Jagar Dorji 2015: ch. 4.

8. See, for example, Taee 2017: 85. Nevertheless, many among them are eyed with suspicion by medical personnel in Bhutan and often also by the Bhutanese media.

9. The nearest biomedical hospital is Lhuntse Dzong Hospital, where only one doctor was operating at the time of my fieldwork in 2010 and 2011.

10. On *zayig (bza' yig)* translated as "edible charms," see Douglas 1978: plates 11–26; Waddell 1985 (1894): 401; Garrett 2009a.

11. On the Nyingma *terma (gter ma)* tradition and a range of "treasure revealers" or *tertön (gter ston)*, see Düdjom Rinpoche 1991, vol. 1: 743–881. It should be noted that *zayig* are also used in Tibetan Bon traditions (see Douglas 1978). On *zayig* under the rubric of "rites for the prevention of contagious diseases and plagues," see Garrett 2009a: 97. On other types of ritual healing and empowerment practices in Tibetan medicine and in tantric Tibetan Buddhism, see Samuel 1999, 2014.

12. Padmasambhava is said to have introduced Indian Buddhism into the Himalayas and Tibet; the Nyingma, or old school, of Tibetan Buddhism also regards him as their founding figure.

13. Tib. *Tertön (gter ston)*. Among the three foremost Nyingma treasure revealers of Bhutan—Dorje Lingpa, Ratna Lingpa, and Pema Lingpa—*zayig* came to represent a whole textual genre in the fourteenth and fifteenth centuries (Garrett 2009a). These three *tertön* were also active in Bhutan and used treasure revealing as a tool for disseminating Buddhism; see also Gayley 2007.

14. The "five degenerations" or "five impurities" (Skt. *pañcakaṣāya*; Tib. *snyigs ma lnga*) lead directly to a decline in human well-being; for example, a shorter life-span (cf. Goldstein 2001: 883, s.v. *tshe snyigs ma*; see also Zhang 1985: 1001, s.v. *snyigs ma lnga*; Düdjom Rinpoche 1991, vol. 2: 144, s.v. "Five Impurities").

15. In the Khoma valley, Ratna Lingpa's lineage is continued within a household to which also belongs a collection of his relics and treasures. On Ratna Lingpa (1404–1479) and his revealed texts on *zayig*, see Garrett 2009a: 91–92.

16. Garrett (2009a: 99) argues further that it makes little sense to count *zayig* as a specialty of so-called tantric medicine because of the latter's vague definition and the ample and varied use of mantra in both Tibetan tantric and medical practices.

17. Douglas (1978) defines these letters as "seed syllables" (*bīja mantra*) originating in "archaic forms of Sanskrit."

18. On *yigkö* (*yig rko*), see Goldstein 2001: 995.

19. *Mantra* (Skt. *dhāraṇī*) or *ngak* (Tib. *sngags*) refers both to spoken words or sounds and their written or printed forms (see also Drungtso 2008: 80). Waddell (1985 [1894]: 401) identifies *zayig* as a type of mantra for healing and classifies its use as a talisman under the rubric of "sacred symbols and charms" commonly used to ward off evil, bad luck, dangerous dogs, and diseases.

20. See Douglas 1978: plates 11–26. Douglas claims that this healing technique goes back to the Indian *Atharvaveda*.

21. Garrett (2009a: 86) argues that the *zayig* tradition has Chinese roots. On analogous Chinese healing practices, see Strickmann 2002: 123–32, 170–79; McBride 2005; *Anthology*, vol. 1, ch. 29 and 45.

22. Bhutanese traditional medicine is a local variant of Sowa Rigpa. On mantra in Tibetan healing practices, see Drungtso 2008.

23. This information was given by the revered late tantric master and teacher Ake Tamdringyal, from Rebgong (Ch. Tongren, Qinghai Province, China) via email communication facilitated by his nephew and received on March 13, 2018.

24. Cf. Pranke 2014; Sárközi 1999.

25. Nyang ban Ting 'dzin bZang po, a student of Vimalamitra, was purportedly active during the reign of the emperor Trisong Detsen (Khri Srong lde btsan; r. ca. 798–815) in Central Tibet. He was associated with the origin of the "Earth Treasure" (*sa gter*) tradition, the masters of which are held to have become manifest as reincarnated beings or *tulku* (*spul sku*), hence his title (Düdjom Rinpoche 1991, vol. 1: 555–56).

26. The author conducted the interviews with Tshampa Tseten first on October 7, 2011, then on January 1, 2012, in Babtong village, Khoma valley. All questions and answers were translated by Dorji Gyaltsen from English into the Dzala language, and vice versa. Additional questions were asked by Dorji Gyaltsen via several subsequent phone calls with Tshampa Tseten.

27. Tshampa Tseten was born in 1956 in Babtong village.

28. Yangma Rinpoche, alias Kunsang Gyurmed, lived at the Yangla Monastery; he died around 1976. When traveling to Amdo, Yangma Rinpoche received religious teachings and healing techniques from Kunsang Gyatsho, a famous Nyingma lama from the area. Kunsang Gyatsho's lineage in turn can be traced back to a famous Tibetan Nyingma

master and *tertön* from the eighteenth century named Kunkyen Jigme Lingpa (1730–1785), well known for his Dzogchen text *Klong chen snying thig*. On this treasure revealer, see *The Treasury of Lives* (www.treasuryoflives.org/biographies/view/Jigme-Lingpa/5457) and the *Buddhist Digital Resource Centre* (www.tbrc.org/#!rid=P314).

29. Kurtö is a neighboring valley of Khoma. Both are village clusters (*gewok*) of Lhuntse district, Eastern Bhutan, a sparsely populated area where even today, many villages can be accessed only by foot.

30. In Tantric Buddhist (and organized Bön) religious practice, "direct instructions" (Skt. *upadeśa*; Tib. *gdams ngag*) consist of empowerment (Tib. *dbang*), oral transmission (Tib. *lung*), and personal instruction (Tib. *khrid*) from the teacher. Additionally, Tshampa Tseten was taught healing with special mantras (*sngags*).

31. *Mo* is a common ritualized divination technique using a rosary or dice. It is used by various healing specialists, as well as by some lamas (*mo pa*), but also by lay people.

32. *Dön* (*gdon*) and *dré* ('*dre*) belong to well-known, large, and varied groups or classes of evil spirits or demons that can attack people and make them sick. They are a pan-Himalayan phenomenon in regions under Tibetan cultural influence and, together with other spirits, such as *nāga* (Tib. *klu*), are also part of the Sowa Rigpa tradition (Samuel 1999, 2007; Millard 2007). On *dré*, popularly known and feared spirits of the diseased in Bhutan (*shi 'dre*, *gson 'dre*), see Choden 2008.

33. The mantra of Dorje Gotrab (*rdo rje go khrab*), or "Diamond Armor Mantra," is perceived as the most powerful panacea mantra for treating all kinds of disease. "Dorje Gotrab" also refers to a collection of mantras (*sNgags 'bum rdo rje go khrab*) that appear to have been revealed by Tertön Dorje Lingpa (1346–1405). Dorje Lingpa also wrote an extensive text on *zayig* (*Za yig nor bu'i bang mdzod*); see Garrett 2009a: 87ff. For his biography, see Düdjom Rinpoche's history of the Nyingma school (1991, vol. 1: 789–92).

34. The correct use of the highly toxic medicinal plant aconite (*bong dkar*) and its many species is one of Tshampa Tseten's specialties, which he also learned from Yangma Rinpoche. This is rare knowledge, as he points out. Tshampa Tseten collects aconite mostly in the ninth and tenth Bhutanese months and includes it in a compound with different types of myrobalan (i.e., chebulic, beleric, and officinalis; Tib. *aru*, *baru*, *kyuru*), which are commonly used in Sowa Rigpa. He also uses a specific *zayig* for general protection against all diseases caused by poison.

35. Known in Sanskrit as *graha*, malevolent planetary spirits (Tib. *gza'*) are perceived as causing *zané* (*gza' nad*, locally also called called *pané*), which is often translated as "epilepsy" or "paralysis." *Gza'* can also designate a distinct class of spirits that belong to the Eight Classes of Gods and Spirits (*lha srin sde brgyad*).

36. There is no direct translation in English for *nyingné* (*snying nad*, lit. "heart disorder"). *Nyingné* designates a complex of syndromes that can be organ related, concern a circulatory or emotional disorder (or social distress), or be related to nerves or an imbalance of the "life-sustaining wind" (*srog 'dzin rlung*), all of which are centered in the area of the heart. Additionally, heart-related disorders are common ailments addressed in Sowa Rigpa and also mentioned in *zayig* texts (Garrett 2009a).

37. Tshampa Tseten's *zayig* seal mantras are identical in name with five mentioned by Drungtso to be recited for addressing most of those diseases (Drungtso 2008: 204).

38. Tantric rituals (*cho ga*) and consecration rituals (*rab gnas*) are common Tibetan practices for invoking tantric deities belonging to a particular tantric ritual cycle and for consecrating sacred objects, such as statues and painted scrolls, to empower them by transferring the deity's power into the object.

39. On longevity rituals and concepts of life-span among Tibetans in the Darjeeling Hills, see Gerke 2012.

40. Most probably, these mantras refer to two particular deities: Pe dkar or Pe har (i.e., the "protector of religion"; Skt. *dharmapāla*, Tib. *chos skyong*) and Dred gong ma (one of four animal-faced goddesses). See de Nebesky-Wojkowitz 1956: 51, 94–133.

41. On the *dön* and *dré* classes of demon referred to here, see note 33.

42. The personal power of an individual, known as *wangtang* (*dbang thang*), is one of several individual energies that humans possess. When low, the person becomes vulnerable and prone to spirit attacks (Cornu 1997: 85–101; Samuel 1999).

43. The Tibetan title reads *Yig rko nyer lnga'i gdam ngag.* Translation into English by Mona Schrempf.

44. This mantra is also said to be used for diseases inflicted by planetary spirits (*gza'*); see Drungtso 2008: 203n1.

45. Cf. Drungtso 2008: 203n2. On *rma rus*, see *rma yi rus zan* in Zhang 1985: 2150; Goldstein 2001: 834.

46. Cf. Drungtso 2008: 203n3.

47. Cf. Drungtso 2008: 203n4.

48. Cf. Drungtso 2008: 203n5.

49. The first partially obscured word may read *thab* or *thub*, though neither relates to a known medical problem.

34. Japanese Buddhist Women's "Way of Healing"

PAULA K. R. ARAI

An ethnographic exploration into the lives of mature and devout Japanese Buddhist women reveals how ritualized activities are a critical tool in their paradigm of healing. I call their approach a "Way of Healing" (yudō), because for them, healing is an orientation to living. It is not about attaining a specific end result. Their daily-life wisdom for responding to a host of challenges, difficulties, and fears is rooted in Zen Buddhist teachings streaming from Dōgen (1200–1253), yet also includes a wide range of practices from esoteric, Pure Land, and home-made sources. Strikingly, these women experience powerful healing through practicing rituals not formally recognized as healing rituals. In a world view in which the interrelatedness of all things is the primary point of reference, healing means to be in harmony with the impermanent web of relationships that constitutes the dynamic universe. Buddhist laywomen, often supported by nuns, respond to some of life's greatest challenges: birth, illness, death, and emotional turmoil. This network of female relationships is the milieu in which the ways of rituals and healing activities in daily life are practiced and transmitted.

The excerpts below are from a series of interviews done in the greater Nagoya area from summer 1998 to spring 2003. The twelve women who generously volunteered to allow their lives to be scrutinized through a scholarly lens are from a distinctive generation in Japanese history. Nine of the twelve women are World War II survivors,[1] and the remaining three were born shortly after the war. Major transformations in Japanese society occurred during this period, including Japan's rise to international economic stature. Women of this generation are the center of their homes. They are the ritual experts, the counselors for the family, and the healers.[2] They understand healing as a relational matter. As they care for others, they attend to themselves with an awareness that this practice is part of a single web of concern.

The Way of Healing of these female Buddhist consociates is most fundamentally a path of retraining themselves to act in harmony with the impermanent, interrelated nature of things. It is not a result of action. Rather, it is a way of acting, seeing, thinking, and "holding one's heart." This Way of Healing is an art form. It is an art of seeking out ways to heal and not suffer. More specifically, it is an art of choosing to be grateful in the face of fear-driven and torment-ridden possibilities. This way of living and interpreting the world, events, the self, and others requires practice and discipline. It is a way that is supported with prayers and nourished with tears. It is more an orientation to living than a clearly delineated and consciously followed course. There are guidelines, but there are no absolutes. It is mostly in hindsight that one can see that there have been consistent values, attitudes, and activities that, when taken as a whole, constitute a way. Although healing is an activity that involves a myriad of factors, ten salient principles emerged from my encounter with the lives of these Buddhist women that constitute my theory of these women's Way of Healing:

1. Experiencing interrelatedness
2. Living body-mind
3. Engaging in rituals
4. Nurturing the self
5. Enjoying life
6. Creating beauty
7. Cultivating gratitude
8. Accepting reality as it is
9. Expanding perspective
10. Embodying compassion

Each principle is distinct. Although there is overlap, there is no redundancy. Each adds a dimension to their healing paradigm. Often one element augments another; for instance, interrelatedness increases one's feelings of thankfulness and heightens one's sense of beauty. This, in turn, commonly sharpens one's experience of enjoyment. Performing rituals sometimes manifests in a deepening of the body–mind connection and results in one taking better care of oneself. Indeed, any factor can initiate an increase in any of the other qualities. The more this happens, the more quickly and thoroughly one can experience healing.

These women's Way of Healing demonstrates the complexity of their lived tradition. My ethnographic data indicate the power rituals can have in fostering an experience of interrelatedness. Focusing on this power illuminates the core of the Buddhist mode of healing. When fully engaged, healing occurs in each act of compassion and every expression of gratitude. My consociates further confirm that rituals help to facilitate healing, because rituals are an experience of the nonbifurcated body-mind (*shinjin*). The rituals they employ show them how to be healers, especially to be healers of their own delusions, which falsely divide and unnecessarily discourage. The difficulty lies in the task of realizing profound interrelatedness in the midst of illness, conflict, misunderstanding, and loneliness. Through assessing these healing activities, it becomes clear that experiencing interrelatedness—not merely having an understanding of it—is the key that unlocks all other elements. Once this occurs, all factors mutually amplify each other, resulting in heightened experiences of healing.

My consociates' practices unfold within a Zen Buddhist world view, but their interest is rarely institutional or philosophical. It is practical. Their practices are simple, accessible, inexpensive, portable, direct, and immediate. Years of disciplined practice are not required to perform or participate; hence, they are accessible, even to the busiest person. The simplicity of the practices also helps keep the cost down. Many can be done at home or on the run. The most important thing to these women is that the effects of a practice are immediate and direct. From calming down in a moment of crisis, to being compassionately embraced despite an avalanche of tragedy, to being cured after a terminal diagnosis, these women have found empowerment for themselves and their families in their domestic practice of Buddhism. These women are conscious to devote time in their daily lives to listen to their hearts. Whether it is chanting *sūtras* for an hour or just quietly gazing out at the trees outside while hanging laundry, they lead ritualized lives that make healing a daily activity.

FURTHER READING

Arai, Paula. 2011. *Bringing Zen Home: The Healing Heart of Japanese Women's Rituals*. Honolulu: University of Hawai'i Press.

Stoltzfus, Michael, Rebecca Green, and Darla Schumm, eds. 2013. *Chronic Illness, Spirituality, and Healing: Diverse Disciplinary Cultural Perspectives*. New York: Palgrave Macmillan.

Traphagan, John. 2004. *The Practice of Concern: Ritual, Well-Being, and Aging in Rural Japan*. Durham, N.C.: Caroline Academic Press.

Vargas-O'Bryan, Ivette, and Zhou Xun, eds. 2014. *Disease, Religion and Healing in Asia: Collaborations and Collisions*. New York: Routledge.

EXCERPTS FROM INTERVIEWS[3]

1. Kawasaki-san on the Power of Healing Water and Chanting

We drink it [sacred water] in the kitchen. We put a little in a cup. Or I put a little in when cooking the rice we all eat. Just one drop at a time. The drop contains the prayers. If someone has a cold, they put it in their tea. [So, if you burn your-self or have a headache,] you do not put it on the spot that hurts. You drink it.

When Grandpa was old and hurt all over because he had been injured in the war, the doctor said that there was nothing more he could do. There was no med-icine to take the pain away. I asked him if he wanted some of the water. So he had it about three or four times, and the pain went away. He died without pain. He would tell people who came he did not have pain.

I cut my foot, and it got infected. I drank, saying, "NAMU AMIDA BUTSU." It never hurt. I had to go get intravenous fluids on an outpatient basis for a couple months. When once I saw the actual cut, I was shocked at the raggedness of the cut. But I never felt pain. I drank one drop in my tea on days when there was to be some treatment. I took a drop, saying, "Please give me favor." It never hurt.[4]

* * *

There were several times my son woke up in the middle of the night crying with a fever, and I fervently chanted, NENPI KANNON RIKI, and he fell back into a peaceful slumber. In the middle of the night, it happens. In the day, he's out play-ing cheerfully. Then suddenly at a time when there's nothing you can do at one or three in the morning, he suddenly wakes up crying. Whether I understand or not, it's not that; I just fervently chant. But then it passes without having to go to the doctor. There are lots of times when there's nothing you can do. The most terrifying time was when he was about four, and he was cleaning his ear with a bamboo ear-cleaning stick. I was thinking it was dangerous, and I warned him to be careful. My husband called for help to carry something heavy, and I went for just a minute, and in that short time, he had pushed the stick into his ear.

There was a scream. I felt my *ki* energy collapse. The ear is one of the worst places for pain! I was so scared. I just chanted, NENPI KANNON RIKI, NENPI KANNON RIKI, NENPI KANNON RIKI. It was late at night, around 9 PM, so we took him to the Red Cross Hospital by car. When we arrived, he just jumped out of the car!

Another time, he was almost hit by a car. He was about five or six. At that time, [the same chant] helped, too. A woman who sees things that cannot be seen with the eye thought he had been hit, too. But she saw Avalokiteśvara stand in front of the car to stop it.

The time it takes for children to grow up is full of terrifying moments. It is not a matter of reason. From others' perspectives, it might look foolish for me to chant, but the reality is he is OK.[5]

2. Yamaguchi-san on Birth and Death

I had a protective amulet when I was pregnant. It made my heart feel strong. I was happy my friend brought me the one she had when she had a safe birth. My husband did the calligraphy "felicitations" for the *hara-obi* cloth wrapped around the lower abdomen of pregnant women. I think it is about how you hold your heart and energy that is the most important.[6]

* * *

I was told I might have uterine cancer. Aoyama Sensei, [abbess of the nunnery I go to for spiritual support,] wrote this [poem about illness being a treasure from the Buddha] for the time that she was hospitalized and about to have an operation because she might have had cancer. I don't think it is easy to think of cancer as a gift from the Buddha. But if it happens, you need to do things to settle your heart. Things you must do for your children, and so on. So you need to live well when you can. If you've had a scare, you can see clearly the things that are important. Even if the body is sick, it does not mean the heart-mind (Jp. kokoro) is. You must keep the heart-mind well.

When I was waiting for the diagnosis about which stage of cancer—1, 2, 3, or 4—I was hanging the futon outside, and a butterfly came. They have very short lives compared to humans. Even if they are going to die that night, they fly around with so much joy. I actually don't know if it's fun—it could be a lot of hard work to fly around—but it looks fun! I thought, the butterfly's life is so much shorter, yet it can fly around all over. So I thought, I, too, must live well when I can. It's the same with fireflies. Live fully until death. I thought of that a lot then.

I didn't fall apart and cry at the time. I have long thought that I would die once, so dying is not so bad. I thought dying in my fifties was a little soon, but when I think clearly, I think it is what it is. When I was given the anesthesia, I said many things to the nurse. I said that I was really scared. When I was doing daily activities, I was fine. When you're in the hospital, you ride along with the flow of the hospital rhythm: this test, that result, [the] next thing, [a] meal, and so on. I was happy to leave the hospital. I went home and waited for a week. I was fine while doing daily activities.

The morning I was to get the results, my feeling got heavy. I wore the prayer beads Aoyama Sensei had given me the whole time, even during the operation. I had the special cleaning cloth [that Aoyama Sensei had imprinted with her calligraphy], too. My feelings about them were, "Please save me!" Aoyama Sensei told me to say the Heart Sūtra when there was nothing more to be done. When I got out of surgery and woke up, I thought, "Oh, yes, Aoyama Sensei said to chant the Heart Sūtra." I was fading in and out, and people would come in and out. So I kept starting over and forgetting where I was [in the chant]. I only got through the whole sūtra once. But it really saved me from thinking of other things. I felt Aoyama Sensei's presence with me. It gave my heart rest to have someone who knows the truth nearby to give me a hand. I wanted someone to know my weakness, and I trusted her. I did everything she told me. I had the prayer beads, the cleaning cloth, the book she gave me, and did what she said. She was a place I could go to, like a birth home for my heart (kokoro no furusato) where I could get support. My mother and sister were with me, too.[7]

I put the cleaning cloth on the pillow where I rested my head in the hospital. In Japan, it is common to have a cloth wrapped around the abdomen, so it helped

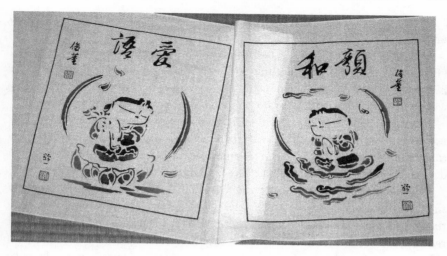

FIGURE 34.1 A CLEANING CLOTH INVOKED FOR HEALING.
Source: Paula K. R. Arai.

me feel settled putting it there, too. Somewhere in my head was Kimura-san's story [about being cured of cancer by Aoyama's cleaning cloth]. I couldn't think my cancer disappeared because the prayer beads and cleaning cloth were there, but it made my heart feel safe. That is what I felt when I received it from Aoyama Sensei. It could have been anything. I did want something I could physically put on my body, although I can't distinguish clearly what is heart and body. It is like a protective amulet, something I could hold on to. It could have been anything. If I had not received anything, I might have asked for something {laughter}.

People told me you don't die from uterine cancer, but people do. It is a cancer. I felt like I could die in peace with [having the things from Aoyama Sensei]. I felt like I had done all I could. Afterward, it is just the results. [. . .] As I went to sleep with one cleaning cloth on my pillow, Aoyama Sensei's prayer beads on my wrist, [and] the other cleaning cloth wrapped around me, my sense of things got big. I could just let it all unfold and sleep well. I did have a feeling that having her prayer beads made me feel like I was not alone.[8]

3. Honda-san on Living with Pain and Gratitude

As you age, your energy gradually declines. So, as my energy declined and when my leg began to hurt, I realized that it was a big mistake to think that humans are living on their own. I thought that it was that we are *receiving* life from somewhere. When you are sad and suffering, you do not just die on your own. Although there are people who do take their own lives, I can't do that, no matter how much I suffer. I began to feel gratitude. I guess it began when my leg began to hurt. For me, it was my leg; for others, it is cancer or something, or they feel pain in their heart. If I had been always healthy, I probably would not feel this happiness.

I cannot judge if I have become a better person because of this, but I think I can say that I have made some progress in being grateful.[9]

When you have health, you get selfish. When you don't have health, you think, if I had health, there would be nothing to complain about. Humans relax upon their health. I felt there was no person I could rely on, because you never know when they will go. I felt empty after [my mother's] funeral [since her death was so sudden].[10]

If you let stress build up, it will be bad for your blood flow. When blood does not flow, many things go wrong with the body. Relaxing is so important. My key to not building stress is not to expect anything. Since I am the only one who can decide, I decide to relax, not build stress, and not be attached to things.[11]

I have learned a lot of things from this illness. Illness is not something you should throw away! I understand this at this age. If I were younger, I would not have thought this way. I would have regretted the illness. The pain is real, but it does not require patience. I have never asked for it to go away. I feel grateful that I have been able to have a good life. Trying to be "patient" builds up stress. Pain is pain, but I don't feel I need patience. I have had this since I was about twenty-seven.[12]

If you think your problems are caused by other people, or that they are other people's responsibility, that is more difficult to live with and painful. I don't like that. It's more difficult and painful if you think of yourself as a sacrificer or a victim. If you feel gratitude, you can begin to see many things. I really think that gratitude is a miraculous medicine! And then your heart becomes light. And other things begin to feel better, too. I sometimes think that my legs becoming bad is a good thing. I have become able to feel all different kinds of things. It is very interesting to see things from the perspective of having bad legs.[13]

NOTES

1. This generation is known for having experienced a difficult youth as a result of living through World War II (Plath 1975: 51–63).

2. In a separate study, Lebra (1984: 289) also found that Japanese elderwomen are the healers in the household.

3. These excerpts were originally published in Arai 2011. They have been slightly edited for inclusion in this volume.

4. Kawasaki interview, December 22, 1998.

5. Kawasaki interview, February 19, 1999.

6. Yamaguchi interview, August 4, 1998.

7. Yamaguchi interview, July 28, 1998.

8. Yamaguchi interview, July 28, 1998.

9. Honda interview, April 3, 1999.

10. Honda interview, April 7, 1999.

11. Honda interview, April 20, 1999.

12. Honda interview, April 20, 1999.

13. Honda interview, April 3, 1999.

35. Conversations About Buddhism and Health Care in Multiethnic Philadelphia

C. PIERCE SALGUERO

This chapter presents edited excerpts from ethnographic interviews conducted at Buddhist temples, meditation centers, and with Buddhist practitioners in the metropolitan area of Philadelphia, Pennsylvania, between 2015 and 2018. These interviews were collected as part of a research project exploring the multifaceted connections between Buddhism and health in Philadelphia across ethnic, racial, and sectarian lines.[1] The study's findings have suggested that Buddhism plays a major, though underappreciated, role in shaping health care in the city among all kinds of practitioners.

At the time of this writing, the ethnographic project currently includes nearly fifty Buddhist institutions, the majority of which are embedded within neighborhoods with a high number of Asian immigrants.[2] In 2016, the U.S. Census Bureau estimated that 7.4 percent of the city's population identify as Asian, up from 6.3 percent in 2010.[3] In the adjacent Montgomery County, north of Philadelphia, where a number of our fieldwork sites are also located, the most recent figure is 5.7 percent. With a population of over six million, the metropolitan area has a large and diverse enough Buddhist population to support a wide range of organizations associated with a number of denominations and cultural–linguistic traditions. Buddhist institutions in the area include Theravāda, Mahāyāna, Vajrayāna/Esoteric, and Zen temples, as well as a range of organizations affiliated with nontraditional forms of Buddhism, such as Won Buddhism, Buddhist Churches of America, and Soka Gakkai. These institutions cater to

Americans of African, Cambodian, Chinese, European, Japanese, Korean, Lao, Taiwanese, Thai, Tibetan, Mongolian, and Vietnamese descent.

Our study has invited the monastic residents, lay leaders, and other representatives or spokespeople for this wide range of Buddhist institutions to tell us how Buddhism relates to health, broadly defined. Through these statements, unstructured follow-up interviews, and participant observation, we have identified a range of culturally specific ways that Buddhism is thought to positively impact physical and mental health. These include practices such as meditation, chanting, prayer, merit-making offerings, and a variety of public and private purification rites. We have also been told about the health care implications of a vegetarian diet, following the lay Buddhist precepts, and living a morally upright life. Interviewees have spoken about the benefits of traditional Asian medical practices—such as acupuncture, massage, scraping, and herbs—which are being offered in temple-supported clinics or informally in the temples themselves. Many of our informants have discussed collaborations with universities, social welfare organizations, or other local groups to organize clinics, fairs, or other health care services for members and their communities. We have also heard that Buddhist organizations provide assistance for recent immigrants to connect with mainstream health care resources; for example, helping with insurance or Medicaid applications, recommending hospitals or doctors, arranging transportation, and offering translation services. More intangibly, we have witnessed how temples serve as community centers that help to connect immigrant families with their home languages, foodways, arts, and other aspects of culture that help to reinforce identity and a sense of belonging. In several cases, our interviewees have expressed that those kinds of activities contribute significantly to overall well-being, especially for refugee communities who have experienced significant collective trauma before coming to the United States.

Spanning these themes and more, the excerpts included below have been chosen to introduce the reader to the diversity of our findings about Buddhism and healing in Philadelphia. While only representing a small minority of the data captured in this project, it is hoped that these excerpts can contribute to illuminating the diverse intersections between Buddhism and health care within the rich multiethnic tapestry of a diverse American urban center. The quotes represent the voices of a range of interviewees from different institutions and contexts, who describe their engagements with Buddhist healing in markedly different ways. Buddhism is sometimes described as a complement, and sometimes as a superior alternative, to surgery and drugs; it is sometimes characterized as primarily mental or spiritual in nature; it sometimes involves ritual, meditation, or simply community solidarity; it sometimes even is characterized as superstition or magic. However, the interviewees all share a conviction that Buddhist practices and perspectives are a source of truly efficacious healing.

FURTHER READING

Cheah, Joseph. 2011. *Race and Religion in American Buddhism: White Supremacy and Immigrant Adaptation*. New York: Oxford University Press.

Hickey, Wakoh S. 2015. "Two Buddhisms, Three Buddhisms, and Racism." In *Buddhism Beyond Borders: New Perspectives on Buddhism in the United States*, edited by Scott A. Mitchell and Natalie E. F. Quli, 35–56. Albany, N.Y.: SUNY Press.

Numrich, Paul D. 2005. "Complementary and Alternative Medicine in America's 'Two Buddhisms.'" In *Religion and Healing in America*, edited by Linda L. Barnes and Susan S. Sered, 343–57. New York: Oxford University Press.

Salguero, C. Pierce. 2019. "Varieties of Buddhist Healing in Multiethnic Philadelphia." *Religions* 10 (1), doi:10.3390/rel10010048.

Wu, Hongyu. 2002. "Buddhism, Health, and Healing in a Chinese Community." The Pluralism Project, Harvard University. http://pluralism.org/wp-content/uploads/2015/08/Wu.pdf.

EXCERPTS FROM INTERVIEWS[4]

1. A Thai American Laywoman on Overcoming Cancer[5]

The Buddha is not God; he's great teacher. He didn't teach anything that's out of this world; he taught things that are in this world. Don't just believe him; practice, and then you know. Chanting, meditation, whatever you do in your daily life: Use it. Use the teaching. That's what I did.

I had non-Hodgkin lymphoma. I had a lesion in the bones of my spine. They said I had to get treatment, so I had radiation and chemotherapy. I didn't have any complications because I meditate every day. I took whatever came. Whatever the sickness or side effect of the chemo was—and I had strong chemo at the time—I took it. And people said, "How come you don't look so sick like other people?" You know what? I think when people are sick, the physical sickness is, like, 50 percent and the mental sickness is, like, 50 percent. So when you don't have the mental sickness, you take what comes. You understand me {laughs}?

So many of these things, science cannot prove. I had interviews with five or six doctors when they decided I had to have back surgery. When I went for the surgery, I meditated right before and after. They said I had to be in the hospital for three weeks. After just one night, I could I walk. I just stayed overnight in the hospital for one night, and then I went home. And I never had any physical therapy, but I walked. I think that proves your mind is more than your body. Mind over body. Sometimes people look so sick, and I don't think it's from cancer. It's from their mental health.

The second time that I had cancer, maybe ten years ago, I had it all over my body, in my organs, everywhere. They said it's cancer. And I asked them, "Do I have to get the treatment again?" They said yes, but I said, "Forget it." I didn't go. I stopped going to see the doctor. I came to the temple only, and I sat in front of the picture of the founder. I talked to him. I said, "If it's my time to go, I'll go. But don't let me suffer." I have faith in him.

Sometimes I could not get up because I had a fever or something, so I would say, "If you want me to go to the temple, you will take me." And it always happened that I felt better. I took a shower, and I came here. It happened all the time. But the thing is, you have to have faith. Faith in the Buddha, in the monks.

Sometimes I have a problem, and I sit and meditate, and then I get to a point that I don't feel pain anymore. I have fibromyalgia. It's a horrible disease. Nothing can take the pain away. But when I meditate, I can chant for one hour, and I meditate afterward for thirty or fifty minutes. My mind is still. It takes the whole pain away, from head to toe. For me, my goal is just to take away the pain, both mental and physical.

2. A Thai American Laywoman on Caring for Monks with Herbal Medicine

Here we have a few monks from Thailand, and I care for them. I've been doing it for thirty, almost forty years now because I am a nurse. They have Medicaid because they're not allowed to work. They have Medicaid just for emergencies. One of the monks went to the hospital for high blood pressure. I took his blood pressure, and I said, "You have to go to the hospital." So, somebody took him. He stayed for three days. And then I told him, "You have to be careful with your food; you have to exercise." They say they do work around the temple, but that's not exercise. You have to exercise on the treadmill or something like that. And I'll say, "Why don't you try this? Try ginger, turmeric." That's what I do every day. Ginger, turmeric, honey, lime juice, something like that. We Thai people have an herb for everything, you know.

We just found out that one of the monks has coronary disease. So last week I mixed a tea for heart disease. We use ginger, a lot of ginger, and boil it with dark mushroom and three dates, which have a lot of calcium in them. We make a big pot like this {gestures with arms}. You drink a couple cups a day. And we can show you that the plaque in the bloodstream is gone.

I have a machine that makes juice, like kale or celery, ginger, and Granny Smith apple. It's easy. I make that every morning for heart problems. Because celery is a diuretic, you know. And we eat a lot of dandelion. And I use the roots, even the flowers. I wash it, and I make a smoothie. And I used to have a bad peptic ulcer, but now it's gone.

3. A Cambodian American Monk on the Role of the Temple in Community Health

In the U.S., we have a lot of good hospitals where people can go. And they fix some kinds of disease. But some of the people from the Cambodian community lack understanding or language. So we can help them, to guide them to where they have to go and how to reach the doctor, especially to get them to understand the importance of getting checkups for their health. You know, not just to come to the temple for the monk's blessing, but to do both.

When they don't understand the language, we find a person to translate for them, to cultivate understanding about the health system in the U.S. Especially the elders. Sometimes they don't have medical care. They're afraid to go the hospital; it costs a lot. So they have to know how to apply for Medicaid or medical insurance for seniors or for people with disabilities. They need more help. They don't speak the language; they don't drive. Sometimes they kind of stress because the younger people go to work or go to school, but they just stay alone at home.

And I think you may know that Cambodians have been through many difficulties in their life after the war. And that's the reason that there are a lot of Cambodians in the U.S., because of the war. We all live separate from family and from our loved ones. And some of us lost their loved ones. Some of us just live alone. So Cambodians face a lot of mental illness and loss of hope.

You know, Cambodia has been a Buddhist country for a thousand years. So Buddhism has become a symbol for Cambodians that can bring people together. It can also teach people peace, forgiveness, and to let go of something that's very destructive. And also at the temple, we're teaching how to do meditation. Meditation is a way to heal mental problems, and also to let people live in peace and harmony, and to understand the reality of what happened in the past, now, and in the future.

Even though we are not living in Cambodia, and we have fled from country to country, still we try really hard to form a community.[6] The reason is that we really need community to support each other. The community comes to feel like our home. So the temple serves as a meeting place where people can come together, and that starts a social connection among Cambodians, and to reach out to the community. And also, the temple is the place to spread information. We provide information about the health system, but not just health. Also culture and belief. When people come to the temple, they feel like it's their home, their country. The temple is the cultural center of Cambodians, to keep or preserve the culture.

4. A Cambodian American Laywoman on When to Seek
Out Lay Ritual Healers

The *achar* [literally, "teacher" or "master"] is not a monk.[7] The monks are always going to have more status than the *achar* because, you know, they live by the Buddhist laws and stuff like that. The *achar*, he's just a regular person who happens to have been a monk before, or he has really studied the Cambodian *Tripiṭaka*. The *achar* leads us with prayer, and they help bless the house and things like that.

They're not rare in Philadelphia, because if you ask any family, they know somebody who knows somebody who knows one. Recently, someone was saying that this girl was possessed, and they called an *achar* to come in, and then the girl got better. There's also a situation in which a fetus is stolen, and they turn it into a spirit animal, and this spirit baby will go and do bad things for whoever took it. It's a black magic thing, like a voodoo doll. The baby will go and look at your enemies, spy for you, or cause problems for your enemies. I've never seen it, but I hear about it a lot. You know, we Cambodians are so superstitious. And that's why we're so afraid. We're always praying, and we'll always have blessing flags on top of our doors, and all these strings on our wrists. And holy water.

How do I decide when to go to a doctor or to the *achar*? If I feel physically sick, I don't go to the *achar*; I just take a medicine for it. Like, if I have a headache, I'm going to take a Tylenol; I don't need to sit there for two or three hours and pray or anything like that. Then, if I feel like there's also bad energy around us, around my family, I'll say my own prayers. I'll light my candles, incense, the whole thing, and kick whatever out. If it's a mental thing, like I feel scared for no reason, then I'll just do that. But, if it's something serious maybe, like cancer or something, then maybe you feel that the extra "oomph" of the *achar's* prayer might help the medicine more.

I mean, it's more spiritual medicine, not physical. If I were going on a trip and I had a bad feeling, like "I don't know if I should get on this plane," I might go to him and get a blessing or a string or something. You know, Americans might go to the doctor for some medicine when they're nervous on the plane. But I might just go to my mom and get a thing of holy water. She'll give me a spray bottle of holy water before my trip just because she's very spiritual. Plus, we don't really want to rely on medicine too much.

5. A German American Practitioner on the
Healing Energies Released in Her Meditation

It's like there are knots in our body. And, since mind and body are not really separate, when we put our attention on them, these knots dissolve. If these knots remain blocked, they manifest finally as physical diseases. But you can reverse the process or prevent diseases from happening. That's my explanation.

There are often people who seem to have a certain energy. That energy comes through their own meditation, and they radiate it out. Because it's life-force, when people are close to them, they also get elevated. They can go into a deep state of meditation very quickly, and some of these people can just heal very quickly.

That just naturally happens. It's a very strong and intense energy, and in the beginning, it's very hard to practice for beginners. But after a while, you gain these . . . {pauses} . . . well, something happens, and your body is filled with life-force. You are in bliss and peace, but you cannot sleep because you have so much energy. It's this energy life-force that is healing. This happens in Zen when you meditate a lot, and it also happens in the *jhanas* [i.e., states of "absorption" induced by Theravāda-style concentration meditation].

6. A Vietnamese American Layman on the Power of Healing Rituals and the "Ultimate Holistic Approach"

We read the *Bhaiṣajyaguru Sūtra* [see *Anthology*, vol. 1, ch. 25] the way it was written, word by word.[8] And after that, when we come toward the end of the ceremony, our resident abbot explains the meaning of the *sūtra* itself. As far as the meaning and the purpose of why we're doing this, spiritually speaking, it's not just to achieve good health for yourself and for your family members. At the end of the day, there's also the collective energy of the whole group that we're trying to spread out.

We are wishing that we are blessed by good health by the Buddha, but also at the same time, to carry on that blessing for everybody else to be fortunate as well. There's a collective field of energy that starts just with your thoughts. The abbot says that when you sit [alone] in meditation, your body doesn't do anything, but when you sit in the presence of a group of many people, that creates a whole collective energy. It's a stillness, a calmness, an inner peace that hopefully can spread out. We don't know how much it can spread, or how far away from the world [it can travel], but that's the ultimate goal or the meaning behind sitting meditation.

If you come to the temple and learn about this spiritual kind of health, you add a layer on to your overall health and protection. I could tell you, "Here's a pill; take it." You might feel well because of how the medication helps you, but in the long run, [the spiritual approach] is more preventive. How do you prevent disease before you have to treat it? I think it's through treating the whole picture—with mental health and spiritual healing—that you will be able to learn over time and help other people.

People without a certain background would say it's a little superstitious: "You're just praying. Whether or not that helps you, you don't know." But I don't think there's any conflict. The West is all about science and technology, which does much of the real work. But if they could see a second complementary layer, cutting deep down and bringing everything together, I think that would be the ultimate holistic approach to achieving wellness. Things might conflict on the superficial level, but when you look deep down, you start finding the connection.

7. A Vietnamese American Layman on the Health Benefits of Bowing

Last week for the Quan Âm [i.e., Avalokiteśvara] event, we did a total of five hundred bows based on the *sūtra*. Each bow represented one of Quan Âm's names. You know how she manifested differently, depending on what sentient beings needed from her? Well, we did five hundred bows for her five hundred different names. It was just like a form of exercise. You know, you make your whole body move, and you sweat a lot.

I know if I am not feeling well, if I do the exercise, I will feel a little bit better. It's like detoxification through perspiration. You could go to the gym or go to a hot spa, and that would kind of be the same, if we're only speaking of the internal science of the body. But this is mind and body. Because when you bow to the Buddha, or a bodhisattva, you focus your mind. You clear your thoughts, and there's only a single-pointed focus. It's just circulation, energy flow, or however you want to put it, but there's also a meaning behind it, spiritually speaking. I heard all this from the master before, but this is also my personal reflection through my own experience. Spiritually, I feel better.

8. An African American Soka Gakkai Practitioner on How Chanting Healed Her Son[9]

At one point, one of my sons started to have epileptic seizures. He was about three, so they could have been febrile seizures, or they could have been epileptic seizures. I talked to my leader, and she told me that I could chant to change his sickness. Even though the principle is that you can change only yourself, someone so close to you as a child is part of your environment, part of you.

I really didn't have confidence, even though I'd been chanting for a number of years, probably five years at that point. I didn't think it would work. But I did it because I trusted my leader. So I kept on chanting and chanting for his seizures.

My mother-in-law, who'd been calling me every week, happens to be a scientist. I couldn't tell her that I was chanting for him to get better because she was serious about her atheism, and she would really not approve of my magical religion. Of course, he also took Dilantin [an anti-seizure medication], and we went to the neurologist and followed all the directions. But, all of a sudden, he started to have a reaction to the medication.

[We went back to] the neurologist, who did all the same tests and said, "Why don't you just discontinue that medication and see if he still needs it?" And he didn't. It was finished. Not only did his illness change after my chanting for about six months, but I didn't ever have to tell my mother-in-law. So the chanting worked out perfectly!

9. A Taiwanese American Chaplain on Her Interactions with Patients in the Hospital

I am from Taiwan, and I came here in 1991. I was born culturally Buddhist. We were into temple worship of Buddha and Guanyin [i.e., Avalokiteśvara]. Then, in 1994, I started to practice meditation with a Pure Land teacher. So I now have a daily meditation practice. And I recite sūtras. Because of reciting the Diamond Sūtra and the Heart Sūtra, that led me to Zen practice from the Japanese tradition. And then, in 2007, I started my chaplaincy training. I'm now a volunteer interfaith chaplain at the hospital.[10]

When I'm walking into the room of a patient, I will concentrate on that person. I don't even think about any other thing, not even, "How should I deal with this patient?" We receive some information from the nurses or others that tells you what has happened to that patient, but I think it's best if you keep yourself blank to directly receive from them, to let them tell you what happened to them. Lots of things are not physical, but more mental. And my meditation practice keeps me focused, concentrated, practicing Zen all the time. Every moment. That's very important.

I don't introduce myself as a Buddhist chaplain right away. I just say, "I am a chaplain, and I've come here to share my energy and strength." Every patient loves that. I might guide a patient to take a deep breath—and see, deep breathing is the very beginning of Buddhist practice—and then to breathe in and out, in and out. I teach the patient to take deep breaths with very gentle air. And I do it with them. If someone asks about meditation, then I will talk more about it. But I think most of the patients, when they are in that kind of circumstance, normally they just want to grab something quick to help themselves, but they are not really deep into it.

Another practice I use is mantra. I learned that when I practiced with my Pure Land teachers. In Pure Land, it is a daily exercise, before and after you recite the sūtra. So I recite those mantras. But I also practice OM MAṆI PADME HŪM, the Tibetan national mantra.

My belief, my goal, is to help everyone to be the way they are. You have to accept everyone the way they are, and then you are just like a lantern. You shine. Some people receive the light; some people don't. But if people receive it, they will appreciate it. In a way, you kind of influence that person with your light, and they transform themselves, and they shine.

NOTES

1. See the project website: www.jivaka.net. Project results are described in more detail in Salguero 2019.

2. On the history of Asian immigration to America, see Takaki 1989; Chan 1991. For critical studies of race, immigration, and Buddhism, see Quli 2009; Cheah 2011: 80–92; Hickey 2015.

3. U.S. Census Bureau. "Quick Facts: Philadelphia County, Pennsylvania, United States." U.S. Census Bureau. www.census.gov/quickfacts/fact/table/philadelphiacountypennsylvani a,US/PST045216.

4. The following are excerpts from interviews conducted with anonymous interviewees by C. Pierce Salguero and undergraduate research assistants. They were conducted in English in various temples and meditation centers around Greater Philadelphia between 2015 and 2018 and have been edited for conciseness as well as for English fluency. Most were previously made available on the project website.

5. The temple in which the following two interviews were conducted is described in more detail in Cadge 2004.

6. For a discussion of Buddhist refugees' acclimation to the United States, see Ong 2003.

7. The importance of lay ritualists, including *achar*, in Cambodian ritual life is discussed in Bertrand 2005; Takahashi 2015.

8. A translation of the Sanskrit version of the *Bhaiṣajyaguru Sūtra* is available in *Anthology*, vol. 1, ch. 25.

9. A study of the history of Soka Gakkai in Japan is available in McLaughlin 2018.

10. For a discussion of interfaith chaplaincy, see Cadge 2013.

GEOGRAPHICAL TABLE OF CONTENTS

GLOSSARY

The following list of key terms with definitions has been compiled collectively by the authors. An attempt has been made to define terms in ways that will be helpful for the current volume, but this glossary is not meant to be definitive for all cultural contexts.

Amitābha Buddha (Jp. Amida): One of the main buddhas of Mahāyāna devotionalism. Amitābha presides over the Pure Land of Utmost Bliss (see below), located to the far west of our own world. This paradise is a favored destination for rebirth; thus, rituals involving Amitābha Buddha have been closely associated with hospice, death, and funerals. His devotees typically focus on chanting a simple mantra paying homage to his name (e.g., in Chinese, NAMO AMITUOFO), which is said to be sufficient cause for rebirth in his Pure Land.

Ānanda: A first cousin of Gautama Buddha and one of his ten principal disciples. Ānanda is said to have had a particularly good memory, and most of the suttas in the Pāli Canon are based on his recitation of the Buddha's discourses.

Avalokiteśvara (Skt.; Ch. Guanyin; Jp. Kannon; Kr. Kwan Um; Tib. Chenrezik; Vtn. Quan Âm): One of the principal bodhisattvas of Mahāyāna Buddhism and the most popularly deity in contemporary East Asian Buddhist practice. Avalokiteśvara—who is mentioned many times in many languages throughout this volume—is, in East Asian traditions, most commonly depicted either in a white-robed feminine form or in an eleven-headed, one-thousand-armed male form. Traditionally, this bodhisattva is connected to Amitābha Buddha (see above) and thus is often said to lead the dead toward rebirth in that buddha's Pure Land of Utmost Bliss (see below). Popularly, the deity is mainly associated with compassion and is invoked as a savior deity who rescues petitioners from calamities of various types (often including illness or impending death).

bardo (Tib.): A Tibetan term that literally means to be "in the middle" or "in between." A "*bardo*-being" is a migrating consciousness in the intermediate state between death and one's next rebirth (see *Anthology*, vol. 1, ch. 5). According to Tibetan medicine, a *bardo*-being must enter in union with the sperm and egg for conception to occur. One well-known Tibetan Buddhist text on *bardo*, known in English as *The Tibetan Book of the Dead*, prepares an individual for death and helps the *bardo*-being achieve a fortunate rebirth, or possibly enlightenment.

Bile: See *tridoṣa*.

Bön (Tib.): Often controversially described as the "shamanistic" faith of pre-Buddhist Tibet, Bön is a distinct Tibetan religious system that developed alongside Buddhism after the latter's arrival in the region. While adherents of Bön claim that it predates Buddhism as a coherent and self-conscious religion by thousands of years, evidence suggests that institutionalized Bön evolved in conversation and competition with Buddhism. Both religions absorbed many features of the pre-Buddhist religious landscape, and today the philosophies, terminology, ritual practices, and institutional structures of Bön and Tibetan Buddhism parallel each other considerably.

Chan (Jp. Zen; Kr. Sŏn): Originally, the word *chan* derived from the Sanskrit term *dhyāna*, meaning "meditative concentration." It was used as a generic term in China for Buddhist meditation. When capitalized and not italicized (likewise with Japanese Zen and Korean Sŏn), it refers to a distinct form of Buddhism that originated in China. Chan claims to represent a wordless teaching not contained within the Buddhist scriptures and is focused on achieving awakening through meditation. Today, the three main Japanese sects are Sōtō, Rinzai, and Ōbaku, with Sōtō being the largest.

ḍākinī (Skt.; Tib. khandroma): In Indo-Tibetan Tantric Buddhism, the term usually refers to a class of enlightened feminine deities who assist practitioners on their spiritual path. Literally meaning "she who goes through space" in Tibetan, *ḍākinī*s appear in forms that are alluring or hideous, and are divided into worldly or enlightened classes. More broadly, the *ḍākinī* points to the conventionally feminine, playful, creative, and revelatory form or display aspect of Buddha-mind or activity. The term is also used as an honorific for particularly accomplished female teachers and practitioners.

dantian (Ch.; Jp. tanden): Literally "elixir fields," these are places within the body that play a special role in breathing and meditation believed to store *qi*. The most important of these is located within the abdomen, behind the navel or slightly below it.

deva (Skt.): The word *deva* refers to the deities of the Hindu–Buddhist pantheon. In Buddhist cosmology, these represent spiritual creatures living in the upper, heavenly abodes of existence, which correspond to the higher levels of rebirth. They are considered very powerful but also benevolent and unable to harm people, unlike inferior spirits such as the territorial spirits.

dhāraṇī (Skt.; Ch. *zhou, shenzhou*): A type of Buddhist incantation or spell typically used to call upon Buddhist deities or to harness their powers. Emphasis is placed on proper pronunciation, as the sound vibrations are its mechanism for efficacy. (For more information, see *Anthology*, vol. 1, ch. 28, 30.) See also mantra.

Dharma (Skt.; Pāli **Dhamma**): Also Buddhadharma. A multivalent Indian term that, when used by Buddhists, most frequently refers to the teachings of the Buddha or to Buddhist doctrine more generally.

Dōgen: 1200–1253. Recognized as the founder of Sōtō Zen in Japan. He founded the monastery, Eihei-ji, in Echizen, Fukui Prefecture. Among other things, Dōgen is famous for his strict monastic discipline, his collection of his philosophical writings *Treasury of the True Dharma Eye* (*Shōbōgenzō*), and his teachings of "just-sitting" (*shikantaza*) and "practice is enlightenment" (*shushōittō*).

Esoteric Buddhism: See Vajrayāna.

feng shui (Ch. *fengshui*): Literally "wind and water." Refers to Chinese geomancy, here meaning primarily the practice of arranging objects in and around architectural spaces according to principles that balance the flow of *qi*, *yin-yang*, and the Five Phases (*wuxing*). Basic guidelines for homes or businesses include details such as where to situate plants or chimes and where to avoid positioning mirrors.

Five Aggregates (Skt. *pañca-skandha*): In Buddhist psychology or philosophy, the five "aggregates" or "accumulations" are the five factors or processes that give rise to sentience: form (*rūpa*), feeling or sensation (*vedanā*), perception (*saṃjñā*), will or intention (*saṃskāra*), and consciousness or discrimination (*vijñāna*).

Five Precepts (Skt. *pañcasīla*): These are the basic moral responsibilities ostensibly upheld by all Buddhist laypersons: to refrain from killing, stealing, sexual misconduct, lying, and intoxicants.

Four Tantras (Tib. **Gyüzhi**): A short title for the *Secret Essence of Ambrosia in Eight Branches: An Instructional Tantra*, the preeminent medical classic of Sowa Rigpa (see below), or traditional Tibetan medicine. This four-volume work contains influences from Persian, Sanskrit, and Chinese medicine, as well as original Tibetan medical concepts. Although the work has traditionally been attributed to either Bhaiṣajyaguru, his emanations, or Yuthok the Elder (ca. eight century), scholars now attribute it to Yuthok Yönten Gönpo (twelfth century) and his students (see discussion in *Anthology*, vol. 1, ch. 62). The relationship between Buddhism and medicine is emphasized in several places, and the text is written in the style of Tantric Buddhist scriptures, which depict a discourse between a realized being and interlocutors. The theories, instructions, and narratives contained in this work have formed the basis of Tibetan medical scholasticism and practice for most of the past millennium.

Gautama (Skt.; Pāli **Gotama**): See Śākyamuni Buddha.

ghosts (Skt. *preta*): Unhappy spirits. In the Buddhist tradition, ghosts are created by karmic debt incurred in life. They are tortured embodiments of unfulfilled longing and desire that are awaiting reincarnation. Throughout Asia, the image of the "hungry ghost" has merged with native conceptions of violent or untended spirits that must be ritually appeased or warded off.

Guanyin: See Avalokiteśvara.

Jōdo Shinshū (Jp.): Also known as Shin Buddhism and True Pure Land Buddhism, this is Japan's largest temple-based Buddhist denomination. Shinran (1173–1263) is regarded as its founder. It emphasizes trust in Amitābha Buddha (see above), rebirth in his Pure Land of Utmost Bliss (see below), and the recitation of his name (Jp. *nenbutsu*).

ki: See *qi*.

kōan (Jp.; Ch. *gong'an*): A Chan Buddhist meditation device in the form of a question or problem that serves as a focal point for a dynamic form of contemplation intended to elicit a nondualistic experience. Originally developed in China, the practice spread to Korea and Japan, from where the Western usage of the term derives.

Kūkai: 774–835. Known posthumously as Kōbō Daishi Kūkai or simply Kōbō Daishi. The Shingon Buddhist tradition credits this Japanese monk as its founder. He trained in China before bringing Esoteric Buddhist practices back to Japan, along with knowledge of Sanskrit linguistics and new architectural and medical practices (on the latter, see *Anthology*, vol. 1, ch. 23). He was also one of Japan's most famous calligraphers and a prolific author, and became a legendary personality as a saintly cultural hero.

lama (Tib.): The Tibetan translation for the Sanskrit *guru*. *Lama* is a general, gender-neutral term used by Tibetans to refer to any trained practitioner of Buddhism who teaches Dharma to others. The lama is central to Tantric Buddhism and serves in this context as an initiator, model, and mentor to disciples. In Tibetan and Himalayan societies, the teachings, charisma, and estates of esteemed lamas have been transferred and institutionalized through lineages based on systems of both hereditary descent and succession through reincarnation.

Mahāyāna (Skt.): Literally the "Great Vehicle," a form of Buddhism that originated several centuries after the lifetime of the Buddha and vocally differentiated itself from earlier forms. Several features that characterized Mahāyāna Buddhism—including an increased emphasis on the doctrines of compassion and emptiness, as well as an expansive pantheon of buddhas and bodhisattvas populating a large number of Buddha-realms throughout the universe—had a direct bearing on its engagement with healing. Whereas early Buddhism saw healing as a noble profession for physicians (see *Anthology*, vol. 1, ch. 20), it remained an unsuitable pursuit for monastics in most situations (see *Anthology*, vol. 1, ch. 10, 11). In Mahāyāna Buddhism, by contrast, healing was considered a much more integral part of the accepted path toward the liberation of all beings (see *Anthology*, vol. 1, ch. 4, 9).

mandala (Skt. *maṇḍala*): "Circle." In Tantric Buddhism specifically, a symbolic circular template representing the perfected mind or cosmos in its entirety. Suggesting a sovereign ruler ensconced in the heart of a fortress, a mandala typically features a central principal deity with or without a consort, surrounded by an array of radiating retinue deities.

mantra (Skt.): Syllables in Sanskrit and other sacred languages written, uttered aloud, intoned mentally, and visualized by Buddhists. As powerful utterances of truth revealed by great realized sages, mantras focus the mind, generate beneficial effects and qualities, and visually and sonically embody various buddhas and deities. See also *dhāraṇī.*

Māra/*māra* (Skt.): In Buddhist cosmology, Māra is a god who rules over the Heaven of Enjoying Others' Creations, at the pinnacle of the desire realm. In Buddhist literature, he and his followers, known collectively as *māras*, are portrayed as single-mindedly focused on obstructing the spread of the Buddhist teachings and leading Buddhist practitioners to violate their ethical and religious discipline.

***nāga* (Tib. *lu*):** In Buddhist mythology, the *nāga* are a class of serpentine beings who dwell in underwater and subterranean palaces. In some contexts, they are regarded as guardians of the Buddhist teachings, whereas in others, they are portrayed as capricious beings responsible for drought and disease. They may also cause illness in humans if disturbed; for example, if humans pollute the lakes, rivers, and streams in which they live.

***nirvāṇa* (Skt.):** Usually translated as "enlightenment" but more correctly meaning "extinguishment," *nirvāṇa* represents the Buddhist aim of escaping *saṃsāra* (the cycle of rebirth; see below).

Original mind (Ch. *benxin*; Jp. *honshin*): Literally "fundamental mind." This term signifies both the everyday working of the mind and Buddha nature. Getting ahold of one's original mind means having full consciousness of reality as it is. The term can also be used to denote one's inner and true self or natural disposition, which is essentially associated with well-being.

Phlegm: See *tridoṣa.*

Pure Land of Utmost Bliss (Skt. Sukhāvatī): A Pure Land established by Amitābha Buddha in the westward direction. Rebirth in one's subsequent life in this location is considered automatically to lead to awakening.

***qi* (Ch.; Jp. *ki*; Kr. *gi*):** A numinous and flowing substance that constitutes and animates all phenomena. It is a central concept in the cosmology and etiology of the Sinitic world, particularly in Confucianism, Daoism, and Chinese medicine. Chinese medicine distinguishes between many forms of *qi*, including forms associated with the five organs. The stagnation, blockage, or imbalance of *qi* causes disease.

qigong: A self-cultivation practice for regulating *qi*, typically done with the conscious intent to direct the flow of *qi* within the body or to exchange *qi* with nature or other living beings. Qigong includes breathing, body postures, movements, and meditation, with the aim of developing the practitioner's physical and mental potential. The term was coined in the mid-twentieth century, but there are various older precursors, such as *taijiquan* and *daoyin* (see also *Anthology*, vol. 1, ch. 52).

Reiki: Literally "numinous *ki*" in Japanese. A transnational form of healing practice that started in early twentieth-century Japan that is currently growing in popularity in the United States and other Western countries. Initiates undergo a ceremony derived from Vajrayāna Buddhist empowerment rituals. Advanced practitioners are taught incantations and symbols that can be used to amplify treatments or treat at a distance.

Śakyamuni Buddha (Skt.): Literally "Sage of the Sakya Clan." Also known by the personal name Siddhārtha Gautama (Skt.) or Siddhattha Gotama (Pāli). This is the individual most often referenced when we talk about "the Buddha." Ostensibly, he was born in present-day Nepal some time in the fifth century BCE. He is said to have founded the first order of Buddhist monks (*sangha*) and to have traveled throughout the Indian subcontinent spreading his teachings. While different schools of Buddhism position him in different successions of Buddhas, all consider themselves to be based on the teachings of this historical figure.

samaya **(Skt.):** Vows of initiation taken during Tantric Buddhist rituals of empowerment, which form a kind of covenant between the practitioner and his or her guru, co-initiates, and tutelary deity. Violation of the vows is believed to hinder the practitioner's spiritual progress.

saṃsāra **(Skt.):** A term used to describe the endless cycle of birth, death, and rebirth. All sentient beings transmigrate through the realms of rebirth (god, demi-god, human, animal, hungry ghost, and animal) based upon the positive and negative karma they accumulate in each life.

Shin Buddhism: See Jōdo Shinshū.

Shingon (Jp.): A tradition of Esoteric or Vajrayāna Buddhism originating in China. Its transmission to Japan is traditionally attributed to Kūkai (see above) in the ninth century.

siddhi **(Skt., also *ṛddhi*):** Literally "attainment" or "accomplishment," *siddhi* refers to so-called supernatural powers developed through ritual practice and meditative discipline. In Vajrayāna Buddhism, *siddhis* are divided into "ordinary/common" and "supreme/uncommon" categories. While ordinary *siddhis* include such abilities as clairvoyance, past-life memory, the transmutation of substances and bodies, bilocation, immortality, command over spirits, and so on, the supreme *siddhi* is described as buddhahood itself.

Sŏn: See Chan.

Sowa Rigpa (Tib.): Literally, "knowledge of healing." The indigenous medical tradition of Tibet, which draws on Persian, Indian, and Chinese concepts, as well as indigenous Tibetan notions of anatomy, health, and illness. This medical tradition is indigenous to the Tibetan cultural areas of the Himalayan region, stretching from Ladakh in Northwest India, northward to Chinese-controlled Tibet and the adjacent provinces, to Bhutan in the east, and Nepal in the south. In India, Sowa Rigpa has, since 2010, been officially recognized by the Indian government as a "system of Indian medicine" alongside Āyurveda, homeopathy, naturopathy, Siddha, Unani, and yoga, affording it a certain amount of protection and availability in different areas. While there is variation in its practice, what is common across geographical regions is its focus on the twelfth-century Tibetan medical text, the *Four Tantras* (see above).

sūtra (Skt.; Pāli *sutta*): A genre of Buddhist canonical texts that contain the authentic teachings attributed to a buddha, most commonly Śakyamuni Buddha. Famous Buddhist *sūtras* mentioned frequently in this volume include the *Heart*, *Diamond*, and *Lotus Sūtras*.

taiji or *taijiquan* (Ch.): Literally "great ultimate" or "great ultimate martial art," referring to the cosmological principle of balancing yin and yang. Commonly transliterated in English as "tai chi," this term collectively refers to a family of martial arts aimed at promoting health. They combine physical movements with breathing techniques designed to maximize *qi* while controlling its circulation through the body (see also qigong).

Tantric Buddhism: See Vajrayāna.

Tendai Buddhism (Jp.; Ch. Tiantai): A form of Buddhism founded in China and brought to Japan by Saichō (767–822 CE). Centered on Mount Hiei, near Kyoto, Japanese Tendai is based on *Lotus Sūtra* devotion, as well as aspects of Esoteric Buddhism and Chan. Tendai was the main form of Japanese Buddhism for centuries, and the founders of Japan's Pure Land, Zen, and Nichiren sects all trained as Tendai monks at Mount Hiei.

Treasure revealers (Tib. *tertön*): Male and female Tibetan Tantric Buddhist visionaries and prophets. By recollecting past lives and engaging in advanced yogic practices, treasure revealers are able to uncover "treasures" hidden under the earth or water, in the sky, or in their own minds. These treasures may take the form of physical relics or encrypted and abridged fragments of texts that treasure revealers decode and then write down. Specific treasure revealers are karmically connected to co-visionary consorts and are destined to reveal particular treasures at particular times. Specific revealed relics and teachings are also understood to be keyed to particular periods, places, and communities. Treasure revelations are an especially important part of the canon and identity of the Old Translation or Nyingma school of Tibetan Buddhism.

tridoṣa (Skt.; Tib. *nyépa*): Typically translated as the "three faults" or "three peccant humors." In early Indian Āyurveda, this triad of Wind, Bile, and Phlegm respectively represented pathogenic excesses of gasses or movement, digestive fluids, and mucus in the body, which were said to be caused by insalubrious diet and behavior (see *Anthology* vol. 1, ch. 4). In the later literature of Āyurveda and Tibetan medicine, Wind, Bile, and Phlegm came to describe the three physiological components of circulation, digestion, and structure, balancing to form the constitution of an individual and causing disease when out of balance. These are frequently encountered in Buddhist texts as primary signs or causes of disease.

Tripiṭaka (Skt.; Pāli *Tipiṭaka*): A collection of authoritative Buddhist texts. Different Buddhist traditions uphold different *Tripiṭaka*s written in different languages and containing different texts or different versions of texts. Literally meaning "Three Baskets," the term refers to the three traditional divisions of the canon into *sūtras* (see above), *vinaya* (i.e., monastic disciplinary texts), and *abhidharma* (i.e., summaries of Buddhist metaphysics, psychology, and philosophy).

Triple Gem (Skt. *triratna*): The Buddha, the Dharma, and the Sangha. Buddhists commonly "take refuge" in the Triple Gem as a declaration of faith in and affiliation with Buddhism.

Vajrayāna (Skt.): Literally "vehicle of the *vajra*," the latter being an indestructible adamantine weapon. The term refers to Esoteric or Tantric Buddhism, a form of Mahāyāna Buddhism that involves complex rites of initiation and which promises full enlightenment in a single human body in one lifetime. In contradistinction to the *sūtras'* focus on renunciation, Tantric Buddhism offers a variety of targeted ritual and meditative methods for transmuting ordinary dualistic experiences and emotions into nondual gnosis. These commonly emphasize reciting mantras, performing *mudrās* (ritualized hand gestures), and visualizing mandalas. However, there is no scholarly consensus on how to definitively distinguish Vajrayāna from other forms of Mahāyāna Buddhism. Part of the problem with clear distinction is that the tradition is called by different names in different contexts. "Esoteric Buddhism" tends to be the preferred English term for East Asian Tantric Buddhism, which serves as a gloss for the Chinese *mijiao* and Japanese *mikkyō*, meaning "secret teachings" or "esoteric teachings." The Sanskrit term *Vajrayāna* (Tib. *dorjé tekpa*) is commonly used in English-language materials discussing Tibet and India, while "secret mantra" (Tib. *sangngak*) is most commonly used in the Tibetan language.

vipassanā (Pāli; Skt. *vipaśyanā*): "Insight meditation," a form of Buddhist meditation that claims to offer practitioners a chance to escape suffering by perceiving the true nature of reality as impermanent, unsatisfactory, and lacking an intrinsic self. It is one of the most popular forms of meditation today throughout the world. It is often contrasted with *śamatha*, or the practice of calming the mind through methods of one-pointed concentration.

Wind (Skt. *vāyu*, *vāta*; Tib. *lung*): A complex term used differently in different Buddhist traditions. In early Indian medicine, Wind is one of the *tridoṣa*, the so-called humors, defects, or constitutional propensities to disease (see above). Wind may also refer to a subtle substance or energy that pervades the body and mind, linking the two together and connecting the human organism with the sensory world. Various therapies are introduced in Buddhist texts to combat Wind ailments (see *Anthology*, vol. 1, ch. 41–43). Especially in Tantric Buddhist traditions, meditations and physical exercises are also elaborated to cultivate the Wind for purposes of spiritual attainment.

yantra: A type of sacred diagram that captures Buddhist magical potency in geometric shapes, written syllables, stylized images of deities and animals, and other symbolic forms. In Southeast Asia, *yantras* are commonly printed on cloth to be hung in the home or business, or carried on the body in the form of amulets or tattoos, in order to ensure protection and prosperity. While yantras are features of contemporary Theravāda Buddhism, they bear certain similarities to Vajrayāna Buddhist practices described in both volumes of this anthology, such as mantras, mandalas, and "edible letters."

Yogācāra: One of the two major schools of Mahāyāna Buddhist philosophy, along with Madhyamaka (see *Anthology*, vol. 1, ch. 6). Yogācāra influenced the understanding of consciousness and karma in most schools of Mahāyāna Buddhism, including Chan, Shingon, Tendai, and Vajrayāna.

Zen: See Chan.

REFERENCES

A ru ra, ed. 2007. *Mkhyen rab nor bu'i sman yig gces btus*. Bod kyi gso ba rig pa'i gna' dpe phyogs bsgrigs dpe tshogs. Vol. 66. Beijing: Mi rigs dpe skrun khang.

Adams, Vincanne. 2007. "Integrating Abstraction: Modernising Medicine at Lhasa's Mentsikhang." In *Soundings in Tibetan Medicine: Historical and Anthropological Perspectives*, edited by Mona Schrempf, 29–43. Leiden: Brill.

Adams, Vincanne, Renqing Dongzhu, and Phuoc V. Le. 2010. "Translating Science: The Arura Medical Group at the Frontiers of Medical Research." In *Studies of Medical Pluralism in Tibetan History and Society: PIATS 2006, Tibetan Studies: Proceedings of the Eleventh Seminar of the International Association for Tibetan Studies, Königswinter 2006*, edited by Sienna R. Craig, et al., 111–36. Andiast, Switzerland: International Institute for Tibetan and Buddhist Studies.

Adams, Vincanne, and Fei-Fei Li. 2008. "Integration or Erasure? Modernizing Medicine at Lhasa's Mentsikhang." In *Tibetan Medicine in the Contemporary World: Global Politics of Medical Knowledge and Practice*, edited by Laurent Pordié, 105–31. London: Routledge.

Adams, Vincanne, Mona Schrempf, and Sienna Craig, eds. 2011. *Medicine Between Science and Religion: Explorations on Tibetan Grounds*. New York: Berghahn.

Ahn, Juhn Y. 2012. "Worms, Germs, and Technologies of the Self—Religion, Sword Fighting, and Medicine in Early Modern Japan." In "Religion and Healing in Japan," edited by Christoph Kleine and Katja Triplett, special issue, *Japanese Religions* 37 (1–2): 93–114.

Akiyama Goan, ed. 1907. *Tanzan oshō zenshū*. Tokyo: Kōyūkan.

American Psychiatric Association. 2013. *Diagnostic and Statistical Manual of Mental Disorders*. 5th ed. Arlington, Va.: American Psychiatric Association.

Anālayo. 2016. *Mindfully Facing Disease and Death: Compassionate Advice from Early Buddhist Texts.* Cambridge: Windhorse.

Andrews, Bridie. 2014. *The Making of Modern Chinese Medicine, 1850–1960.* Vancouver: University of British Columbia Press.

Andrews, Roy Chapman. 1921. *Across Mongolian Plains.* New York: D. Appleton.

Anonymous. 1829. *Yakkun Nattannawā: A Cingalese Poem, Descriptive of the Ceylon System of Demonology, to Which Is Appended The Practices of a Capua or Devil Priest, as Described by a Buddhist, and Kolan Nattannawa: A Cingalese Poem, Descriptive of the Characters Assumed by Natives of Ceylon in a Masquerade.* London: Oriental Translation Fund.

Anonymous. 1891. *Demon Worship and Other Superstitions in Ceylon.* Madras: Christian Vernacular Education Society.

Anonymous. 1896. *The Advantages of Devil Ceremonies—Yak Piḷivetvala Prayojanaya.* Colombo: Wesleyan Methodist Mission Press Colombo and the Ceylon Religious Tract Society.

Anonymous. 1970. "Nanbanji kōhaiki." In *Nihon shisō tōsō shiryō*, vol. 10, edited by Washio Junkyō, 281–308. Tokyo: Meichōkankōkai.

Arai, Paula. 2011. *Bringing Zen Home: The Healing Heart of Japanese Women's Rituals.* Honolulu: University of Hawaiʻi Press.

——. 2019. *Painting Enlightenment: Healing Poetic Meditations on the Art and Science Visions of the Heart Sūtra—The Buddhist Art of Iwasaki Tsuneo.* Boulder, Colo.: Shambhala.

Arasaratnam, Sinnappah. 1996. *Ceylon and the Dutch, 1600–1800: External Influences and Internal Change in Early Modern Sri Lanka.* Brookfield, Vt.: Variorum.

Aris, Michael. 1979. *Bhutan: The Early History of a Himalayan Kingdom.* Warminster, UK: Aris and Phillips.

——. 1986. *Sources for the History of Bhutan.* Wien: Arbeitskreis für Tibetische und Buddhistische Studien, Universität Wien.

Aung-Twin, Maitrii. 2010. "Healing, Rebellion, and the Law: Ethnologies of Medicine in Colonial Burma, 1928–1932." *Journal of Burma Studies* 14 (1): 151–86.

Avertin, Gyurmé, trans. 2012. "A Powerful Pith Instruction to Abstain from Tobacco, the Tenacious Demon Plaguing People of Degenerate Times." Lotsawa House. www.lotsawa house.org/tibetan-masters/jigdral-tutop-lingpa/pith-instruction-to-abstain-from -tobacco.

Baer, Ruth A. 2014. *Mindfulness-Based Treatment Approaches: Clinician's Guide to Evidence Base and Applications.* 2nd ed. London: Academic.

Bahir, Cody R. 2013. "Buddhist Master Wuguang's (1918–2000) Taiwanese Web of the Colonial, Exilic and Han." *Electronic Journal of East and Central Asian Religions* 1 (1): 81–93.

Baigalma, Ürjingiin. 2006. *Mongolyn Ulamjlalt Anagaakh Ukhaany Onoshlogo.* Ulaanbaatar: Khutaibilg Töv.

Baker, Don. 1994. "Monks, Medicine, and Miracles: Health and Healing in the History of Korean Buddhism." *Korean Studies* 18 (1): 50–75.

Baker, Ian. 2017. "Yoga and Physical Culture in Vajrayāna Buddhism and Dzogchen, with Special Reference to Tertön Pema Lingpa's 'Secret Key to the Winds and Channels.'" In *Mandala of Twenty-First Century Perspectives: Proceedings of the International Conference on Tradition and Innovation in Vajrayana Buddhism*, edited by Dasho Karma Ura, Dorji Penjore, and Chhimi Dem, 54–101. Thimphu: Centre for Bhutan Studies.

Bamber, Scott. 1987. "Metaphor and Illness Classification in Traditional Thai Medicine." *Asian Folklore Studies* 46: 179–95.

——. 1998. "Medicine, Food and Poison in Traditional Thai Healing." *Osiris* 13: 339–53.

Bass, Jacquelynn. 2004. *Buddha Mind in Contemporary Art*. Berkeley: University of California Press.

Bdud-'joms 'jigs-bral ye-shes rdo-rje. 1979. *The Collected Writings and Revelations of H. H. Bdud-'joms Rin-po-che 'Jigs-bral-ye-'ses-rdo-rje*. Kalimpong: Dupjung Lama.

Becker, Carl B. 1993. *Breaking the Circle: Death and the Afterlife in Buddhism*. Carbondale: Southern Illinois University Press.

Bell, Charles. 1928. *The People of Tibet*. Oxford: Oxford University Press.

Berman, Michael. 2018. "Religion Overcoming Religions: Suffering, Secularism, and the Training of Interfaith Chaplains in Japan." *American Ethnologist* 45 (2): 228–40.

Bernstein, Gail Lee, 1991. *Recreating Japanese Women, 1600–1945*. Berkeley: University of California Press.

Berounský, Daniel. 2013. "Demonic Tobacco in Tibet." *Mongolo-Tibetica Pragensia* 6 (2): 7–34.

Bertrand, Didier. 2005. "The Therapeutic Role of Khmer Mediums (*kru boramei*) in Contemporary Cambodia." *Mental Health, Religion and Culture* 8 (4): 309–27.

Beyer, C. 1907. "About Siamese Medicine." *Journal of the Siam Society* 4 (1): 1–22.

Bianchi, Ester. 2004. "The Tantric Rebirth Movement in Modern China: Esoteric Buddhism Revivified by the Japanese and Tibetan Traditions." *Acta Orientalia Academiae Scientiarum Hungarica* 57 (1): 31–54.

Biegel, Gina M., Kirk Warren Brown, Shauna L. Shapiro, and Christine M. Schubert. 2009. "Mindfulness-Based Stress Reduction for the Treatment of Adolescent Psychiatric Outpatients: A Randomized Clinical Trial." *Journal of Consulting and Clinical Psychology* 77 (5): 855–66.

Blum, Mark. 2013. *The Nirvana Sutra*. Berkeley: BDK English Tripitaka.

Blum, Mark, and Robert F. Rhodes. 2011. *Cultivating Spirituality: A Modern Shin Buddhist Anthology*. Albany, N.Y.: SUNY Press.

Bodiford, William. 1996. "Zen and the Art of Religious Prejudice: Efforts to Reform a Tradition of Social Discrimination." *Japanese Journal of Religious Studies* 23 (1–2): 1–27.

Bogin, Benjamin. 2008. "The Dreadlocks Treatise: On Tantric Hairstyles in Tibetan Buddhism." *History of Religions* 48 (2): 85–109.

Bokenkamp, Stephen R. 2008. "*Fu*." In *The Encyclopedia of Taoism*, 2 vols., edited by Fabrizio Pregadio, vol. 1, 35–38. New York: Routledge.

Bold, Sharavyn. 2006. *Mongolyn ulamjlalt agagaakh ukhaany tüükh*. Ulaanbaatar: Admon.

Bowers, John Z. 1970. *Western Medical Pioneers in Feudal Japan*. Baltimore, Md.: John Hopkins University Press.

Boxer, Charles Ralph. 1951. *The Christian Century in Japan, 1549–1650*. Berkeley: University of California Press.

Boyd, James W. 1971. "Symbols of Evil in Buddhism." *Journal of Asian Studies* 31 (1): 63–75.

Brac de La Perrière, Bénédicte, Guillaume Rozenberg, and Alicia Turner, eds. 2014. *Champions of Buddhism: Weikza Cults in Contemporary Burma*. Singapore: NUS Press.

Bradley, Dan Beach. 1967. Reprint. "Siamese Practice of Medicine (*Bangkok Calendar*, 1865)." *Sangkhomsat parithat* 5 (3): 83–94.

Brauen-Dolma, Martin. 1985. "Millenarianism in Tibetan Religion." In *Soundings in Tibetan Civilization*, edited by Barbara Nimri Aziz and Matthew Kapstein, 245–56. New Delhi: Manohar.

Braun, Erik. 2013. *The Birth of Insight: Meditation, Modern Buddhism and the Burmese Monk Ledi Sayadaw*. Chicago: University of Chicago Press.

Brown, Michael F. 1997. *The Channeling Zone: American Spirituality in an Anxious Age*. Cambridge, Mass.: Harvard University Press.

Brun, Viggo. 1990. "Traditional Manuals and the Transmission of Knowledge in Thailand." In *The Master Said: To Study and . . .*, edited by Birthe Arendrup, Simon Heilesen, and Jens Ostergård Petersen, 43–65. Copenhagen: East Asian Institute, University of Copenhagen.

Brun, Viggo, and Trond Schumacker. 1987. *Traditional Herbal Medicine in Northern Thailand*. Bangkok: White Lotus.

Bruun, Ole. 2003. *Fengshui in China: Geomantic Divination Between State Orthodoxy and Popular Religion*. Honolulu: University of Hawai'i Press.

Bu, Liping. 2015. "The Patriotic Health Movement and China's Socialist Reconstruction: Fighting Disease and Transforming Society, 1950–80." In *Public Health and National Reconstruction in Post-war Asia: International Influences, Local Transformations*, edited by Liping Bu and Ka-che Yip. London: Routledge.

Burcusa, Stephanie L., and William G. Iacono. 2007. "Risk for Recurrence in Depression." *Clinical Psychology Review* 27 (8): 959–85.

Buswell, Robert E. 1992. *The Zen Monastic Experience: Buddhist Practice in Contemporary Korea*. Princeton, N.J.: Princeton University Press.

Byams pa 'phrin las. 1996. "Bod kyi gso rig rgyud bzhi'i nang don mtshon pa'i sman thang bris cha'i skor la rags tsam dpyad pa." In *Byams pa 'phrin las kyi gsung rtsom phyogs bsgrigs*, 370–81. Beijing: krung go'i bod kyi shes rig dpe skrun khang.

——. 2000. Reprint. *Gangs ljongs gso rig bstan pa'i nyin byed rim byon gyi rnam thar phyogs bsgrigs*. Beijing: Mi rigs dpe skrun khang.

Cadge, Wendy. 2004. *Heartwood: The First Generation of Theravada Buddhism in America*. Chicago: University of Chicago Press.

——. 2013. *Paging God: Religion in the Halls of Medicine*. Chicago: University of Chicago Press.

Carlson, Linda E. 2012. "Mindfulness-Based Interventions for Physical Conditions: A Narrative Review Evaluating Levels of Evidence." *ISRN Psychiatry* 2012: 651583. https://doi.org/10.5402/2012/651583.

Casanova, José. 2006. "Rethinking Secularization: A Global Comparative Perspective." *The Hedgehog Review* 8 (Spring/Summer): 7–22.

Cavanagh, Kate, Clara Strauss, Lewis Forder, and Fergal Jones. 2014. "Can Mindfulness and Acceptance be Learnt by Self-Help? A Systematic Review and Meta-analysis of Mindfulness and Acceptance-Based Self-Help Interventions." *Clinical Psychology Review* 34 (2): 118–29.

Chan, Sucheng. 1991. *Asian Americans: An Interpretive History*. Boston: Twayne.

Chandler, Stuart. 2004. *Establishing a Pure Land on Earth: The Fo Guang Buddhist Perspective on Modernization and Globalization*. Honolulu: University of Hawai'i Press.

Chang, Chia-Feng. 2002. "Disease and Its Impact on Politics, Diplomacy, and the Military: The Case of Smallpox and the Manchus (1613–1795)." *Journal of the History of Medicine and Allied Sciences* 57 (2): 177–97.

Changlyu. 2014. *Ziran shiwu zhenduan shu*. Gaoxiong, Taiwan: Ciyin Magazine.

Chao, Yüan-ling. 2009. *Medicine and Society in Late Imperial China: A Study of Physicians in Suzhou, 1600–1850*. New York: Peter Lang.

Cheah, Joseph. 2011. *Race and Religion in American Buddhism: White Supremacy and Immigrant Adaptation*. New York: Oxford University Press.

Chen, Carolyn. 2008. *Getting Saved in America: Taiwanese Immigration and Religious Experience*. Princeton, N.J.: Princeton University Press.

Chenagtsang, Nida. 2014a. "Sngags kyi bcos thabs ni bod lugs gso rig gi yan lag med du mi rung ba zhig yin 1–3." http://bod.sorig.net/?p=32.

——. 2014b. "Sman sngags zung 'brel gyi nyams zhib dgos pa'i bsam tshul 'ga'. http://bod.sorig .net/?p=154.

——. 2015. *Mirror of Light: A Commentary on Yuthok's Ati Yoga*. Vol. 1. Portland, Oreg.: Sky.

Chervenkova, Velizara. 2017. *Japanese Psychotherapies: Silence and Body-Mind Interconnectedness in Morita, Naikan and Dohsa-hou*. Singapore: Springer.

Chiesa, Alberto, and Alessandro Serretti. 2009. "Mindfulness-Based Stress Reduction for Stress Management in Healthy People: A Review and Meta-analysis." *The Journal of Alternative and Complementary Medicine* 15 (5): 593–600.

Chilson, Clark. 2018. "Naikan: A Meditation Method and Psychotherapy." *Oxford Research Encyclopedias: Religion*. https://doi.org/10.1093/acrefore/9780199340378.013.570.

Chiu, Angela S. 2017. *The Buddha in Lanna: Art, Lineage, Power, and Place in Northern Thailand*. Honolulu: University of Hawai'i Press.

Cho, Eunsu, ed. 2012. *Korean Buddhist Nuns and Laywomen: Hidden Histories, Enduring Vitality*. Albany, N.Y.: SUNY Press.

Cho, Sungtaek. 2002. "Buddhism and Society: On Buddhist Engagement with Society." *Korea Journal* 42 (4): 119–36.

Choden, Kunzang. 2008. "The Malevolent Spirits of sTang valley (Bumthang): A Bhutanese Account." *Revue d'Etudes Tibétaines* 15: 313–30.

Choi, Michael Hyun. 2010. *Orijinol Mansin: An Ethnography of Shaman Life in South Korea*. Cambridge, Mass.: Harvard University Press.

Chokevivat, Vichai, and Anchalee Chuthaputhi. 2005. "The Role of Thai Traditional Medicine in Health Promotion." In *Proceedings of the Sixth Global Conference on Health Promotion*. Bangkok: Department for the Development of Thai Traditional and Alternative Medicine, Ministry of Public Health.

Christian, William A. Jr. 1989. *Person and God in a Spanish Valley*. Princeton N.J.: Princeton University Press.

Clark, Barry. 1995. *The Quintessence Tantras of Tibetan Medicine*. Ithaca, N.Y.: Snow Lion.

Clart, Philip, and Gregory Adam Scott. 2014. *Religious Publishing and Print Culture in Modern China: 1800–2012*. Boston: De Gruyter.

Clausen, Søren. 2000. "Early Modern China: A Preliminary Postmortem." Working Paper 84–00. Centre for Cultural Research, University of Aarhus.

Clifford, Terry. 1989. *Tibetan Buddhist Medicine and Psychiatry: The Diamond Healing*. Irthlingbor-
ough, UK: Crucible, Aquarian.

Coderey, Céline. 2011. "Les maîtres du 'reste': La quête d'équilibre dans les conceptions et les
pratiques thérapeutiques en Arakan (Birmanie)," Ph.D. diss., University of Aix-Marseille.

——. 2014. "Healing Through *Weikza*: Therapeutic Cults in the Arakanese Context." In *Champions
of Buddhism: Weikza Cults in Contemporary Burma*, edited by Bénédicte Brac de la Perrière,
Guillaume Rozenberg, and Alicia Turner, 164–87. Singapore: NUS Press.

——. 2017. "The (Buddhist) Grammar of Healing. Building Therapeutic Efficacy in the Pluralistic
Context of Rakhine, Myanmar." *Asian Medicine* 12: 1–32.

——. 2018. "Immortal Medicine: Understanding the Resilience of Burmese Alchemic Practice,"
Medical Anthropology. https://doi.org/10.1080/01459740.2018.1550756

Cogan, Gina. 2014. *The Princess Nun: Bunchi, Buddhist Reform, and Gender in Early Edo Japan*.
Cambridge, Mass.: Harvard University Press.

Cohen, Paul T. 2001 "Buddhism Unshackled: The Yuan 'Holy Man' Tradition and the Nation-
State in the Tai World." *Journal of South East Asian Studies* 32 (2): 227–47.

——. 2010. "Local Leaders and the State in Thailand." In *Tracks and Traces: Thailand and the Work of
Andrew Turton*, edited by Philip Hirsch and Nicholas Tapp, 39–46. Amsterdam: Amsterdam
University Press.

Cook, Joanna. 2010. *Meditation in Modern Buddhism: Renunciation and Change in Thai Monastic Life*.
Cambridge, Mass.: Cambridge University Press.

——. 2016. "Mindful in Westminster: The Politics of Meditation and the Limits of Neoliberal
Critique." *HAU: Journal of Ethnographic Theory* 6 (1): 141–61.

Cooper, Michael, ed. 1965. *They Came to Japan: An Anthology of European Reports on Japan, 1543-1640*.
Berkeley: University of California Press.

Cornu, Philippe. 1997. *Tibetan Astrology*. Boston: Shambala.

Costanza, Robert, Brendan Fisher, Saleem Ali, Caroline Beer, Lynne Bond, Roelof Boumans,
Nicolas L. Danigelis, Jennifer Dickinson, Carolyn Elliott, Joshua Farley, Diane Elliott Gayer,
Linda MacDonald Glenn, Thomas Hudspeth, Dennis Mahoney, Laurence McCahill, Bar-
bara McIntosh, Brian Reed, S. Abu Turab Rizvi, Donna M. Rizzo, Thomas Simpatico, and
Robert Snapp. 2007. "Quality of Life: An Approach Integrating Opportunities, Human
Needs, and Subjective Well-Being." *Ecological Economics* 61 (2–3): 267–76.

Costanza, Robert, Maureen Hart, Stephen Posner, and John Talberth. 2009. "Beyond GDP: The
Need for New Measures of Progress." *Pardee Papers* no. 4. Boston: Frederick S. Pardee
Center for the Study of the Longer-Range Future, Boston University. www.bu.edu
/pardee/files/documents/PP-004-GDP.pdf.

Covell, Stephen. 2005. *Japanese Temple Buddhism: Worldliness in a Religion of Renunciation*. Honolulu:
University of Hawai'i Press.

Craig, Sienna. 2012. *Healing Elements: Efficacy and the Social Ecologies of Tibetan Medicine*. Berkeley:
University of California Press.

Crane, Rebecca S., and Willem Kuyken. 2013. "The Implementation of Mindfulness-Based
Cognitive Therapy: Learning from the UK Health Service experience." *Mindfulness* 4 (3):
246–54.

Crozier, Ralph C. 1968. *Traditional Medicine in Modern China: Science, Nationalism, and the Tensions of
Cultural Change*. Cambridge, Mass.: Harvard University Press.

Cuevas, Bryan. 2008. *Travels in the Netherworld: Buddhist Popular Narratives of Death and the Afterlife in Tibet.* Oxford: Oxford University Press.

——. 2009. "The 'Calf's Nipple' (*Be'u bum*) of Ju Mipam ('Ju Mi pham): A Handbook of Tibetan Ritual Magic." In *Tibetan Ritual*, edited by José Ignacio Cabezón, 165–86. Oxford: Oxford University Press.

Cuomu, Mingji. 2010. "Qualitative and Quantitative Research Methodology in Tibetan Medicine: The History, Background and Development of Research in Sowa Rigpa." In *Medicine Between Science and Religion: Explorations on Tibetan Grounds*, edited by Vincanne Adams, Mona Schrempf, and Sienna R. Craig, 245–63. New York: Berghahn.

Cush, Denise. 1996. "British Buddhism and the New Age." *Journal of Contemporary Religion* 11 (2): 195–208.

Dai-Ichi Life Insurance Institute (Kotani Midori, chief researcher). 2006. "Zenkoku no 40-sai kara 74-sai made no danjō 1000-mei ni kiita *Nichijōsei ni okeru shūkyōteki kōdō to ishiki chōsa*. *Dai-Ichi Seimei News Takuhaibin*, June.

Davies, Gloria, L. 2013. *Lu Xun's Revolution: Writing in a Time of Violence.* Cambridge, Mass.: Harvard University Press.

Davis, Daphne M., and Jeffrey A Hayes. 2011. "What Are the Benefits of Mindfulness? A Practice Review of Psychotherapy-Related Research." *Psychotherapy* 48 (2), 198–208.

De Michelis, Elizabeth. 2004. *A History of Modern Yoga: Patanjali and Western Esotericism.* London: Continuum.

De Nebesky-Wojkowitz, René. 1956. Reprint. *Oracles and Demons of Tibet: The Cult and Iconography of the Tibetan Protective Deities.* Taipei: SMC.

De Vibe, Michael, Arild Bjørndal, Elizabeth Tipton, and Karianne Thune Hammerstrøm. 2012. "Mindfulness-Based Stress Reduction (MBSR) for Improving Health, Quality of Life, and Social Functioning in Adults." *Campbell Systematic Reviews* 2012 (3). https://doi.org/10.4073/csr.2012.3.

DeCaroli, Robert. 2004. *Haunting the Buddha: Indian Popular Religions and the Formation of Buddhism.* New York: Oxford University Press.

DeHart, Jonathan. August 5, 2013. "Bhutan's New PM Tshering Tobgay Questions the Politics of Happiness." *The Diplomat.* https://thediplomat.com/2013/08/bhutans-new-pm-tshering-tobgay-questions-the-politics-of-happiness/.

Dharmachakra Translation Committee. 2006. *Deity, Mantra, and Wisdom: Development Stage Meditation in Tibetan Buddhist Tantra.* Ithaca, N.Y.: Snow Lion.

Di Cosmo, Nicola. 2012. "From Alliance to Tutelage: A Historical Analysis of Manchu–Mongol Relations Before the Qing Conquest." *Frontiers of History in China* 7 (2): 175–97.

Dickman, Henry. 1863. "Treatment of Diseases by Charms, as Practised by the Singhalese in Ceylon." *Transactions of the Ethnological Society of London* 2: 140–46.

Ding Fubao. 1920. *Foxue cuoyao.* Shanghai: Yixue shuju.

Djurdjevic, Goran. 2014. *India and the Occult: The Influence of South Asian Spirituality on Modern Western Occultism.* New York: Palgrave Macmillan.

Doctor, Andreas. 2005. *Tibetan Treasure Literature: Revelation, Tradition, and Accomplishment in Visionary Buddhism.* Ithaca, N.Y.: Snow Lion.

Dorje, Gyurme. 1991. "The rNying-ma Interpretation of Commitment and Vow." *The Buddhist Forum* 2: 71–95.

Dorjee, Pema. 2005. *The Spiritual Medicine of Tibet: Heal Your Spirit, Heal Yourself.* London: Watkins.

Douglas, Nik. 1978. *Tibetan Tantric Charms and Amulets.* New York: Dover.

Dreyfus, Georges. 2003. *The Sound of Two Hands Clapping: The Education of a Tibetan Buddhist Monk.* Berkeley: University of California Press.

Drungtso, Tsering Thakchoe. 2008. *Healing Power of Mantra: The Wisdom of Tibetan Healing Science.* Dharamshala, India: Drungtso.

DuBois, Thomas David. 2005. *The Sacred Village: Social Change and Religious Life in Rural North China.* Honolulu: University of Hawai'i Press.

——. 2008. "Manchukuo's Filial Sons: States, Sects and the Adaptation of Graveside Piety." *East Asian History* 36: 3–28.

Düdjom Rinpoche, Jikdrel Yeshe Dorje. 1991. *The Nyingma School of Tibetan Buddhism: Its Fundamentals and History,* translated and edited by Gyurme Dorje and Matthew Kapstein. Boston: Wisdom.

Ebisawa Arimichi. 1944. *Kirishitan no shakai katsudō oyobi Nanban igaku.* Tokyo: Fuzanbō.

——, trans. 1964. *Nanbanji kōhaiki, Jakyō taii, Myōtei mondo, Ha deusu.* Tokyo: Heibonsha.

Edou, Jérôme. 1996. *Machig Labdrön and the Foundations of Chöd.* Ithaca, N.Y.: Snow Lion.

Eglauer, Anton. 1794. *Die Missionsgeschichte späterer Zeiten, oder, Gesammelte Briefe der katholischen Missionare aus allen Theilen der Welt. Ein wichtiger Beytrag zur Natur-, Länder- und Völkerkunde, vorzüglich aber zur christlichen Erbauung. Der Briefe aus Ostindien erster-[dritter] Theil.* 3 vols. Augsburg: N. Doll.

Elison, George. 1973. *Deus Destroyed: The Image of Christianity in Early Modern Japan.* Cambridge, Mass.: Harvard University Press.

Elman, Benjamin A. 2001. *From Philosophy to Philology: Intellectual and Social Aspects of Change in Late Imperial China.* Rev. ed. Los Angeles: University of California, Los Angeles, Asian Pacific Monograph Series.

——. 2005. *On Their Own Terms: Science in China, 1550-1900.* Cambridge, Mass.: Harvard University Press.

——. 2011. "Early Modern or Late Imperial Philology? The Crisis of Classical Learning in Eighteenth Century China." *Frontiers of History in China* 6: 3–25.

——, ed. 2015. *Antiquarianism, Language, and Medical Philology: From Early Modern to Modern Sino-Japanese Medical Discourses.* Leiden: Brill.

Elverskog, Johan. 2006. *Our Great Qing: The Mongols, Buddhism and the State in Late Imperial China.* Honolulu: University of Hawai'i Press.

Emmerick, Ronald Eric. 1977. "Sources of the rGyud-bzhi." *Zeitschrift der Deutschen Morgenländischen Gesellschaft* 3 (Supplement, Deutscher Orientalistentag vom 28. Sept. bis 4. Okt. 1975 in Frieburg i. Br.): 1135–42.

England, Richard W. 1998. "Measurement of Social Well-Being: Alternatives to Gross Domestic Product." *Ecological Economics* 25: 89–103.

Eppsteiner, Fred, ed. 1988. *The Path of Compassion: Writing Socially Engaged Buddhism.* Berkeley, Calif.: Parallax.

Epstein, Mark, and Sonam Topgay. 1982. "Mind and Mental Disorders in Tibetan Medicine." *ReVision: A Journal of Consciousness and Change* 9 (1): 67–79.

Esposito, Monica. 2008. "Sanguan." In *The Encyclopedia of Daoism,* edited by Fabrizio Pregadio, 835–36. New York: Routledge.

Fang, Xiaoping. 2012. *Barefoot Doctors and Western Medicine in China*. Rochester, N.Y.: University of Rochester Press.

Feltus, George Haws, ed. 1936. *Abstract of the Journal of Rev. Dan Beach Bradley, M.D., Medical Missionary in Siam, 1835-1873*. Cleveland, Ohio: Pilgrim Church.

Ferguson, John P., and E. Michael Mendelson. 1981. "Masters of the Buddhist Occult: The Burmese Weikzas." *Contributions to Asian Studies* 16: 62–80.

Ford, James L. 2002. "Jokei and the Rhetoric of 'Other-Power' and 'Easy Practice' in Medieval Japanese Buddhism." *Japanese Journal of Religious Studies* 29 (1–2): 67–106.

Foster, Kenelm, and Silvester Humphries, trans. 1954. *Aristotle's De Anima: In the Version of William of Moerbeke and the Commentary by St. Thomas of Aquinas*. New Haven, Conn.: Yale University Press.

Foxeus, Niklas. 2011. "The Buddhist World Emperor's Mission: Millenarian Buddhism in Postcolonial Burma." Ph.D. diss., Stockholm University, Stockholm.

——. 2016. "'I Am the Buddha, the Buddha Is Me': Concentration Meditation and Esoteric Modern Buddhism in Burma/Myanmar." *NUMEN* 63 (4): 411–45.

Fróis, Luís, Georg Schurhammer, and Ernst Arthur Voretzsch, trans. 1926. *Die Geschichte Japans (1549-1578)*. Leipzig: Verlag der Asia major.

Fróis, Luís, and Josef Wicki, eds. 1976–84. *Historia de Japam*. 5 vols. Lisboa: Presidência do Conselho de Ministros, Secretaria de Estado da Cultura, Direcção-Geral do Património Cultural, Biblioteca Nacional de Lisboa.

Furth, Charlotte. 2007. "Producing Medical Knowledge Through Cases: History, Evidence, and Action." In *Thinking with Cases: Specialist Knowledge in Chinese Cultural History*, edited by Charlotte Furth, Judith T. Zeitlin, and Ping-chen Hsiung, 125–51. Honolulu: University of Hawai'i Press.

Furuta Shōkin. 1980. "Hara Tanzan to jikken Bukkyō-gaku." *Nihon Daigaku Seishin Bunka Kenkyūjo Kyōiku Seidō Kenkyūjo kiyō* 11: 145–67.

Ga, Yang. 2010. "The Sources for the Writing of the Rgyud Bzhi, Tibetan Medical Classic." Ph.D. diss., Harvard University.

——. 2014. "The Origin of the *Four Tantras* and an Account of Its Author, Yuthog Yonten Gonpo." In *Bodies in Balance: The Art of Tibetan Medicine*, edited by Theresia Hofer, 154–77. Seattle: Rubin Museum of Art, New York, and University of Washington Press.

Garcia, José Manuel, 1997. *Cartas que os padres e irmãos da Companhia de Iesus escreuerão dos Reynos de Iapão y China aos da mesma Companhia da India, y Europa, des do anno de 1549 atè o de 1580* [Facsimile of edition published as "Em Evora por Manoel de Lyra. Anno de MDXCVIII" (1598)]. 2 vols. Maia: Castoliva.

Garrett, Frances. 2009a. "Eating Letters in the Tibetan Treasure Tradition." *Journal of the International Association of Buddhist Studies* 32 (1–2): 85–114.

——. 2009b. "The Alchemy of Accomplishing Medicine (*sman sgrub*): Situating the Yuthok Heart Essence (*G.yu thog snying thig*) in Literature and History." *Indian Philosophy* 37: 207–30.

Garrett, Frances, and Vincanne Adams. 2008. "The Three Channels in Tibetan Medicine with a Translation of Tsultrim Gyaltsen's 'A Clear Explanation of the Principle Structure and Location of the Circulatory Channels as Illustrated in the Medical Paintings.'" *Traditional South Asian Medicine* 8: 86–114.

Gayley, Holly. 2007. "Patterns in the Ritual Dissemination of Padma Gling pa's Treasures." In *Bhutan: Tradition and Changes*, edited by John Ardussi and Françoise Pommaret, 97–119. Leiden: Brill.

——. 2017. *Love Letters from Golok: A Tantric Couple in Modern Tibet*. New York: Columbia University Press.

Gelder, Stuart, and Roma Gelder. 1965. *The Timely Rain: Travels in New Tibet*. New York: Monthly Review.

Gerke, Barbara. 2012. *Long Lives and Untimely Deaths: Life-Span Concepts and Longevity Practices Among Tibetans in the Darjeeling Hills, India*. Leiden: Brill.

——. 2014. "The Art of Tibetan Medical Practice." In *Bodies in Balance: The Art of Tibetan Medicine*, edited by Theresia Hofer, 16–31. Seattle: Rubin Museum of Art, New York, and University of Washington Press.

Germano, David. 1997. "Food, Clothes, Dreams, and Karmic Propensities." In *Religions of Tibet in Practice*, edited by Donald S. Lopez Jr, 221–40. Princeton, N.J.: Princeton University Press.

Gill, Tom, Brigitte Steger, and David H. Slater, eds. 2013. *Japan Copes with Calamity: Ethnographies of the Earthquake, Tsunami and Nuclear Disasters of March 2011*. Bern: Peter Lang.

Gimello, Robert M., Robert E. Buswell, and Richard D. McBride. 2014. *The State, Religion, and Thinkers in Korean Buddhism*. Seoul: Dongguk University Press.

Givel, Michael. 2015. "Mahayana Buddhism and Gross National Happiness in Bhutan." *International Journal of Wellbeing* 5 (2): 14–27.

Goldstein, Melvyn C. 1989. *A History of Modern Tibet, 1913-1951: The Demise of the Lamaist State*. Berkeley: University of California Press.

——, ed. 2001. *The New Tibetan-English Dictionary of Modern Tibetan*. Berkeley: University of California Press.

——. 2007. *A History of Modern Tibet*. Vol. 2, *The Calm Before the Storm, 1951-1955*. Berkeley: University of California Press.

Goleman, Daniel, and Richard J. Davidson. 2017. *Altered Traits: Science Reveals How Meditation Changes Your Mind, Brain, and Body*. New York: Penguin.

Gooneratne, Dandris De Silva. 1865. "On Demonology and Witchcraft in Ceylon." *Journal of the Ceylon Branch of the Royal Asiatic Society* 4 (13): 1–117.

Goossaert, Vincent. 2013. "The Local Politics of Festivals: Hangzhou, 1850–1950," *Daoism Religion, History & Society* 5: 57–80.

——. 2019. "Doing Historical–Anthropological Fieldwork in Jiangnan: Gazetteers, Newspapers, and Real Life." In *Out of the Archive: A Fieldwork Research Reader on Modern Chinese History*, edited by Thomas DuBois and Jan Kiely. London: Routledge.

Goyal, Madhav, Sonal Singh, Erica M. S. Sibinga, Neda F. Gould, Anastasia Rowland-Seymour, Ritu Sharma, Zackary Berger, Dana Sleicher, David D. Maron, Hasan M. Shihab, Padmini D. Ranasinghe, Shauna Linn, Shonali Saha, Eric Bass, and Jennifer A. Haythornthwaite. 2014. "Meditation Programs for Psychological Stress and Well-Being: A Systematic Review and Meta-analysis." *Journal of the American Medical Association, Internal Medicine* 174 (3): 357–68.

Graf, Tim. 2016. "Buddhist Responses to the 3.11 Disasters in Japan." In *Disasters and Social Crisis in Contemporary Japan: Political, Religious, and Cultural Responses*, edited by Mark Mullins and Nakano Koichi, 156–81. Basingstoke: Palgrave Macmillan.

Grayson, James H. 2013. *Korea: A Religious History*. New York: Routledge.

Griffiths, Paul. 1981. "Buddhist Hybrid English: Some Notes on Philology and Hermeneutics for Buddhologists." *Journal of the International Association of Buddhist Studies* 4 (2): 17–32.

Gu, Mingyuan. 2013. *Cultural Foundations of Chinese Education*. Boston: Brill.

Guest, Kenneth. 2003. *God in Chinatown: Religion and Survival in New York's Evolving Immigrant Community*. New York: New York University Press.

Gutierrez, Cathy. 2015. *Handbook of Spiritualism and Channeling*. Leiden: Brill.

Gyatso, Desi Sangyé. 2010. *Mirror of Beryl: A Historical Introduction to Tibetan Medicine*, translated by Gavin Kilty. Somerville, Mass.: Wisdom.

Gyatso, Janet. 1999. *Apparitions of Self: The Secret Autobiographies of a Tibetan Visionary*. Princeton, N.J.: Princeton University Press.

——. 2004. "The Authority of Empiricism and the Empiricism of Authority: Medicine and Buddhism in Tibet on the Eve of Modernity." *Comparative Studies of South Asia, Africa and the Middle East* 24 (2): 83–96.

——. 2015. *Being Human in a Buddhist World: An Intellectual History of Medicine in Early Modern Tibet*. New York: Columbia University Press.

Haas, Hans. 1904. *Geschichte des Christentums in Japan: Fortschritte des Christentums unter dem Superioriat des P. Cosmo de Torres*. Supplement Bd. 5, 7, der "Mittheilungen" der Deutschen Gesellschaft für Natur- und Völkerkunde Ostasiens. Vol. 2. Tokyo: Buchdruck der Rikkyo Gakuin.

Hackett, Paul G. 2013. *Theos Bernard, the White Lama: Tibet, Yoga, and American Religious Life*. New York: Columbia University Press.

Hall, David L., and Roger T. Ames. 1987. *Thinking Through Confucius*. Albany, N.Y.: SUNY Press.

Halliwell, Ed. 2010. *Mindfulness Report*. London: Mental Health Foundation.

Hammerstrom, Erik J. 2012. "Early Twentieth-Century Buddhist Microbiology and Shifts in Chinese Buddhism's 'Actual Canon,'" *Theology and Science* 10: 3–18.

——. 2015. *The Science of Chinese Buddhism: Early Twentieth-Century Engagements*. New York: Columbia University Press.

Hanegraaff, Wouter. 1998. *New Age Religion and Western Culture: Esotericism in the Mirror of Secular Thought*. Albany, N.Y.: SUNY Press.

Hanson, Marta E. 2011. *Speaking of Epidemics in Chinese Medicine: Disease and the Geographic Imagination in Late Imperial China*. New York: Routledge.

Hara Tanzan. 1988 [1885]. *Daijōkishinron ryō yaku shōgi kōgi*. Tokyo: Banshōin Kōunji.

Hardacre, Helen. 2007. "Aum Shinrikyō and the Japanese Media: The Pied Piper Meets the Lamb of God." *History of Religions* 47 (2–3): 171–204.

Hardiman, David, and Projit Bihari Mukharji. 2012. *Medical Marginality in South Asia: Situating Subaltern Therapeutics*. London: Routledge.

Harding, Christopher, Iwata Fumiaki, and Yoshinaga Shin'ichi, eds. 2014. *Religion and Psychotherapy in Modern Japan*. London: Routledge.

Harrington, Ann. 2008. *The Cure Within: A History of Mind-Body Medicine*. New York: W. W. Norton.

Hashimoto, Akira. 2014. "Psychiatry and Religion in Modern Japan: Traditional Temple and Shrine Therapies." In *Religion and Psychotherapy in Modern Japan*, edited by Christopher Harding, Iwata Fumiaki, and Yoshinaga Shin'ichi, 51–75. London: Routledge.

Hattori, Tōrō. 1971. *Muromachi Azuchi Momoyama jidai igaku-shi no kenkyū*. Tokyo: Yoshikawa kōbunkan.

Hayashi Razan. 1979. "Sōzoku zenki." In *Hayashi Razan bunshū*, edited by Kyōto shisekikai. Tokyo: Perikansha.

Heelas, Paul. 1996. *The New Age Movement: Religion, Culture and Society in the Age of Postmodernity*. Cambridge, Mass.: Blackwell.

Helderman, Ira P. 2016. "Drawing the Boundaries Between 'Religion' and 'Secular' in Psychotherapists' Approaches to Buddhist Traditions in the United States." *Journal of the American Academy of Religion* 84 (4): 937–72.

Heruka [Chenagtsang], Nida, and Yeshe Drolma. 2015. *Rten 'brel sngags bcos rig pa*. Beijing: Mi rigs dpe skrun khang.

Heuschert, Dorothea. 1998. "Legal Pluralism in the Qing Empire: Manchu Legislation for the Mongols." *The International History Review* 20 (2): 310–24.

Hickey, Wakoh S. 2010. "Meditation as Medicine: A Critique." *CrossCurrents* 60 (2):168–84.

——. 2015. "Two Buddhisms, Three Buddhisms, and Racism." In *Buddhism Beyond Borders: New Perspectives on Buddhism in the United States*, edited by Scott A. Mitchell and Natalie E. F. Quli, 35–56. Albany, N.Y.: SUNY Press.

Hinrichs, T. J., and Linda L. Barnes. 2013. *Chinese Medicine and Healing: An Illustrated History*. Cambridge, Mass.: Harvard University Press.

Hirota, Dennis. 2014. "Christian Tradition in the Eyes of Asian Buddhists: The Case of Japan." In *The Oxford Handbook of Christianity in Asia*, edited by Felix Wilf, 411–27. Oxford: Oxford University Press.

Hofer, Theresia. 2011. "Changing Representations of the Female Tibetan Medical Doctor Khandro Yangkar (1907–1973)." In *Buddhist Himalayas: Studies in Religion, History and Culture*, vol. 1, edited by Alex McKay and Anna Balicki-Dengjongpa, 99–122. Gangtok: Namgyal Institute of Tibetology.

Hofer, Theresia, and Knud Larsen. 2014. "Pillars of Tibetan Medicine: The Chagpori and the Mentsikhang Institutes in Lhasa." In *Bodies in Balance: The Art of Tibetan Medicine*, edited by Theresia Hofer, 257–67. Seattle: University of Washington Press.

Holmes-Tagchungdarpa, Amy. 2017. "Beyond Living Buddhas, Snowy Mountains and Mighty Mastiffs: Imagining Tibetan Buddhism in Contemporary China's Mediascape." In *Religion and Media in China: Insights and Case Studies from the Mainland, Taiwan, and Hong Kong*, edited by Stefania Travagnin, 256–74. New York: Routledge.

Hopkins, Donald. 2002. *The Greatest Killer*. Chicago: University of Chicago Press.

Hori Ichirō. 1968. *Folk Religion in Japan: Continuity and Change*. Chicago: Chicago University Press.

Horner, I. B. 2000. *The Book of the Discipline (Vinaya-Piṭaka)*. Vol. 4, *Mahāvagga*. Oxford: Pāli Text Society.

Houtman, Gustaaf. 1990. "Traditions of Buddhist Practices in Burma." Ph.D. diss., School of Oriental and African Studies, University of London.

Huang Xianian, ed. 2006. *Minguo Fojiao qikan wenxian jicheng*. 209 vols. Beijing: Quanguo tushuguan wenxian suowei fuzhi zhongxin.

Huber, Toni. Forthcoming. *Source of Life: Revitalization Rites and Bon Shamans in Bhutan and the Eastern Himalayas*. Vienna: Austrian Academy of Sciences.

Huntington, C. W. Jr. 2015. "The Triumph of Narcissism: Theravāda Buddhist Meditation in the Marketplace." *Journal of the American Academy of Religion*, 83 (3): 624–48.

Inoue Enryō. 1901. "Wakubyō dōgen-ron." *Enryō zuihitsu*, 13. Tokyo: Tetsugakukan.

Inoue, Katsuhito. 2014. "Meiji-Era Academic Philosophy and Its Lineage: Monism of the True Form and Organismic Philosophy." *Kokusai tetsugaku kenkyū* 3: 271–89.

Irwin, Anthony Lovenheim. 2017. "Partners in Power and Perfection: *Khrubas*, Construction, and *Khu Barami* in Chiang Rai, Thailand." In *Charismatic Monks of Lanna Buddhism*, edited by Paul T. Cohen, 87–114. Copenhagen: Nordic Institute of Asian Studies Press.

Ishii, Yoneo. 1986. *Sangha, State, and Society: Thai Buddhism in History*. Honolulu: University of Hawai'i Press.

Jacobson, Eric. 2002. "Panic Attack in a Context of Comorbid Anxiety and Depression in a Tibetan Refugee." *Culture, Medicine and Psychiatry* 26 (2): 259–79.

——. 2007. "Life-Wind Illness in Tibetan Medicine: Depression, Generalised Anxiety, and Panic Attack." In *Soundings in Tibetan Medicine: Historical and Anthropological Perspectives. Proceedings of the Tenth Seminar of the International Association of Tibetan Studies (PIATS), Oxford, 2003*, edited by Mona Schrempf, 225–46. Leiden: Brill.

Jacoby, Sarah. 2015. *Love and Liberation: Autobiographical Writings of the Tibetan Buddhist Visionary Sera Khandro*. New York: Columbia University Press.

Jaffe, Richard M. 2010. *Neither Monk nor Layman: Clerical Marriage in Modern Japanese Buddhism*. Honolulu: University of Hawai'i Press.

Jagar Dorji, ed. 2015. *The Intangible Cultural Heritage of Bhutan*. Thimphu: Research and Media Division, National Library and Archives of Bhutan.

Japanese Naikan Medical Association and Japanese Naikan Association, eds. 2013. *Naikan Therapy: Techniques and Principles for Use in Clinical Practice*. Fukuoka: Daido Gakkan.

Jigmed. 2009. *Mongol anaġakhu ukhaġan-u teükhe bolon erten-u surbalǰi bičig-yin sinǰilege*. Ulaanbaatar: Soyombo.

Jinkhene Dagaj Yavakh Khuuly. 2004. *Dürem: 1913–1918*. Edited and transliterated into Cyrillic by Bayarsaikhan. Ulaanbaatar: University of Mongolia.

Joffe, Ben. 2017. "Interview with Dr Nida Chenagtsang on Tibetan Tantra and Medicine." *A Perfumed Skull*. https://perfumedskull.com/2017/02/18/interview-with-dr-nida-chenagtsang -on-tibetan-tantra-and-medicine.

Johnston, William D. 2016. "Buddhism Contra Cholera: How the Meiji State Recruited Religion Against Epidemic Disease." In *Science, Technology, and Medicine in the Modern Japanese Empire*, edited by David G. Wittner and Philip C. Brown, 62–78. London: Routledge.

Jones, Noa. 2014. "Buddhism in Bhutanese Education." In *Global Perspectives in Spirituality and Education*, edited by Jacqueline Watson, Marian de Souza, and Ann Trousdale, 153–65. New York: Routledge.

Joo, Ryan Bongseok. 2011. "Countercurrents from the West: 'Blue-Eyed' Zen Masters, Vipassanā Meditation, and Buddhist Psychotherapy in Contemporary Korea." *Journal of the American Academy of Religion* 79 (3): 614–38.

Jordt, Ingrid. 2007. *Burma's Mass Lay Meditation Movement: Buddhism and the Cultural Construction of Power*. Athens: Ohio University Press.

Josephson, Jason Ānanda. 2012. *The Invention of Religion in Japan*. Chicago: University of Chicago Press.

Kabat-Zinn, Jon. 1990. *Full Catastrophe Living: How to Cope with Stress, Pain and Illness Using Mindfulness Meditation*. New York: Delacorte.

——. 1994. *Wherever You Go There You Are: Mindfulness Meditation in Everyday Life*. New York: Hyperion.

Kang, Xiaofei. 2006. *The Cult of the Fox: Power, Gender and Popular Religion in Late Imperial and Modern China*. New York: Columbia University Press.

Kapferer, Bruce. 1983. *A Celebration of Demons: Exorcism and the Aesthetics of Healing in Sri Lanka*. Bloomington: Indiana University Press.

——. 1997. *The Feast of the Sorcerer: Practices of Consciousness and Power*. Chicago: University of Chicago Press.

Kasai, Kenta. 2016. "Introducing Chaplaincy to Japanese Society: A Religious Practice in Public Space." *Journal of Religion in Japan* 5 (2–3): 246–62.

Kasamatsu, Akira, and Tomio Hirai. 1966. "An Electroencephalographic Study on the Zen Meditation (Zazen)." *Psychiatry and Clinical Neurosciences* 20 (4): 315–36.

Kawahara Ryuzō. 2003. "Naikanhō no kokusai ni mukete." *Seishin shinkeigaku zasshi* 105 (8): 988–93.

Kendall, Laurel. 1985. *Shamans, Housewives, and Other Restless Spirits: Women in Korean Ritual Life*. Honolulu: University of Hawai'i Press.

——. 1998. "Who Speaks for Korean Shamans When Shamans Speak of the Nation?" In *Making Majorities: Constituting the Nation in Japan, Korea, China, Malaysia, Fiji, Turkey, and the United States*, edited by Dru C. Gladney, 55–72. Stanford, Conn.: Stanford University Press.

——. 2009a. "Shifting Intellectual Terrain: 'Superstition' Becomes 'Culture' and 'Religion.'" In *Shamans, Nostalgias, and the IMF: South Korean Popular Religion in Motion*, 1–33. Honolulu: University of Hawai'i Press.

——. 2009b. "The Global Reach of Gods and the Travels of Korean Shamans." In *Transnational Transcendence: Essays on Religion and Globalization*, edited by Thomas J. Csordas, 305–26.

Kendall, Laurel, Yang Jongsung, and Yoon Yul Soo. 2015. *God Pictures in Korean Contexts: The Ownership and Meaning of Shaman Paintings*. Honolulu: University of Hawai'i Press.

Keown, Damien. 2003. *A Dictionary of Buddhism*. Oxford: Oxford University Press.

Keyes, Charles. 1971. "Buddhism and National Integration in Thailand." *Journal of Asian Studies* 30 (3): 551–67.

Khempo Sodargye. 2013. *Mysteries of the World According to Buddhism*. New York: Bodhi Institute of Compassion and Wisdom.

Khenpo Phuntsok Tashi. 2004. "The Role of Buddhism in Achieving Gross National Happiness." In *Gross National Happiness and Development: Proceedings of the First International Conference on Operationalization of Gross National Happiness*, edited by Karma Ura and Karma Galay, 483–95. Thimphu, Bhutan: Centre for Bhutan Studies.

Khenpo Sodargye. 2008. "Xiyan zhi guohuan." *KhenpoSodargye.org*. http://www.zhibeifw.com/va/1a31e78b-c2fa-11e7-b81c-1c1b0d070cdb/. Archived at https://web.archive.org/web/20180703145508/https://www.zhibeifw.com/va/1a31e78b-c2fa-11e7-b81c-1c1b0d070cdb/, last accessed July 3, 2018.

Khoury, Bassam, Tania Lecomte, Brandon A. Gaudiano, and Karine Paquin. 2013. "Mindfulness Interventions for Psychosis: A Meta-analysis." *Schizophrenia Research* 150 (1): 176–84.

Kim, Dong-kyu. 2012. "Reconfiguration of Korean Shamanic Ritual: Negotiating Practices Among Shamans, Clients, and Multiple Ideologies." *Journal of Korean Religions* 3 (2): 11–37.

Kim, Kwang-Ok. 1993. "The Religious Life of the Urban Middle Class." *Korea Journal* 33 (4): 5–33.

Kim, Taegon. 1999. "Definition of Korean Shamanism." In *Culture of Korean Shamanism*, edited by Chun Shinyong, 9–44. Seoul: Kimpo College Press.

Kimura Kiyotaka. 2001. "Hara Tanzan to 'Indo tesugaku' no tanjō: kindai Nihon Bukkyōshi no ichidanmen." *Indo tetsugaku Bukkyōgaku kenkyū* 49 (2), 533–41.

King, Winston L. 1980. *Theravada Meditation: The Buddhist Transformation of Yoga*. University Park: Pennsylvania State University Press.

——. 1986. *Death Was His Kōan: The Samurai-Zen of Suzuki Shōsan*. Berkeley, Calif.: Asian Humanities Press.

Kingston, Jeff, ed. 2012. *Natural Disaster and Nuclear Crisis in Japan: Response and Recovery After Japan's 3/11*. London: Routledge.

Kitagawa, Joseph Mitsuo. 1989. "Buddhist Medical History." In *Healing and Restoring: Health and Medicine in the World's Religious Traditions*, edited by Lawrence E. Sullivan, 9–32. New York: Macmillan.

Kitsuse, John. 1965. "Moral Treatment and Reformation of Inmates in Japanese Prisons." *Psychologia* 8: 9–23.

Klautau, Orion. 2008. "Against the Ghosts of Recent Past: Meiji Scholarship and the Discourse on Edo-Period Buddhist Decadence." *Japanese Journal of Religious Studies* 35 (2): 263–303.

——. 2012. *Kindai Nihon shisō toshite no Bukkyō shigaku*. Kyoto: Hōzōkan.

Kloos, Stephan. 2010. "Tibetan Medicine in Exile: The Ethics, Politics and Science of Cultural Survival." Ph.D. diss., University of California, San Francisco, and University of California, Berkeley.

Knecht, Peter. 2003. "Aspects of Shamanism." In *Shamans in Asia*, edited by Clark Chilson and Peter Knecht, 1–30. London: RoutledgeCurzon.

Kohn, Livia, ed. 1981. *Taoist Meditation and Longevity Techniques*. Michigan Monographs in Chinese Studies 61. Ann Arbor: Center for Chinese Studies, University of Michigan.

——, ed. 2000. *Daoism Handbook*. Leiden: Brill.

——. 2006. "Yoga and Daoyin." In *Daoist Body Cultivation*, edited by Livia Kohn. Magdalena, N. Mex.: Three Pines.

Komjathy, Louis. 2013. *The Daoist Tradition: An Introduction*. London: Bloomsbury Academic.

Korom, Frank. 1997. "'Editing' Dharmaraj: Academic Genealogies of a Bengali Folk Deity." *Western Folklore* 56 (1): 51–77.

Kratoska, Paul H., ed. 2001. *South East Asia: Colonial History*. 6 vols. London: Routledge.

K'uei-chi. 2001. *A Comprehensive Commentary on the* Heart Sutra, translated by Shih Heng-ching and Dan Lusthaus. Moraga, Calif.: BDK America.

Kuriyama, Shigehisa. 1999. *The Expressiveness of the Body and the Divergence of Greek and Chinese Medicine*. New York: Zone.

Kuroita Katsumi and Kokushi taikei henshūkai, eds. 1981–1982. *Tokugawa jikki*, Kokushi taikei. Tokyo: Yoshikawa kōbunkan

Kuyken, Willem, Sarah Byford, Rod S. Taylor, Ed Watkins, Emily Holden, Kat White, Barbara Barrett, Richard Byng, Alison Evans, Eugene Mullan, and John D. Teasdale. 2008. "Mindfulness-Based Cognitive Therapy to Prevent Relapse in Recurrent Depression." *Journal of Consulting and Clinical Psychology* 76 (6): 966–78.

Kyle, Richard. 1995. *The New Age Movement in American Culture*. Lanham, Md.: University Press of America.

Lang, Karen. 2003. *Four Illusions: Candrakīrti's Advice for Travelers on the Bodhisattva Path*. Oxford: Oxford University Press.

Langer, Susanne. 1957. *Problems of Art: Ten Philosophical Lectures*. New York: Scribner.

Langford, Jean M. 2002. *Fluent Bodies: Ayurvedic Remedies for Postcolonial Imbalance*. Durham, N.C.: Duke University Press.

Laufer, Berthold. 1924. *Tobacco and Its Use in Asia*. Anthropology Leaflet no. 18. Chicago: Field Museum of Natural History.

Laures, Johannes. 1951. *Die Anfänge der Mission von Miyako*. Missionswissenschaftliche Abhandlungen und Texte. Münster: Aschendorff.

Lebra, Takei Sugiyama. 1984. *Japanese Women: Constraint and Fulfillment*. Honolulu: University of Hawai'i Press.

Leuchtenberger, Jan C. 2013. *Conquering Demons: The 'Kirishitan,' Japan, and the World in Early Modern Japanese Literature*. Ann Arbor: University of Michigan, Center for Japanese Studies.

Leung, Angela Ki-che. 1997. "Medical Learning from the Song to the Ming." In *The Song-Yuan-Ming Transition in Chinese History*, edited by Paul Jakov Smith and Richard von Glahn, 374–98. Cambridge, Mass.: Harvard University Press.

Lewis, James R., and J. Gordon Melton, eds. 1992. *Perspectives on the New Age*. Albany, N.Y.: SUNY Press.

Lha mo skyid. 2010. *Bod kyi gso rig skor gyi shes bya dris len blo gsal nyer mkho*. Beijing: Mi rigs dpe skrun khang.

Li, Wei-tsu. 1954. "On the Cult of the Four Sacred Animals (*Szu Ta Men*) in the Neighbourhood of Peking." *Folklore Studies* 7: 1–94.

Lin, Irene. 1996. "Journey to the Far West: Chinese Buddhism in America." *Amerasia Journal* 22: 106–32.

Lin, Noel Yuan. 2001. "Finding Buddha in the West: An Ethnographic Study of a Chinese Buddhist Community in North Carolina." Master's thesis, University of North Carolina at Chapel Hill.

Lindahl, Jared R., Nathan E. Fisher, David J. Cooper, Rochelle K. Rosen, and Willoughby B. Britton. 2017. "The Varieties of Contemplative Experience: A Mixed-Methods Study of Meditation-Related Challenges in Western Buddhists." *PLoS One* 12 (5): e0176239. https://doi.org/10.1371/journal.pone.0176239.

Ling, Trevor. 1978. "Buddhist Bengal, and After," in *History and Society: Essays in Honor of Professor Niharranjan Ray*, edited by Debiprasad Chattopadhyaya, 317–25. Calcutta: Bagchi.

Liu, Guohui, and Henry McCann. 2016. *Discussion of Cold Damage (Shang Han Lun): Commentaries and Clinical Applications*. Philadelphia, Pa.: Singing Dragon.

Liu, Xun. 2012. "Scientizing the Body for the Nation: Chen Yingning and the Reinvention of Daoist Inner Alchemy in 1930s Shanghai." In *Daoism in the Twentieth Century: Between Eternity and Modernity*, edited by David A. Palmer, 154–72. Berkeley: University of California Press.

Liu Zuyi and Sun Guangrong, eds. 2002. *Zhongguo lidai mingyi mingshu*. Beijing: Zhongyi guji chubanshe.

Lobsang-Samrübnima. 2008 [1817]. *Getülgegči degedü blam-a adiltǧal ügei ačitu Bogda Sumadi Šila Širi Badr-a-yin gegein-ü eirünghei-yin jokhiol namtar-i tobči-yin tedüi egülegsen süsüg-ün linqu-a-yi müsiyelgegči naran-u gerel degedü mör-i geyigülün üildügči khemegdekhü orošiba*, translated by Jurmeddanzan. Khokhot: People's Press Bureau of Inner Mongolia.

Lobsang Tsültim. 1785. *Ba sam sman mar bya tshul bzhugs so*. Xylographic print, folios 1–8. Authors' private collection.

Lobsang Wangyal. 2007. *My Life, My Culture: Autobiography and Lectures on the Relationship Between Tibetan Medicine, Buddhist Philosophy and Tibetan Astrology and Astronomy*, translated by Bhuchung D. Sonam and Dhondup Tsering. Dharamsala: Paljor.

Loizzo, Joseph J., Leslie J. Blackhall, and Lobsang Rapgay. 2009. "Tibetan Medicine: A Complementary Science of Optimal Health." *Annals of the New York Academy of Sciences* 1172 (1): 218–30.

Lopez, Donald S. Jr. 2001. *The Story of Buddhism: A Concise Guide to Its History and Teachings*. New York: Harper.

——. 2008. *Buddhism and Science: A Guide for the Perplexed*. Chicago: University of Chicago Press.

Lord, Donald C. 1969. *Mo Bradley and Thailand*. Grand Rapids, Mich.: Eerdmans.

Low, Morris, ed. 2005. *Building a Modern Japan: Science, Technology, and Medicine in the Meiji Era and Beyond*. New York: Palgrave Macmillan.

Lu, Huitzu. 2002. "Women's Ascetic Practices during the Song." *Asia Major* 15 (1): 73–108.

Lu, Yan. 2004. *Re-understanding Japan: Chinese Perspectives, 1895–1945*. Honolulu: University of Hawai'i Press.

Lü, Yingfan. 1984. "Yu Chang." In *Qingdai Renwu Zhuankao*. Vol. 3, edited by Qingshi bianjihui, 273–79. Beijing: Zhonghua shuju.

Lusthaus, Dan. 2004. "Yogācāra School." In *Encyclopedia of Buddhism*, edited by Robert E. Buswell Jr., 914–21. New York: Macmillan Reference.

Lutz, Antoine, John Dunne, and Richard J. Davidson. 2007. "Meditation and the Neuroscience of Consciousness: An Introduction." In *The Cambridge Handbook of Consciousness*, edited by Philip David Zelazo, Morris Moscovitch, and Evan Thompson, 499–553. Cambridge: Cambridge University Press.

Ma, S. Helen, and John D. Teasdale. 2004. "Mindfulness-Based Cognitive Therapy for Depression: Replication and Exploration of Differential Relapse Prevention Effects." *Journal of Consulting and Clinical Psychology* 72 (1): 31–40.

Ma gcig lab sgron. 2003. *Machik's Complete Explanation: Clarifying the Meaning of Chöd; A Complete Explanation of Casting Out the Body as Food*, translated by Sarah Harding. Ithaca, N.Y.: Snow Lion.

Macdonald, Keith Norman. 1879. *The Practice of Medicine Among the Burmese, Translated from Original Manuscripts, with an Historical Sketch of the Progress of Medicine, from the Earliest Times*. Edinburgh: Maclachlan and Stewart.

Mao Juntong and Ding Guangdi. 1992. "Yu Chang." In *Zhongyi Gejia Xueshuo*, edited by Qiu Peiran and Ding Guangdi, 592–601. Beijing: Renmin weisheng chubanshe.

Masini, Federico. 1993. *The Formation of Modern Chinese Lexicon and Its Evolution Toward a National Language*. Rome: Department of Oriental Studies, University of Rome.

Matthieu, Ricard. 2001. *The Quantum and the Lotus: A Journey to the Frontiers Where Science and Buddhism Meet*. New York: Crown.

Maxey, Trent E. 2014. *The "Greatest Problem": Religion and State Formation in Meiji Japan*. Cambridge, Mass.: Harvard University Press.

McBride, Richard D. 2005. "Dhāraṇī and Spells in Medieval Sinitic Buddhism." *Journal of the International Association of Buddhist Studies* 28 (1): 85–114.

McCrone, Paul, Sujith Dhanasiri, Anita Patel, Martin Knapp, and Simon Lawton-Smith. 2008. *Paying the Price: The Cost of Mental Health Care in England to 2026*. London: King's Fund.

McDaniel, Justin. 2008. *Gathering Leaves and Lifting Words: Histories of Buddhist Monastic Education in Laos and Thailand*. Chiang Mai: Silkworm.

McKay, Alex. 2004. "British–Indian Medical Service Officers in Bhutan, 1905–1947: A Historical Outline." In *The Spider and the Piglet: Proceedings of the First International Seminar on Bhutan Studies*, edited by Karma Ura and Sonam Kinga, 137–59. Thimphu: Centre for Bhutan Studies.

——. 2005a. " 'The Birth of a Clinic'? The IMS Dispensary in Gyantse (Tibet), 1904–1910." *Medical History* 49: 135–54.

——. 2005b. " 'It Seems He Is an Enthusiast About Tibet': Lieutenant-Colonel James Guthrie, OBE (1906–71)." *Journal of Medical Biography* 13 (3): 128–35.

——. 2005–06. " 'An Excellent Measure': The Battle Against Smallpox in Tibet, 1904–47." *The Tibet Journal* 30/31 (4/1): 119–30.

——. 2007a. *Their Footprints Remain: Biomedical Beginnings Across the Indo-Tibetan Frontier*. Amsterdam: Amsterdam University Press.

——. 2007b. "Himalayan Medical Encounters: The Establishment of Biomedicine in Tibet and in Indian Exile." In *Soundings in Tibetan Medicine: Historical and Anthropological Perspectives*, edited by Mona Schrempf, 9–27. Leiden: Brill.

McKibben, Bill. 2007. *Deep Economy: The Wealth of Communities and the Durable Future*. New York: Time Books.

McLaughlin, Levi. 2013a. "What Have Religious Groups Done After 3.11? Part 1: A Brief Survey of Religious Mobilization after the Great East Japan Earthquake Disasters." *Religion Compass* 7 (8): 294–308.

——. 2013b. "What Have Religions Done After 3.11? Part 2: From Religious Mobilization to 'Spiritual Care.' " *Religion Compass* 7 (8): 309–25.

——. 2016. "Hard Lessons Learned: Tracking Media Presentations of Religion and Religious Mobilizations After the 1995 and 2011 Disasters in Japan." *Asian Ethnology* 75 (1): 105–37.

——. 2018. *Soka Gakkai's Human Revolution: The Rise of a Mimetic Nation in Modern Japan*. Honolulu: University of Hawai'i Press.

McMahan, David L., and Erik Braun, eds. 2017. *Meditation, Buddhism, and Science*. New York: Oxford University Press.

McManus, Freda, Christina Surawy, Kate Muse, Maria Vazquez-Montes, and J. Mark G. Williams. 2012. "A Randomized Clinical Trial of Mindfulness-Based Cognitive Therapy Versus Unrestricted Services for Health Anxiety (Hypochondriasis)." *Journal of Consulting and Clinical Psychology* 80 (5): 817–28.

McVeigh, Brian. 2017. *The History of Japanese Psychology: Global Perspectives, 1875–1950*. London: Bloomsbury Academic.

Mendelson, E. Michael. 1963. "Observations on a Tour in the Region of Mount, Central Burma." *France-Asie* 19 (179): 780–807.

Messner, Angelika C. 2000. "Emotions in Late Imperial Chinese Medical Discourse: A Preliminary Report." *Ming Qing Yanjiu* 9: 197–215.

——. 2006a. "Emotions, Body, and Bodily Sensations Within an Early Field of Expertise Knowledge in China." In *From Skin to Heart: Perceptions of Emotions and Bodily Sensations in Traditional Chinese Culture*, edited by Paolo Santangelo and Ulrike Middendorf, 41–66. Wiesbaden: Otto Harrassowitz.

——. 2006b. "Making Sense of Signs: Emotions in Chinese Medical Texts." In *Love, Hatred, and Other Passions: Questions and Themes on Emotions in Chinese Civilization*, edited by Paolo Santangelo and Donatella Guida, 91–109. Leiden: Brill.

——. 2016. *Zirkulierende Leidenschaft*. Köln: Böhlau.

Metcalf, Franz Aubrey. 2002. "The Encounter of Buddhism and Psychology." In *Westward Dharma: Buddhism Beyond Asia*, edited by Charles S. Prebish and Martin Baumann, 348–64. Berkeley: University of California Press.

Meyer, Ferdinand. 1998. *The History and Foundations of Tibetan Medicine*. New York: Rizzoli.

Mgon po skyabs. 2008. *Gso rig dpyad rtsom kun+da dgyes pa'i zla zer*. Beijing: Mi rigs dpe skrun khang.

Michel, Wolfgang. 2001. "On the Reception of Western Medicine in Seventeenth Century Japan." In *Higashi to nishi no iryōbunka*, edited by Yoshida Tadashi and Fukase Yasuaki, 3–17. Kyoto: Shibunkaku shuppan.

Millard, Colin. 2007. "Tibetan Medicine and the Classification and Treatment of Mental Illness." In *Soundings in Tibetan Medicine: Historical and Anthropological Perspectives. Proceedings of the Tenth Seminar of the International Association of Tibetan Studies (PIATS), Oxford, 2003*, edited by Mona Schrempf, 247–82. Leiden: Brill.

Millioud, Alfred. 1895a. "Histoire du convent catholique de Kyōto (1568–85): préface." *Revue de l'histoire des religions* 31: 270–91.

——. 1895b. "Histoire du convent catholique de Kyōto (1568–85) (Suite et fin)." *Revue de l'histoire des religions* 32: 23–55.

Mindfulness All-Party Parliamentary Group. 2015. *Mindful Nation UK*. London: The Mindfulness Initiative. www.themindfulnessinitiative.org.uk/images/reports/Mindfulness-APPG -Report_Mindful-Nation-UK_Oct2015.pdf.

Ministry of Health. n.d. *National Health Policy*. Thimphu, Bhutan: Ministry of Health. www .health.gov.bt/wp-content/uploads/moh-files/2015/11/National-Health-Policy.pdf.

Mitra, Amalendu. 1972. *Rarher Sanskriti O Dharma Thakur*. Calcutta: Firma KL Mukhopadhyay.

Miyata, Taisen. 1999. *Ajiakan: A Manual for the Esoteric Meditation*. Los Angeles: Koyasan Beikoku Betsuin.

Moffat, Abbot Low. 1961. *Mongkhut, the King of Siam*. Ithaca, N.Y.: Cornell University Press.

Mollier, Christine. 2008. *Buddhism and Taoism Face to Face: Scripture, Ritual, and Iconographic Exchange in Medieval China*. Honolulu: University of Hawai'i Press.

Moran, Joseph F. 1993. *The Japanese and the Jesuits: Alessandro Valignano in Sixteenth-Century Japan*. London: Routledge.

Morgan, David. 2005. *The Sacred Gaze: Religious Visual Culture in Theory and Practice*. Berkeley: University of California Press.

Mthu-stobs gling-pa. 2013. *Gter chos*. 10 vols. Chengdu: Si khron bod yig dpe rnying 'tshol bsdu rtsom sgrig khang.

Mukharji, Projit Bihari. 2016a. *Doctoring Traditions: Ayurveda, Small Technologies and Braided Sciences*. Chicago: University of Chicago Press.

——. 2016b. "Feringhee Dharma: Augustinians, Amerindians and a Bengali Deity in an Early Modern Iberian World," *South Asian History and Culture* 7 (1): 37–54.

Muller, A. Charles. 1999. *The Sutra of Perfect Enlightenment: Korean Buddhism's Guide to Meditation (with Commentary by the Son Monk Kihwa)*. Albany, N.Y.: SUNY Press.

——, ed. 2018. *Digital Dictionary of Buddhism*. www.buddhism-dict.net/ddb/.

Mullholland, Jean. 1979. "Thai Traditional Medicine: Ancient Thought and Practice in a Thai Context." *Journal of the Siam Society* 67 (2): 80–115.

——. 1988. "Ayurveda, Congenital Disease and Birthdays in Thai Traditional Medicine." *Journal of the Siam Society* 76: 174–82.

Murase Masamitsu. 2012. "Kanwa kea byōtō ni okeru shūkyōsha no katsudō no genjō: bihāra ni okeru bihārasō." *Nihon bukkyō shakai fukushigaku nenpō* 43.

National Collaborating Centre for Mental Health. 2010. *Depression in Adults with a Chronic Physical Health Problem: Treatment and Management*. NICE Clinical Guidelines no. 91. Leicester and London: British Psychological Society and Royal College of Psychiatrists.

Nattier, Jan. 1992. "The *Heart Sūtra*: A Chinese Apocryphal Text?" *Journal of the International Association of Buddhist Studies* 15 (2): 153–223.

Naylor, Chris, Michael Parsonage, David McDaid, Martin Knapp, Matt Fossey, and Amy Galea. 2012. *Long-Term Conditions and Mental Health: The Cost of Co-morbidities*. London: King's Fund.

Ng, On-cho. 2003. "The Epochal Concept of 'Early Modernity' and the Intellectual History of Late Imperial China." *Journal of World History* 14: 37–61.

NHS England. July 11, 2013. *The NHS Belongs to the People: A Call to Action*. NHS England. www.england.nhs.uk/2013/07/call-to-action/.

Nomura, Akiko. 2000. *Ōoku no saishō: Ona no tsubone*. Tokyo: Sōbunsha.

Numrich, Paul D. 2005. "Complementary and Alternative Medicine in America's 'Two Buddhisms.' " In *Religion and Healing in America*, edited by Linda L. Barnes and Susan S. Sered, 343–57. Oxford: Oxford University Press.

Nyoshul Khenpo, Jamyang Dorje. 2005. *A Marvelous Garland of Rare Gems: Biographies of Masters of Awareness in the Dzogchen Lineage*, translated by Richard Barron. Junction City, Calif.: Padma.

Obeyesekere, Gananath. 1969. "The Ritual Drama of the Sanni Demons: Collective Representations of Disease in Ceylon." *Comparative Studies in Society and History* 11 (2): 174–216.

——. 1970. "The Idiom of Demonic Possession: A Case Study." *Social Science & Medicine* 4: 97–111.

Ochi. 1996. *Chahar Géshé Lobsang Tsültim*. Khailaar: Inner Mongolia National Printing.

Oda Tokuno. 1917. *Bukkyō Daijiten*. Tokyo: Ōkura shuten.

Okabe Takeshi. 2012. "Higashi Nihon daishinsai to kanwa kea: zaitaku to hisai no genba kara kangaeru." *Kanwa kea* 22 (1): 6–10.

Okuno Shūji. 2013. *Mitori sensei no yuigon*. Tokyo: Bungei Shunjū.

Olson, Grant A. 1992. "Thai Cremation Volumes: A Brief History of a Unique Genre of Literature." *Asian Folklore Studies* 51 (2): 279–94.

Onda Akira. 2002. "The Development of Buddhist Psychology in Modern Japan." In *Awakening and Insight: Zen Buddhism and Psychotherapy*, edited by Polly Young-Eisendrath and Shoji Muramoto, 235–44. New York: Routledge.

O'Neal, Halle. 2018. *Word Embodied: The Jeweled Pagoda Mandalas in Japanese Buddhist Art*. Cambridge, Mass.: Harvard University Press.

Ong, Aihwa. 2003. *Buddha Is Hiding: Refugees, Citizenship, the New America*. Berkeley: University of California Press.

Ong, Saraphanmathurot. 1969. "*Banthuek pathom het thi dai phop lae kan pan lo rup boromakhuru phaet Chiwaka Komaraphat*." In *Winyan mi ching rue mai lae prawat boromakhuru Chiwaka Komaraphat*, 17–26. Bangkok: Wat Makutakasat.

Orzech, Charles D., Richard K. Payne, and Henrik H. Sørensen. 2011. "Introduction: Esoteric Buddhism and the Tantras in East Asia: Some Methodological Considerations." In *Esoteric Buddhism and the Tantras of East Asia*, edited by Charles D. Orzech, Henrik H. Sørensen, and Richard K. Payne, 1–18. Leiden: Brill.

Ōshita Daien. 2005. *Iyashi iyasareru supirichuarukea: iryō, fukushi, kyōiku ni ikasu bukkyō no kokoro*. Tokyo: Igakushoin.

——. 2006. "Mikkyō to supirichuaru kea." In *Koyasan daigaku sensho kankokai*, vol. 3, edited by Gendai ni mikkyō wo tō, 112–23. Kōyacho, Japan: Kōyasan. University Anthology Publication Committee, Kōyasan University.

——. 2010. *Keya to taijin enjō ni ikasu meisō ryōhō*. Tokyo: Igakushoin.

——. 2016a. *Rinshō meisō hō: kokoro to shintai ga yomigaeru yottsu no mesoddo*. Tokyo: Nippon Kangokyōkai Shuppansha.

——. 2016b. *Mikkyō tairaku ni ikiru waza: tōgō meisō ga anata wo kaeru*. Tokyo: Nippon Hyoronsha.

Ospina, Maria B., Kenneth Bond, Mohammad Karkhaneh, Lisa Tjosvold, Ben Vandermeer, Yuanyuan Liang, Liza Bialy, Nicola Hooton, Nina Buscemi, Donna M. Dryden, and Terry P. Klassen. 2007. *Meditation Practices for Health: State of the Research*. Evidence Reports/ Technology Assessments, no. 155. Rockville, Md.: Agency for Healthcare Research and Quality.

Ownby, David, Vincent Goossaert, and Ji Zhe, eds. 2017. *Making Saints in Modern China*. New York: Oxford University Press.

Oyunchimeg. 2002. *Encyclopaedia of Mongolology: Medicine*. Khuh hot: People's Press Bureau of Inner Mongolia.

Ozawa-de Silva, Chikako. 2006. *Psychotherapy and Religion in Japan: The Japanese Introspective Practice of Naikan*. London: Routledge.

——. 2015. "Mindfulness of the Kindness of Others: The Contemplative Practice of Naikan in Cultural Context." *Transcultural Psychiatry* 52 (4): 524–42.

Palmer, David A. 2007. *Qigong Fever: Body, Science, and Utopia in China*. New York: Columbia University Press.

Paramore, Kiri. 2009. *Ideology and Christianity in Japan*. Abingdon, Oxon: Routledge.

Parfionovitch, Yuri, Gyurme Dorje, and Fernand Meyer, eds. 1991–92. *Tibetan Medical Paintings: Illustrations to the Blue Beryl Treatise of Sangye Gyamtso*. 2 vols. London: Serindia.

Park, Jin Y., ed., 2012. *Makers of Modern Korean Buddhism*. Albany, N.Y.: SUNY Press.

Park, Sung Hyun, Seoung Yun Sung, and Mi San Mi San. 2016. "A Mixed-Methods Study of the Psychological Process of Loving-Kindness Meditation and Its Effects on Heart-Smile Meditation Participants." *Korean Psychological Association Journal: Counseling and Psychotherapy* 28 (2). https://doi.org/10.23844/kjcp.2016.05.28.2.395.

Parry, Richard Lloyd. 2017. *Ghosts of the Tsunami: Death and Life in Japan's Disaster Zone*. New York: Farrar, Strauss and Giroux.

Patton, Thomas Nathan. 2012. "In Pursuit of the Sorcerer's Power: Sacred Diagrams as Technologies of Potency." *Contemporary Buddhism* 13 (2): 213–31.

——. 2016a. "Buddhist Salvation Armies as Vanguards of the Sāsana: Sorcerer Societies in Twentieth-Century Burma." *The Journal of Asian Studies* 75 (4): 1083–1104.

——. 2016b. "The Wizard King's Granddaughters: Burmese Buddhist Female Mediums, Healers, and Dreamers." *Journal of the American Academy of Religion* 84 (2): 430–65.

——. 2018. *The Buddha's Wizards: Magic, Healing and Protection in Burmese Buddhism*. New York: Columbia University Press.

Perdue, Peter. 2005. *China Marches West: The Qing Conquest of Central Eurasia*. Cambridge, Mass.: Harvard University Press.

Piet, Jacob, and Esben Hougaard. 2011. "The Effect of Mindfulness-Based Cognitive Therapy for Prevention of Relapse in Recurrent Major Depressive Disorder: A Systematic Review and Meta-analysis." *Clinical Psychology Review* 31 (6): 1032–40.

Pike, Sarah M. 2004. *New Age and Neopagan Religions in America*. New York: Columbia University Press.

Pittman, Don A. 2001. *Toward a Modern Chinese Buddhism: Taixu's Reforms*. Honolulu: University of Hawai'i Press.

Planning Commission Secretariat, Royal Government of Bhutan. 2000. *Bhutan National Human Development Report 2000: Gross National Happiness and Human Development—Searching for Common Ground*. Thimphu, Bhutan: Planning Commission Secretariat, Royal Government of Bhutan. http://hdr.undp.org/sites/default/files/bhutan_2000_en.pdf.

Plath, David. 1975. "The Last Confucian Sandwich Becoming Middle Aged." In *Adult Episodes in Japan*, edited by David Plath, 51–63. Leiden: Brill.

Poceski, Mario. 2009. *Chinese Religions: The eBook*. Providence, Utah: Journal of Buddhist Ethics Online Books.

Potkin, Fanny. March 31, 2016. "For Unbanked Populations, the Future of Banking Is Pocket-Size: A Dispatch from the Streets of Myanmar." *How We Get to Next*. https://howweget tonext.com/for-unbanked-populations-the-future-of-banking-is-pocket-size -c18fcf1a4acb.

Powers, John. 1995. *Introduction to Tibetan Buddhism*. Boulder, Colo.: Snow Lion.

Pozdneyev, Aleksei Matveevich. 1971. *Mongolia and the Mongols*. Vols. 1–2, translated by John Roger Show and Dale Plank, and edited by John R. Krueger. Uralic and Altaic Series, Vols. 61–61/2. Bloomington: Indiana University Press.

——. 1980. *Sketches of Life of Buddhist Monasteries and Buddhist Clergy in Mongolia*. Seattle: University of Washington Press.

Pranke, Patrick. 1995. "On Becoming a Buddhist Wizard." In *Buddhism in Practice*, edited by Donald S. Lopez, 343–58. Princeton, N.J.: Princeton University Press.

Pranke, Patrick. 2010 [2011]. "On Saints and Wizards—Ideals of Human Perfection and Power in Contemporary Burmese Buddhism." *Journal of the International Association of Buddhist Studies* 33 (1–2): 453–88.

——. 2014. "On Saints and Wizards: Ideals of Human Perfection in Contemporary Burmese Buddhism." In *Champions of Buddhism: Weikza Cults in Contemporary Burma*, edited by

Bénédicte Brac de la Perrière, Guillaume Rozenberg, and Alicia Turner, 3–31. Singapore: National University of Singapore Press.

Pregadio, Fabrizio. 2008. "Dantian." In *The Encyclopedia of Daoism*, edited by Fabrizio Pregadio, 302–3. New York: Routledge.

Prothero, Stephen R. 1996. *The White Buddhist: The Asian Odyssey of Henry Steel Olcott*. Bloomington: Indiana University Press.

Puaksom, Davisakd. 2007. "Of Germs, Public Hygiene, and the Healthy Body: The Making of the Medicalizing State in Thailand." *Journal of Asian Studies* 66 (2): 311–44.

Purser, Ronald E., David Forbes, and Adam Burke, eds. 2016. *Handbook of Mindfulness: Culture, Context, and Social Engagement*. Switzerland: Springer.

Qian Qianyi. 2001 [1658]. "Yu Jiayan *yimen falü zu*." In *Qian Muzhai Quanji*, vol. 5, edited by Qian Zhonglian, 718. Shanghai: Shanghai guji chubanshe.

Quli, Natalie E. 2009. "Western Self, Asian Other: Modernity, Authenticity, and Nostalgia for 'Tradition' in Buddhist Studies." *Journal of Buddhist Ethics* 16: 18.

Reader, Ian. 2000. *Religious Violence in Contemporary Japan: The Case of Aum Shinrikyō*. Honolulu: University of Hawai'i Press.

Rechung Rinpoche. 1973. *Tibetan Medicine: Illustrated in Original Texts*. Berkeley: University of California Press.

Reed, Christopher A. 2004. *Gutenberg in Shanghai: Chinese Print Capitalism, 1876–1937*. Vancouver: UBC Press.

Reff, Daniel T., Richard K. Danford, and Robin Gill, eds. 2014. *The First European Description of Japan, 1585: A Critical English-Language Edition of* Striking Contrasts in the Customs of Europe and Japan *by Luis Fróis, S.J*. London: Routledge.

Rigyal, Samdrup, and Alyson Prude. 2017. "Buddhism in Contemporary Bhutan." In *The Oxford Handbook of Contemporary Buddhism*, edited by Michael Jerryson, 61–78. Oxford: Oxford University Press.

Ritzinger, Justin. 2017. *Anarchy in the Pure Land: Reinventing the Cult of Maitreya in Modern Chinese Buddhism*. New York: Oxford University Press.

Rogaski, Ruth. 2004. *Hygienic Modernity: Meanings of Health and Disease in Treaty-Port China*. Berkeley: University of California Press.

Rozenberg, Guillaume. 2001. "Thamanya : enquête sur la sainteté dans la Birmanie contemporaine." Ph.D. diss., École des Hautes Études en Sciences Sociales, Paris.

——. 2010. *Les immortels: Visages de l'incroyable en Birmanie bouddhiste*. Vannes: Éditions Sully.

——. 2015. *The Immortals: Faces of the Incredible in Buddhist Burma*. Honolulu: Hawai'i University Press.

Salguero, C. Pierce. 2009. "The Buddhist Medicine King in Literary Context: Reconsidering an Early Medieval Example of Indian Influence on Chinese Medicine and Surgery." *History of Religions* 48 (3): 183–210.

——. 2014a. "Medicine." *Oxford Bibliographies Online: Buddhism*. Last updated March 28, 2018. https://doi.org/10.1093/obo/9780195393521-0140.

——. 2014b. *Translating Buddhist Medicine in Medieval China*. Philadelphia: University of Pennsylvania Press.

——. 2015a. "Reexamining the Categories and Canons of Chinese Buddhist Healing." *Journal of Chinese Buddhist Studies* 28: 35–66.

——. 2015b. "Toward a Global History of Buddhism and Medicine." *Buddhist Studies Review* 32 (1): 35–61.

——. 2016. *Traditional Thai Medicine: Buddhism, Animism, Yoga, Ayurveda.* Revised edition. Bangkok: White Lotus.

——. 2017. "Honoring the Teachers, Constructing the Lineage: A *Wai Khru* Ritual Among Healers in Chiang Mai, Thailand." In *Translating the Body: Medical Education in Southeast Asia*, edited by Hans Pols, C. Michele Thompson, and John Harley Warner, 295–318. Singapore: National University of Singapore Press.

——. 2018. "'This Fathom-Long Body': Bodily Materiality and Ascetic Ideology in Medieval Chinese Buddhist Scriptures." *Bulletin of the History of Medicine* 92: 237–60.

——. 2019. "Varieties of Buddhist Healing in Multiethnic Philadelphia." *Religions* 10 (1), doi:10.3390/rel10010048. https://www.mdpi.com/2077-1444/10/1/48

Samuel, Geoffrey. 1993. *Civilized Shamans: Buddhism in Tibetan Societies.* Washington, D.C.: Smithsonian Institution Press.

——. 1999. "Religion, Health and Suffering Among Contemporary Tibetans." In *Religion, Health and Suffering*, edited by John R. Hinnells and Roy Porter, 85–110. London: Kegan Paul International.

——. 2001. "Tibetan Medicine in Contemporary India: Theory and Practice." In *Healing Powers and Modernity: Traditional Medicine, Shamanism, and Science in Asian Studies*, edited by Linda H. Connor and Geoffrey Samuel, 247–68. London: Bergin and Garvey.

——. 2007. "Spirit Causation and Illness in Tibetan Medicine." In *Soundings in Tibetan Medicine: Anthropological and Historical Perspectives*, edited by Mona Schrempf, 213–24. Leiden: Brill.

——. 2014. "Healing in Tibetan Buddhism." In *The Wiley Blackwell Companion to East and Inner Asian Buddhism*, edited by Mario Poceski, 278–96. Chichester, UK: John Wiley.

Samuels, Jeffrey, Justin Thomas McDaniel, and Mark Michael Rowe, eds. 2016. *Figures of Buddhist Modernity in Asia.* Honolulu: University of Hawai'i Press.

Sangyé Gyatso. 1691. *Man ngag lhan thabs.* Xylographic print.

Sarfati, Liora. 2016. "Shifting Agencies Through New Media: New Social Statuses for Female South Korean Shamans." *Journal of Korean Studies* 21 (1): 179–211.

Sárközi, Alice. 1999. "The Magic of Writing Edible Charms." *Studia Orientalia* 87: 227–34.

Sastri, Haraprasad. 1894. "Remnants of Buddhism in Bengal." *Proceedings of the Asiatic Society of Bengal (January–December 1893)*: 135–38.

——. 1897. *Discovery of Living Buddhism in Bengal.* Calcutta: Hare.

Schäfer, Dagmar. 2011. *The Crafting of the Ten Thousand Things: Knowledge and Technology in Seventeenth-Century China.* Chicago: University of Chicago Press.

Scheid, Volker. 2013. "Transmitting Chinese Medicine: Changing Perceptions of Body, Pathology, and Treatment in Late Imperial China." *Asian Medicine* 8 (2): 299–360.

——. 2017. "Promoting Free Flow in the Networks: Reimagining the Body in Early Modern Suzhou." *History of Science* 56 (2): 131–67.

——. Forthcoming. *Renaissance and Enlightenment in Seventeenth Century East Asia: The View from Medicine.* Oxford: Berghahn.

Schilling, Konrad. 1931. "Das Schulwesen der Jesuiten in Japan (1551–1614)." Ph.D. diss. Münster: Regensbergschen Buchdruckerei.

Schmidt, Stefan. 2014. "Opening Up Meditation for Science: The Development of a Meditation Classification System." In *Meditation-Neuroscientific Approaches and Philosophical Implications*, edited by Stefan Schmidt and Harald Walach, 137–52. Switzerland: Springer.

Schober, Juliane. 1980. "On Burmese Horoscopes." *The South East Asian Review* 10 (1): 43–56.

——. 1988. "The Path to Buddhahood: The Spiritual Mission and Social Organisation of Mysticism in Contemporary Burma." *Crossroads* 4 (1): 13–30.

Schopen, Gregory. 2017. "The Training and Treatment of an Indian Doctor in a Buddhist Text." In *Buddhism and Medicine: An Anthology of Premodern Sources*, edited by C. Pierce Salguero, 184–204. New York: Columbia University Press.

Schoppa, R. Keith. 2000. *The Columbia Guide to Modern Chinese History*. Columbia Guides to Asian History. New York: Columbia University Press.

Schrempf, Mona. 2011. "Between Mantra and Syringe: Healing and Health-Seeking Behaviour in Contemporary Amdo." In *Medicine Between Science and Religion: Explorations on Tibetan Grounds*, edited by Vincanne Adams, Mona Schrempf, and Sienna Craig, 157–84. New York: Berghahn.

——. 2015a. "Becoming a Female Ritual Healer in East Bhutan." *Revue d'Etudes Tibétaines* 34: 189–213.

——. 2015b. "Fighting Illness with Gesar—A Healing Ritual from Eastern Bhutan." In *Tibetan and Himalayan Healing: An Anthology for Anthony Aris*, edited by Charles Ramble and Ulrike Rösler, 621–30. Oxford: Oxford University Press.

——. 2015c. "Spider, Soul, and Healing in Eastern Bhutan." In *From Bhakti to Bon: Festschrift for Per Kværne*, edited by Hanna Havnevik and Charles Ramble, 481–97. Oslo: Institute for Comparative Research in Human Culture.

Schrempf, Mona, and Nicola Schneider, eds. 2015. "Women as Visionaries, Healers and Agents of Social Transformation in the Himalayas, Tibet, and Mongolia," *Revue d'Etudes Tibétaines* 34 (special issue): 1–217.

Schurhammer S. J., Georg. 1928. *Das kirchliche Sprachproblem in der japanischen Jesuitenmission des 16 und 17 Jahrhunderts: ein Stück Ritenfrage*. Tokyo: Deutsche Gesellschaft für Natur- und Völkerkunde Ostasiens.

Schütte, S. J., and Josef Franz. 1951. *Valignanos Missionsgrundsätze für Japan. Von der Ernennung zum Visitator bis zum ersten Abschied von Japan (1573-1582), I Teil: Das Problem (1573-1580)*, Rome: Edizioni di storia e letteratura.

——. 1958. *Valignanos Missionsgrundsätze für Japan. Von der Ernennung zum Visitator bis zum ersten Abschied von Japan (1573-1582), II. Teil Die Lösung (1580-1582)*. Rome: Edizioni di storia e letteratura.

Scott, David. 1994. *Formations of Ritual: Colonial and Anthropological Discourses on the Sinhala Yaktovil*. Minneapolis: University of Minnesota Press.

Scott, Gregory A. 2015. "Navigating the Sea of Scriptures: The Buddhist Studies Collectanea, 1918-1923." In *Religious Publishing and Print Culture in Modern China, 1800-2012*, edited by Philip Clart and Gregory Adam Scott, 91–138. Boston: De Gruyter.

Segal, Zindel V., J. Mark G. Williams, and John D. Teasdale. 2013. *Mindfulness-Based Cognitive Therapy for Depression*. 2nd ed. New York: Guilford.

Seigle, Cecilia Segawa, and Linda H. Chance. 2014. *Ōoku: The Secret World of the Shogun's Women*. Amherst, N.Y.: Cambria.

Shahar, Meir. 2008. *The Shaolin Monastery: History, Religion, and the Chinese Martial Arts*. Honolulu: University of Hawaiʻi Press.

Shahidullah, Muhammad. 1966. *Buddhist Mystic Songs, Oldest Bengali and Other Eastern Vernaculars*. Dhaka: Bangla Academy.

Shakya, Tsering. 2000. *The Dragon in the Land of Snows : A History of Modern Tibet Since 1947*. New York: Penguin Compass.

Sharf, Robert H. 1995. "The Zen of Japanese Nationalism." In *Curators of the Buddha: The Study of Buddhism Under Colonialism*, edited by Donald S. Lopez, 107–60. Chicago: University of Chicago Press.

——. 2002. *Coming to Terms with Chinese Buddhism: A Reading of the Treasure Store Treatise*. Honolulu: University of Hawaiʻi Press.

——. 2015. "Is Mindfulness Buddhist? (And Why It Matters)." *Transcultural Psychiatry* 52 (4): 470–84.

Shiba Keiko. 1994. *Aizu-han no onnatachi: buke shakai o ikitai jūnin no joseizō*. Tokyo: Kōbunsha.

Shimazono Susumu. 2004. "From Religion to Psychotherapy." In *From Salvation to Spirituality: Popular Religious Movements in Modern Japan*, 212–25. Melbourne: Trans Pacific.

Shinmura, Taku. 2013. *Nihon bukkyō no iryōshi*. Tokyo: Hōsei daigaku shuppankyoku.

Sigerist, Henry E. 1928–32. *Kyklos: Jahrbuch des Instituts für Geschichte der Medizin an der Universität Leipzig*. 4 vols. Leipzig: Georg Thieme.

Sihlé, Nicolas. 2013. *Rituels bouddhiques de pouvoir et de violence: la figure du tantriste tibétain*. Turnhout: Brepols.

Singha, Maniklal. 1979. *Rārher Mantrajān*. Bishnupur, India: New Minerva.

Singleton, Nicola, Alison Lee, and Howard Meltzer. 2002. *Psychiatric Morbidity Among Adults Living in Private Households, 2000: Technical Report*. London: Office for National Statistics.

Sinor, Denis. 1997. *Inner Asia: History, Civilization, Languages*. 3rd ed. The Hague: Mouton.

Sivin, Nathan. 2015. *Health Care in Eleventh-Century China*. New York: Springer.

Slouber, Michael. 2017. *Early Tantric Medicine: Snakebite, Mantras, and Healing in the Garuda Tantras*. Oxford: Oxford University Press.

Soshin-ni. 1916. "Soshin-ni kōhōgo." In *Kinsei bukkyō shūsetsu*, edited by Mitamura Engyo, 266–90. Tokyo: Kokusho kankōkai.

——. 1925. "Soshin-ni hōgo." In *Kokubun tōhō bukkyō sōsho*. Part 2, vol. 2, edited by Washio Junkyō, 211–47. Tokyo: Tōhō shoin.

Specia, Megan, and Paul Mozur. October 27, 2017. "A War of Words Puts Facebook at the Center of Myanmar's Rohingya Crisis." *New York Times*. http://www.nytimes.com/2017/10/27/world/asia/myanmar-government-facebook-rohingya.html.

Spek, Annelies A., Nadia C. van Ham, and Ivan Nyklícek. 2013. "Mindfulness-Based Therapy in Adults with an Autism Spectrum Disorder: A Randomized Controlled Trial." *Research in Developmental Disabilities* 34 (1): 246–53.

Spiro, Melford Elliot. 1967. *Burmese Supernaturalism. A Study in the Explanation of Reduction of Suffering*. New York: Prentice-Hall.

——. 1971. *Buddhism and Society: A Great Tradition and Its Burmese Vicissitudes*. London: George Allen and Unwin.

Stein, Rolf A. 1979. "Religious Taoism and Popular Religion from the Second to Seventh Centuries." In *Facets of Taoism: Essays in Chinese Religion*, edited by Anna K. Seidel and Holmes H. Welch, 53–81. New Haven, Conn.: Yale University Press.

Stoltzfus, Michael, Rebecca Green, and Darla Schumm, eds. 2013. *Chronic Illness, Spirituality, and Healing: Diverse Disciplinary Cultural Perspectives.* New York: Palgrave Macmillan.

Stone, Jacqueline. 1995. "Medieval Tendai *Hongaku* Thought and the New Kamakura Buddhism." *Japanese Journal of Religious Studies* 22 (1–2): 17–48.

Strauss, Clara, Kate Cavanagh, Annie Oliver, and Danelle Pettman. 2014. "Mindfulness-Based Interventions for People Diagnosed with a Current Episode of an Anxiety or Depressive Disorder: A Meta-analysis of Randomised Controlled Trials." *PLoS One* 9 (4): e96110.

Strickmann, Michael. 2002. *Chinese Magical Medicine,* edited by Bernard Faure. Stanford, Conn.: Stanford University Press.

Sturge, E. A. 1884. "Notes from Special Correspondents: Siamese Theory and Practice of Medicine." *Philadelphia Medical Times* 15 (October 18, 1884): 51–52.

Sueki Fumihiko. 2006. "Soshin-ni: chōsaku to shisō." In *Nihonjin no shūkyō to shomin shinkō,* edited by Tamamuro Fumio, 350–72. Tokyo: Yoshikawa kōbunkan.

Sung, Seoung Yun, Sung Hyun Park, and Mi San Mi San. 2016. "A Qualitative Research on Experience of Heart Smile Meditation." *Bulgyohang-nyeongu* 28 (2): 395.

Sutcliffe, Steven J. 2003. *Children of the New Age: A History of Spiritual Practices.* London: Routledge.

Sutherland, Gail Hinich. 1991. *The Disguises of the Demon: The Development of the Yakṣa in Hinduism and Buddhism.* Albany, N.Y.: SUNY Press.

Suwaki Hiroshi. 1979. "Naikan and Danshukai for the Treatment of Japanese Alcoholic Patients." *British Journal of Addiction* 74: 15–19.

Suzuki, Daisetz T., and Richard M. Jaffe. 2018. *Zen and Japanese Culture.* Princeton, N.J.: Princeton University Press.

Swearer, Donald K. 2004. *Becoming the Buddha: The Ritual of Image Consecration in Thailand.* Princeton, N.J.: Princeton University Press.

Taee, Jonathan. 2017. *The Patient Multiple: An Ethnography of Healthcare and Decision-Making in Bhutan.* New York: Berghahn.

Takahashi Miwa. 2015. "Food Supply in Cambodian Buddhist Temples: Focusing on the Roles and Practices of Lay Female Ascetics." *Southeast Asian Studies* 4 (2): 233–58.

Takaki, Ronald. 1989. *A History of Asian Americans: Strangers from a Different Shore.* Boston: Little, Brown.

Takamatsu Tetsuyū. 2006. "Shukyō to iryō: kanwa iryō to shukyōsha no hatasu yakuwari." In *Koyasan daigaku sensho kankokai,* vol. 3, edited by Gendai Ni Mikkyō Wo Tō, 98–109. Kōyacho, Japan: Kōyasan.

Takemoto Takehiro. 1994. *Naikan to igaku.* Ibusuki-shi: Naikan Kenshūjo.

Takemura Makio. 2017. "Kindai nihon bukkyō no ichibamen: Inoue Enryō no bukkyō fukkō katsudō ni tsuite." *Shūkyō Tetsugaku Kenkyū* 34: 29–43.

Tamiya Masashi. 2007. *"Bihāra" no teishō to tenkai.* Tokyo: Gakubunsha.

Tanahashi, Kazuaki. 2011. *The* Heart Sutra: *A Comprehensive Guide to the Classic of Mahayana Buddhism.* Boulder, Colo.: Shambhala.

Taniyama Yōzō. 2005. "Bihāra to wa nani ka? Ōyō bukkyōgaku no shiten kara." *Pārigaku bukkyō bunkagaku* 19: 33–41.

——. 2008. "Supirichuaru kea ni okeru sosen sūhaiteki sokumen: kinshin no kojin e no tsuibo." *Rinshō shiseigaku* 13 (1): 58–64.

——. 2009. "Supirichuaru kea o kō kangaeru: supirichuaru kea to shūkyōteki kea." *Kanwa kea* 19 (1): 28–30.

——. 2013. "'Kokoro no sōdanshitsu' no sono ato to rinshō shūkyōshi." In *Shūkyō to gendai ga wakaru hon 2013*, edited by Watanabe Naoki, 26–31. Tokyo: Heibonsha.

——. 2014. "Supirichuaru kea no ninaite to shite no shūkyōsha: bihārasō to rinshō shūkyōshi." In *Supirichuaru kea*, edited by Kamata Tōji, 125–43. Sagamihara: Being Net.

Taube, Manfred. 1981. *Beiträge zur Geschichte der medizinischen Literatur Tibets*. Sankt Augustin: VGH Wissenschaftsverlag.

Tawney, Richard H. 1931. *Equality*. London: G. Allen and Unwin.

——. 2009 [1920]. *The Acquisitive Society*. Charleston, S.C.: BiblioLife.

Teasdale, John D., Zindel V. Segal, J. Mark G. Williams, Valerie A. Ridgeway, Judith M. Soulsby, and Mark A. Lau. 2000, "Prevention of Relapse/Recurrence in Major Depression by Mindfulness-Based Cognitive Therapy." *Journal of Consulting and Clinical Psychology* 68 (4): 615–23.

Temkin, Owsei. 1977. *The Double Face of Janus and Other Essays in the History of Medicine*. Baltimore, Md.: Johns Hopkins University Press.

Tennent, James Emerson. 1998. *Christianity in Ceylon*. New Delhi: Asian Educational Services.

Tenzin Choedrak, and Gilles van Grasdorff. 2000. *The Rainbow Palace*. London: Bantam.

Tenzin Gyatso. 2005. *Essence of the* Heart Sutra: *The Dalai Lama's Heart of Wisdom Teachings*. Somerville, Mass.: Wisdom.

Terwiel, B. J. 1984. *A History of Modern Thailand 1767-1942*. New York: University of Queensland Press.

Thich Nhat Hanh. 2017. *The Other Shore: A New Translation of the* Heart Sūtra. Berkeley, Calif.: Parallax.

Toda, Dylan Luers. Forthcoming. "Hara Tanzan (1819–1892), The Gist of Indian Philosophy." In *Buddhism and Modernity: Sources from Nineteenth-Century Japan*, edited by Orion Klautau and Hans Martin Krämer.

Tosa, Keiko. 1996. "A Consideration of *Weikza* Belief in Burma: The Meaning of *Làwki* and *Làwkoktăra* for the *Gaìng*." *Mizokugaku Kenkyu* 61 (2): 215–42.

——. 2005. "The Chicken and the Scorpion: Rumor, Counter Narratives, and the Political Uses of Buddhism." In *Burma at the Turn of the 21st Century*, edited by Monique Skidmore, 154–74. Honolulu: University of Hawai'i Press.

——. 2009. "The Cult of Thamanya Sayadaw: The Social Dynamism of a Formulating Pilgrimage Site." *Asian Ethnology* 68 (2): 239–64.

——. 2014. "From Bricks to Pagodas: *Weikza* Specialists and the Rituals of Pagoda-Building." In *Champions of Buddhism: Weikza Cults in Contemporary Burma*, edited by Bénédicte Brac de la Pierrière, Guillaume Rozenberg, and Alicia Turner, 113–39. Singapore: NUS Press.

Tran Duy Hieu, Venerable [Thich Nhuan An]. 2008. "A Study of Annam-Nikaya in Thailand." Master's thesis, Mahachulalongkornrajavidyalaya University.

Traphagan, John. 2004. *The Practice of Concern: Ritual, Well-Being, and Aging in Rural Japan*. Durham, N.C.: Caroline Academic.

Tsui, Bonnie. 2009. *American Chinatown: A People's History of Five Neighborhoods*. New York: Free Press.

United Nations. 2011. "Happiness Should Have Greater Role in Development Policy—UN Member States." *UN News*. https://news.un.org/en/story/2011/07/382052#.WmzfVBh7EXo, last accessed July 19, 2018.

Unno, Taitetsu. 2006. "Naikan Therapy and Shin Buddhism." In *Buddhism and Psychotherapy Across Cultures*, edited by Mark Unno, 159–168. Somerville, Mass.: Wisdom.

——. 2010. *River of Fire, River of Water: An Introduction to the Pure Land Tradition of Shin Buddhism*. New York: Random House.

Unschuld, Paul U. 2003. *Huang Di Nei Jing Su Wen: Nature, Knowledge, Imagery in an Ancient Chinese Medical Text*. Berkeley: University of California Press.

——. 2010. *Medicine in China: A History of Ideas*. Berkeley: University of California Press.

Upham, Edward. 1829. *The History and Doctrine of Buddhism, Popularly Illustrated, with Notices of the Kappooism, or Demon Worship, and of the Bali, or Planetary Incantations, of Ceylon*. London: R. Ackermann.

Ura, Karma, Sabina Alkire, Tshoki Zangmo, and Karma Wangdi. 2012. *An Extensive Analysis of GNH Index*. Thimphu, Bhutan: Centre for Bhutan Studies. www.grossnationalhappiness. com/wp-content/uploads/2012/10/An%20Extensive%20Analysis%20of%20GNH%20 Index.pdf.

Ura, Karma, and Karma Galay. 2004. *Gross National Happiness and Development: First International Seminar on Operationalization of Gross National Happiness*. Thimphu: Centre for Bhutan Studies.

Urban, Hugh B. 2007. *Tantra: Sex, Secrecy, Politics, and Power in the Study of Religion*. Delhi: Motilal Banarsidass.

——. 2015. *New Age, Neopagan, and New Religious Movements: Alternative Spirituality in Contemporary America*. Oakland: University of California Press.

Valignano, Alessandro, and José Luis Alvarez-Taladriz, eds. 1954. *Sumario de las cosas de Japón (1583), Adiciones del Sumario de Japón (1592)*. Tokyo: Sophia University.

Van Dam, Nicholas T., Marieke K. van Vugt, David R. Vago, Laura Schmalzl, Clifford Saron, Andrew Olendzki, Ted Meissner, Sara W. Lazar, Catherine Kerr, Jolie Gorchov, Kieran Fox, Brent Field, Willoughby B. Britton, Julie A. Brefczynski-Lewis, and David E. Meyer. 2018. "Mind the Hype: A Critical Evaluation and Prescriptive Agenda for Research on Mindfulness and Meditation." *Perspectives on Psychological Science* 13 (1): 36–61.

Van Esterik, John L. 1977. "Cultural Interpretation of Canonical Paradox: Lay Meditation in a Central Thai Village." Ph.D. diss., University of Illinois.

Van Vleet, Stacey. 2011. "Children's Healthcare and Astrology in the Nurturing of a Central Tibetan Nation-State, 1916–24." *Asian Medicine* 6 (2): 348–86.

Varela, Francisco. 1991. *The Embodied Mind: Cognitive Science and Human Experience*. Cambridge, Mass.: MIT Press.

Vargas-O'Bryan, Ivette, and Zhou Xun, eds. 2014. *Disease, Religion and Healing in Asia: Collaborations and Collisions*. New York: Routledge.

Victoria, Brian Daizen. 2006. *Zen at War*. 2nd ed. London: Rowman and Littlefield.

Von Schiefner, F. Anton. 1906. *Tibetan Tales Derived from Indian Sources*. London: Trübner.

Vos, Fritz. 1991. "From God to Apostate: Medicine in Japan Before the Caspar School." In *Red-Hair Medicine: Dutch-Japanese Medical Relations*, edited by H. Beukers, 19–26. Amsterdam: Rodopi.

Waddell, L. Austin. 1985 [1894]. *Buddhism and Lamaism of Tibet*. Darjeeling: Oxford Book and Stationery.

Wales H. G. Quaritch. 1933. "Siamese Theory and Ritual Connected with Pregnancy, Birth and Infancy." *Journal of the Royal Anthropological Institute of Great Britain and Ireland* 63: 441–51.

Wallace, B. Alan, ed. 2003. *Buddhism and Science: Breaking New Ground.* New York: Columbia University Press.

Wallace, Robert K. 1970. "Physiological Effects of Transcendental Meditation." *Science* 167 (3926): 1751–54.

Wallace, Vesna A. 2012. "The Method-and-Wisdom Model of the Medical Body in Traditional Mongolian Medicine." *Arc—The Journal of the Faculty of Religious Studies, McGill University* 40: 1–22.

Wangmo, Tashi, and John Valk. 2012. "Under the Influence of Buddhism: The Psychological Well-Being Indicators of GNH." *Journal of Bhutan Studies* 26: 53–81.

Watts, Jonathan S., and Yoshiharu Tomatsu, eds. 2012. *Buddhist Care for the Dying and Bereaved.* Somerville, Mass.: Wisdom.

Weisberg, Daniel. 1984. "The Practice of 'Dr' Paep: Continuity and Change in Indigenous Healing in Northern Thailand." *Social Science and Medicine* 18 (2): 117–28.

Wellcome, Henry. 1913. *The History of Inoculation and Vaccination for the Prevention and Treatment of Disease.* London: Burroughs Welcome.

Weller, Robert P., C. Julia Huang, Keping Wu, and Fan Lizhu. 2018. *Religion and Charity the Social Life of Goodness in Chinese Societies.* Cambridge: Cambridge University Press.

Whitney, William D. 1856. "Additions to the Library and Cabinet." *Journal of the American Oriental Soceiety* 5: xxv–xxxviii.

Williams, Duncan Ryūken. 2005. *The Other Side of Zen: A Social History of Sōtō Zen; Buddhism in Tokugawa Japan.* Princeton, N.J.: Princeton University Press.

Williams, J. Mark G., and Jon Kabat-Zinn, eds. 2011. "Mindfulness: Diverse Perspectives on its Meaning, Origins, and Multiple Applications at the Intersection of Science and Dharma," Special issue, *Contemporary Buddhism* 12 (1): 1–18.

Wilson, Constance Marilyn. 1970. "State and Society in the Reign of King Mongkut, 1851–1868: Thailand on the Eve of Modernization." Ph. D. diss., Cornell University.

Wilson, Jeff. 2008. " 'Deeply Female and Universally Human': The Rise of Kuan-yin Worship in America." *Journal of Contemporary Religion* 23 (3): 285–306.

——. 2014. *Mindful America: The Mutual Transformation of Buddhist Meditation and American Culture.* New York: Oxford University Press.

Winder, Marianne. 2001. "Vaiḍūrya." In *Studies on Indian Medical History*, edited by Gerrit Jan Meulenbeld and D. Wujastyk, 85–94. New Delhi: Motilal Banarsidass.

Winfield, Pamela. 2013. *Icons and Iconoclasm in Japanese Buddhism: Kukai and Dogen on the Art of Enlightenment.* New York: Oxford University Press.

Wirz, Paul. 1954. *Exorcism and the Art of Healing in Ceylon.* Leiden: Brill.

World Health Organization. 2011. *ICD-10: International Statistical Classification of Diseases and Related Health Problems.* 10th revision. Geneva: World Health Organization.

Wu, Emily S. 2013. *Traditional Chinese Medicine in the United States: In Search of Spiritual Meaning and Ultimate Health.* Lanham, Md.: Lexington.

Wu, Hongyu. 2002. "Buddhism, Health, and Healing in a Chinese Community." *The Pluralism Project.* http://pluralism.org/wp-content/uploads/2015/08/Wu.pdf.

Wuguang. 1996. *Yujia yangsheng shu yu mimi dao.* Kaohsiung: Paise wenhua.

——. 1999. *Cangsang huiyilu.* Kaohsiung: Handwritten manuscript.

Wyatt, David K. 2003. *Thailand: A Short History*. 2nd ed. New Haven, Conn.: Yale University Press.

Yang, Mayfair Mei-hui. 1994. *Gifts, Favors and Banquets: The Art of Social Relationship in China*. Ithaca, N.Y.: Cornell University Press.

Yeshi Dönden. 1986. *Health Through Balance: An Introduction to Tibetan Medicine*, translated by Jeffrey Hopkins. Ithaca, N.Y.: Snow Lion.

——. 2000. *Healing from the Source: The Science and Lore of Tibetan Medicine*, translated by B. Alan Wallace. Ithaca, N.Y.: Snow Lion.

Yingyong Taoprasert. 2005. "The Revitalising and Restoring of Lanna Traditional Medicine and Medicinal Herbs: Final Report on the Sub-regional Experts Meeting on Intangible Cultural Heritage." *Sub-Regional Experts Meeting in Asia on Intangible Cultural Heritage: Safeguarding and Inventory-Making Methodologies (Bangkok, Thailand, 13–16 December 2005)*. https://www.accu.or .jp/ich/en/pdf/c2005subreg_RP1.pdf.

Yoeli-Tlalim, Ronit. 2010. "Tibetan 'Wind' and 'Wind' Illnesses: Towards a Multicultural Approach to Health and Illness." *Studies in History and Philosophy of Science Part C: Studies in History and Philosophy of Biological and Biomedical Sciences* 41: 318–24.

Yonemoto, Marcia. 2016. *The Problem of Women in Early Modern Japan*. Oakland, Calif.: University of California Press.

Yoon, Seung Yong. 2012. "The Movement to Reform Korean Buddhism and the Limits Thereof." *Korea Journal* 52 (3): 35–63.

Yoshimoto, Ishin. 1965. *Naikanhō*. Tokyo: Shunjusha.

Yoshinaga Shin'ichi. 2006. "Hara Tanzan no shinrigaku-teki Zen: sono shisō to rekishi-teki eikyō." *Jintai Kagaku* 15 (2): 5–13.

——. 2015. "The Birth of Japanese Mind Cure Methods." In *Religion and Psychotherapy in Modern Japan*, edited by Christopher Harding, Fumiaki Iwata, and Shin'ichi Yoshinaga, 76–102. New York: Routledge.

Yu Chang. 1999a [1648]. "*Shang lun pian*." In *Yu Jiayan yixue quanshu*, edited by Chen Yi, 1–96. Beijing: Zhongguo zhongyiyao chubanshe.

——. 1999b [1658]. "*Yimen falü*." In *Yu Jiayan Yixue Quanshu*, edited by Chen Yi, 175–368. Beijing: Zhongguo zhongyiyao chubanshe.

Yü, Chün-fang. 2001. *Kuan-Yin: The Chinese Transformation of Avalokitesvara*. New York: Columbia University Press.

Zhang Yisun, ed. 1985. *Bod rgya tshig mdzod chen mo*. 3 vols. Beijing: Minzu chubanshe.

Zhe, Ji. 2016. "Comrade Zhao Puchu: Bodhisattva Under the Red Flag." In *Making Saints in Modern China*, edited by David Ownby, Vincent Goossaert, and Ji Zhe, 312–48. Oxford: Oxford University Press.

Zupanov, Ines G. 2006. "Goan Brahmans in the Land of Promise: Missionaries, Spies and Gentiles in Seventeenth and Eighteenth Century Sri Lanka." In *Portugal—Sri Lanka: 500 Years*, edited by Jorge Flores, 171–210. Wiesbaden: Harrassowitz and the Calouste Gulbenkian Foundation.

Zysk, Kenneth G. 1998. *Asceticism and Healing in Ancient India: Medicine in the Buddhist Monastery*. Delhi: Motilal Banarsidass.

CONTRIBUTORS

Paula K. R. Arai holds the Urmila Gopal Singhal Professorship in Religions of India at Louisiana State University and earned her Ph.D. at Harvard University. The recipient of two Fulbright grants, she is the author of *Women Living Zen: Japanese Sōtō Buddhist Nuns* (1999), *Bringing Zen Home: The Healing Heart of Japanese Buddhist Women's Rituals* (2011), and *Painting Enlightenment: Healing Visions of the* Heart Sūtra—*The Buddhist Art of Iwasaki Tsuneo* (2019).

Cody R. Bahir received his Ph.D. in Asian studies from Leiden University. Currently, he is the Sheng Yen Postdoctoral Scholar in Chinese Buddhism at the University of California, Berkeley. His research focuses on the magical aspects of contemporary Chinese religiosity. From 2011 to 2017, he lived in Taiwan, conducting fieldwork throughout the island.

Jenny Bright completed her Ph.D. at the University of Toronto in the Department for the Study of Religion and through the Collaborative Specialization in Women's Health program at the Dalla Lana School of Public Health. She researches the intersection of religion, medicine, gender, and politics in Tibetan medical literature produced in contemporary China. She is currently working on a book that examines gender and sexuality in contemporary Tibetan medical works, which speak to biomedical ideas of hormones and their relation to Tibetan medicine.

Joshua Capitanio received his Ph.D. from the University of Pennsylvania in 2008 and is currently the public services librarian at Stanford University's East Asia Library. His research focuses on the role of the body in the ritual practices of Buddhism and Daoism.

Kin Cheung is an assistant professor of Asian religions at Moravian College. He researches contemporary Buddhism, including the effect of Buddhist-based meditation on the brain and senses of self, the practical implications of Buddhist ethics, the relationship between Buddhism and mindfulness, and the involvement of Buddhist institutions in China's stock market.

Clark Chilson is an associate professor in the Department of Religious Studies at the University of Pittsburgh, where he teaches Asian religions and Buddhist psychology. His publications include *Secrecy's Power: Covert Shin Buddhists in Japan and Contradictions of Concealment* (2014) and articles on spiritual care and Naikan in Japan.

Céline Coderey is a medical anthropologist and a research fellow at the Asia Research Institute of the National University of Singapore. Her research covers several aspects of the "therapeutic field" in Myanmar: the institutionalization of traditional medicine, the governance of medical products, the accessibility of biomedical services, and practices of divination and alchemy.

Joanna Cook is a reader in anthropology at University College London. She is the author of *Meditation in Modern Buddhism: Renunciation and Change in Thai Monastic Life* (2010). Her current research focuses on mindfulness-based initiatives and civil society in the United Kingdom.

Susannah Deane is a British Academy postdoctoral research fellow in the Department of Religion and Theology at the University of Bristol. Her research focuses on Tibetan perspectives on mental health, illness, and healing within Tibetan communities in Tibetan areas of the People's Republic of China and in exile.

Thomas David DuBois is a scholar of modern Chinese history and religion. He has taught at universities in the United States, Singapore, and Australia. His most recent book is *Empire and the Meaning of Religion in Northeast Asia* (2017).

Assunta Hunter is a medical anthropologist with an interest in the modernization and professionalization of traditional medicine systems. She has written about changes in the education of traditional medicine practitioners in Thailand and works at the Department of General Practice at the University of Melbourne.

Anthony Lovenheim Irwin received his Ph.D. in Asian Religions from the Department of Asian Languages and Cultures at the University of Wisconsin–Madison. He writes about Buddhist temple building in northern Thailand and the social and ethical resonance of craft and construction as a religious activity.

Ben P. Joffe was born and raised in South Africa and is a doctoral candidate in anthropology at the University of Colorado, Boulder. His research focuses on the globalization of Tibetan religion and culture and the transnational circulation of esoteric knowledge and practices.

Lina Koleilat is a Ph.D. student at the Australian National University. Her research focuses on the social justice activism of religious groups in South Korea. She obtained an M.A. in Korean Studies from Yonsei University and an M.S.Sc. in International Studies from the National University of Singapore.

William A. McGrath is a visiting assistant professor of religious studies at Manhattan College, where he teaches courses on Asian religions. His research primarily concerns the historical intersections of religious and medical traditions in Tibet and China.

Alexander McKinley earned a BA in religious studies from Grinnell College in 2008, a Master of Theological Studies from Harvard Divinity School in 2012, and a Ph.D. in religion and modernity from Duke University in 2018. He researches the interactions among different religious traditions in Sri Lanka. Recent publications include: "The Sacred Second: Religious Moments in a Colombo Marketplace" in *Culture and Religion* and "The Spacing of Pilgrimage: Two Journeys to Sri Pada in Sinhala Verse" in *SAGAR: A South Asia Research Journal*.

Levi McLaughlin is an associate professor in the Department of Philosophy and Religious Studies at North Carolina State University. He received his Ph.D. from Princeton University. He is a co-author and co-editor of *Kōmeitō: Politics and Religion in Japan* (2014), a co-editor of a special issue of *Asian Ethnology* (2016), and the author of *Soka Gakkai's Human Revolution: The Rise of a Mimetic Nation in Modern Japan* (2019).

David L. McMahan is the Charles A. Dana Professor of Religious Studies at Franklin & Marshall College in Lancaster, Pennsylvania. He is the author of *Empty Vision: Metaphor and Visionary Imagery in Mahāyāna Buddhism* (2002) and *The Making of Buddhist Modernism* (2008), the editor of *Buddhism in the Modern World* (2012), and a co-editor of *Meditation, Buddhism, and Science* (2017).

Nathan Jishin Michon is a doctoral candidate at the Institute of Buddhist Studies in Berkeley, California, and a Fulbright scholar and research assistant at Tōhoku University in Sendai, Japan. He specializes in Buddhist chaplaincy, both in practice and as a subject of research. He also studies contemporary Japanese religion and Shingon Buddhism. He is a co-editor of *A Thousand Hands: A Guidebook to Caring for Your Buddhist Community* (2016), among other works.

Projit Bihari Mukharji is an associate professor in the history and sociology of science at the University of Pennsylvania. He is the author of *Nationalizing the Body: The Medical Market, Print and Daktari Medicine* (2011) and *Doctoring Traditions: Ayurveda,*

Small Technologies, and Braided Sciences (2016) and a co-editor of *Crossing Colonial Historiographies: Histories of Colonial and Indigenous Medicines in Transnational Perspective* (2010) and *Medical Marginality in South Asia: Situating Subaltern Therapeutics* (2013).

Minjung Noh is a Ph.D. candidate in the Department of Religion at Temple University with a specialization in religion and gender and in Korean Christianity in North America. She currently teaches in the Department of Religion and the Gender, Sexuality, and Women's Studies program at Temple University.

Batsaikhan Norov is a researcher and practitioner of traditional Mongolian medicine who runs a clinic in Oxford, United Kingdom. He has earned degrees in traditional medicine and has lectured at the Health Sciences University of Mongolia. He has an interest in medical treatises written by Mongolian scholars in the Tibetan language.

Charles Jamyang Oliphant of Rossie studied Tibetan religions, language and culture at the University of Oxford. His thesis examined the Tibetan medical practice of rejuvenation. He has travelled extensively in Asia and leads tours to religious sites throughout the continent. He enjoys researching, lecturing and publishing on different aspects of Himalayan religion, medicine and history.

Thomas Nathan Patton is an assistant professor of Buddhist studies and Southeast Asia in the Department of Asian and International Studies and the associate director of the Southeast Asia Research Centre at the City University of Hong Kong. He is the author of *The Buddha's Wizards: Magic, Protection, and Healing in Burmese Buddhism* (2018) and has also published articles on lived religion in Myanmar.

C. Pierce Salguero is an interdisciplinary humanities scholar interested in the role of Buddhism in the cross-cultural exchange of medical ideas. He earned a Ph.D. in the history of medicine from the Johns Hopkins University School of Medicine and teaches Asian history, religion, and culture at Penn State University's Abington College, in Philadelphia, Pennsylvania. He is the author of numerous books and articles on Buddhism and medicine, and the editor in chief of the journal *Asian Medicine*.

Volker Scheid is visiting professor of East Asian medicines at the University of Westminster, London. His academic research focuses on the development and transformation of Chinese medicine from the seventeenth century to the present and its integration into contemporary health care practices. He is also a practitioner of Chinese medicine and a leading authority on the history and use of Chinese medicine formulas.

Mona Schrempf is a social and cultural anthropologist affiliated with the China Center at the University of Kiel and the Central Asian Seminar at the Humboldt University of Berlin. She specializes in ethnographies related to Tibetan and other

Asian medical knowledge systems as well as performing arts. Her work also includes ritual healing practices, alternative medicine, and the role of science and biomedicine in Tibetan and Himalayan communities in Bhutan, China, India, Europe, and transnationally.

Gregory Adam Scott is lecturer in Chinese culture and history at the University of Manchester. His work examines Buddhism in modern China, print culture, and sacred spaces.

Justin B. Stein is a Japan Society for the Promotion of Science postdoctoral research fellow at Bukkyō University. His research focuses on religious practices, ideas, and organizations that have spanned Japan and the United States, particularly Hawaii, including Buddhism and Reiki. He holds a Ph.D. in religious studies from the University of Toronto.

Katja Triplett holds a Ph.D. in the study of religions, Japanese linguistics, and anthropology from Marburg University and is currently associated with the Humanities Centre for Advanced Studies "Multiple Secularities—Beyond the West, Beyond Modernities" at the University of Leipzig. Her current research explores Buddhism and medicine in premodern Japan.

Batchimeg Usukhbayar is part of a hematology research team in Oxford, United Kingdom. With a background in Mongolian–Tibetan traditional medicine, she enjoys contributing to projects on the theoretical and practical issues of traditional medicine that take an integrative approach to health care.

Vesna A. Wallace is a professor of Buddhist studies in the Department of Religious Studies at the University of California, Santa Barbara, where she teaches South and Inner Asian religious traditions and the Sanskrit language. Her research and publications focus on Indian Buddhist tantric traditions and Mongolian Buddhism.

Emily S. Wu specializes in Daoism and folk religions in the Chinese diasporas, particularly their intersection with popular contemporary healing practices. She is the author of *Traditional Chinese Medicine in the United States: In Search of Spiritual Meaning and Ultimate Health* (2013) and serves as a co-chair of the *Religions, Medicines, and Healing* group at the American Academy of Religion.

INDEX